THE FINAL
FRCA

Structured Oral Examination – A Complete Guide

BOBBY KRISHNACHETTY

and

DARSHINDER SETHI

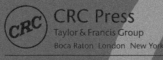

CRC Press
Taylor & Francis Group
Boca Raton London New York

CRC Press is an imprint of the
Taylor & Francis Group, an **informa** business

CRC Press
Taylor & Francis Group
6000 Broken Sound Parkway NW, Suite 300
Boca Raton, FL 33487-2742

© 2016 by Bobby Krishnachetty and Darshinder Sethi
CRC Press is an imprint of Taylor & Francis Group, an Informa business

No claim to original U.S. Government works

Printed on acid-free paper
Version Date: 20150710

International Standard Book Number-13: 978-1-909368-25-5

Visit the Taylor & Francis Web site at
http://www.taylorandfrancis.com

and the CRC Press Web site at
http://www.crcpress.com

CONTENTS

FOREWORD   vii
PREFACE   ix
LIST OF CONTRIBUTORS   xi
ACKNOWLEDGEMENT   xii
INTRODUCTION   xiii

SECTION 01

Clinical Viva   1
01.1   Long case: Epilepsy and learning difficulties   2
01.2   Short case: Complete heart block   7
01.3   Short case: Nutrition in ICU   11
01.4   Short case: Electroconvulsive therapy   14

Basic Science Viva   19
01.5   Anatomy: Liver and spleen   20
01.6   Physiology: Brainstem death   26
01.7   Pharmacology: Anaesthesia in Parkinson's disease   30
01.8   Physics: Magnetic resonance imaging   33

SECTION 02

Clinical Viva   37
02.1   Long case: Foreign body aspiration in a child   38
02.2   Short case: Anaesthesia for lung resection   42
02.3   Short case: Amniotic fluid embolism   45
02.4   Short case: Postoperative eye pain   47

Basic Science Viva   51
02.5   Anatomy: Spinal cord blood supply   52
02.6   Physiology: Pneumoperitoneum   56
02.7   Pharmacology: Drugs used in malignancy   58
02.8   Physics: Sodalime   61

SECTION 03

Clinical Viva   65
03.1   Long case: Pregnant woman with diabetic ketoacidosis   66
03.2   Short case: ICU weakness   72
03.3   Short case: Consent issues   75
03.4   Short case: WPW syndrome   78

Basic Science Viva   **81**

03.5   Anatomy: Cranial nerve monitoring   82
03.6   Physiology: Apnoea physiology   85
03.7   Pharmacology: Comparing volatile agents   87
03.8   Physics: Intracranial pressure monitoring   89

SECTION 04

Clinical Viva   **93**

04.1   Long case: Guillain Barre syndrome   94
04.2   Short case: Intrauterine fetal death   99
04.3   Short case: Eisenmenger's syndrome   101
04.4   Short case: Myotonic dystrophy   104

Basic Science Viva   **107**

04.5   Anatomy: Mediastinum   108
04.6   Physiology: Cerebral circulation   110
04.7   Pharmacology: Serotonin   112
04.8   Physics: Monitoring in scoliosis surgery   115

SECTION 05

Clinical Viva   **119**

05.1   Long case: Abdominal aortic aneurysm for EVAR   120
05.2   Short case: Fracture mandible   127
05.3   Short case: Rheumatoid arthritis   130
05.4   Short case: Inadvertent dural puncture   134

Basic Science Viva   **137**

05.5   Anatomy: Caudal block   138
05.6   Physiology: Preeclampsia   142
05.7   Pharmacology: Tricyclic antidepressants   147
05.8   Physics: Osmolarity   149

SECTION 06

Clinical Viva   **151**

06.1   Long case: Pregnant woman with aortic stenosis   152
06.2   Short case: Hoarseness and microlaryngoscopy   161
06.3   Short case: Head injury   164
06.4   Short case: Chronic obstructive pulmonary disease   168

Basic Science Viva   **171**

06.5   Anatomy: Coronary circulation   172
06.6   Physiology: Liver disease   177
06.7   Pharmacology: Drugs used for secondary prevention   180
06.8   Physics: Scavenging   182

SECTION 07

Clinical Viva **185**
07.1   Long case: Child for fundoplication   186
07.2   Short case: Epidural abscess   192
07.3   Short case: Cardiomyopathy   194
07.4   Short case: Autonomic dysreflexia   200

Basic Science Viva **203**
07.5   Anatomy: Pleura   204
07.6   Physiology: Denervated heart   209
07.7   Pharmacology: Hypotensive drugs   213
07.8   Physics: Renal replacement therapy   217

SECTION 08

Clinical Viva **221**
08.1   Long case: Patient with valve replacements for urgent surgery   222
08.2   Short case: Supraventricular tachycardia   230
08.3   Short case: Cystic fibrosis   233
08.4   Short case: Pneumothorax   236

Basic Science Viva **239**
08.5   Anatomy: Pituitary   240
08.6   Physiology: Ventilator associated pneumonia   247
08.7   Pharmacology: Anticholinesterase   250
08.8   Physics: Humidity/temperature   253

SECTION 09

Clinical Viva **257**
09.1   Long case: Acute cervical spine subluxation   258
09.2   Short case: Diseases of red cell morphology   264
09.3   Short case: Permanent pacemaker   269
09.4   Short case: Bleeding tonsil   271

Basic Science Viva **275**
09.5   Anatomy: Paravertebral block   276
09.6   Physiology: Pulmonary hypertension   282
09.7   Pharmacology: Target controlled infusion   285
09.8   Physics: Cardiac output monitoring   289

SECTION 10

Clinical Viva **293**
10.1   Long case: Mediastinal mass   294
10.2   Short case: Preoperative anaemia   301
10.3   Short case: Cholesteatoma   304
10.4   Short case: Cardiac risk stratification   306

Basic Science Viva   **309**
10.5   Anatomy: Intraosseous anatomy   310
10.6   Physiology: Chronic regional pain syndrome   314
10.7   Pharmacology: Anticoagulants and bridging   317
10.8   Physics: Peripheral nerve monitoring   319

Appendix 1   **323**
Appendix 2   **345**
Appendix 3   **373**
Appendix 4   **379**
Appendix 5   **383**
Appendix 6   **391**

Index   **399**

FOREWORD

The Structured Oral Examination (SOE) has undergone considerable development since it was introduced more than a decade ago. It is intended to test an understanding of safe practice of anaesthesia. This component of the FRCA examination process combines a vast curriculum of clinical anaesthesia with the clinical application of basic sciences. Add the daunting task of facing unknown examiners in the viva, and this proves to certainly be the biggest professional challenge that any aspiring anaesthetist would have been confronted with, up to that stage in their career.

Good preparation for the examination is crucial to a successful outcome. Answering intimidating questions while thinking on one's feet, does not come naturally for any candidate, and has to be practiced. This exam preparation book, *The Final FRCA Structured Oral Exam – a Complete Guide*, is exactly what its name says. This is an excellent guide to polish the candidate who has successfully passed their written exams.

The editors of this book, Bobby Krishnachetty and Darshinder Sethi, are both College Tutors for the Royal College of Anaesthetists, and are well-experienced leaders in trainee education and preparation of candidates for FRCA Exams. In addition, the other contributors to the book are all young anaesthetists who have recently been exposed to the challenge of the FRCA SOE. This group is therefore perfectly equipped to share their important examination preparation experience.

Together they have compiled this book comprising ten sections, over a wide range of possible examination topics. Each section starts with a long clinical case followed by three different short scenarios. A viva section then follows, with four topics covering applied anatomy, physiology, pharmacology, and physics/monitoring. The case scenarios as well as the viva topics are problem-based and supported by evidence. All the section topics are presented with numerous possible examination questions, accompanied by well-prepared answers. Plenty of basic diagrams and special investigations are included, which if reproduced during the real exam, will definitely impress any examiner.

A real valuable resource is the six appendices covering such important areas like ECG interpretation, patient risk scoring systems, as well as risk stratification indices, and blood result interpretation. In addition there is one appendix with a list and short explanation of recent important clinical trials, which when quoted during the exam, will definitely have a positive influence on examiner judgment!

The SOE arrives rapidly after the FRCA written examination and time to revise the full syllabus is limited. I believe that the educational material in this book is up-to-date, and presented in such a way that it will identify gaps in areas of clinical knowledge. It provides the candidate with the important practice of answering appropriate, but uncomfortable questions. I can strongly recommend this book to both teacher and candidate preparing for the FCA SOE.

Justiaan Swanevelder
Professor and Head of Department of Anaesthesia
Health Sciences Faculty
University of Cape Town
South Africa

Previous Examiner for Royal College of Anaesthesia Primary and Final Examinations – 2003–2012

Present Examiner for the Faculty of Anaesthesia, College of Medicine of South Africa – 2012–present

PREFACE

We have conducted the Darent Final FRCA course in Kent for 3 years, and it was during this period that we felt motivated to write this book as a way of contributing to a wider audience preparing for the exam. We have collected a vast database of questions from our trainees who sit the exam, and the book reflects a variety of commonly asked themes.

The style of questions mimics the exam, and we have added tutorials for ECG interpretation and radiology, which will benefit trainees immensely in their preparation.

We have spent several months researching the subject material in an effort to make it as evidence-based and the references as up-to-date as possible. We would like to express our gratitude and appreciation to our colleagues who have contributed to the publication of this book.

We sincerely hope this book will be a valuable addition to the FRCA exam preparation and that anaesthetic trainees will find the book highly useful.

BK
DSS

LIST OF CONTRIBUTORS

Oliver Blightman
Specialist Registrar in Anaesthetics
South East School of Anaesthesia

Oliver Boney
Specialist Registrar in Anaesthetics
Barts and the London School of Anaesthesia

Parminder S Chaggar
Senior Registrar in Cardiology
University Hospital of South Manchester

Dinesh Das
Specialist Registrar in Anaesthetics
Central London School of Anaesthesia

Geetha Gunaratnam
Specialist Registrar in Anaesthetics
Barts and the London School of Anaesthesia

Francoise Iossifidis
Consultant Anaesthetist
Darent Valley Hospital

Sidath Liyanage
Consultant Radiologist
Southend University Hospital

Queenie Lo
Specialist Registrar in Anaesthetics
Barts and the London School of Anaesthesia

Sanjay Parmar
Consultant Anaesthetist
Darent Valley Hospital

Jenny Townsend
Specialist Registrar in Anaesthetics
Barts and the London School of Anaesthesia

Ali Zaman
Specialist Registrar in Radiology
Southend University Hospital

ACKNOWLEDGEMENT

Dr Mike Cadogan of Life in the FASTLANE
Lifeinthefastlane.com

For permitting the use of important X-rays and ECG from their collection

Dr William Herring of Learning Radiology
learningradiology.com

For permitting the use of X-rays from their collection

INTRODUCTION

Confucius (c. 551 – c. 479 BC)
There's a place in the brain for knowing what cannot be remembered.

Clinical Long case
The 10-min preparation time is usually short for getting things ready. Use it wisely!

First part of the question will be about summarising and discussing the investigation results. Write down your punchy summary so you have a confident start. Find the abnormal investigations, think why they are abnormal, derive possible reasons etc. Anaemia is one such example… almost always expect them to ask you the causes of anaemia if the patient is anaemic.

Second part would be the anaesthetic management of the patient. Prepare your answers with the possible headings in mind.

Preoperative
- Is it emergency or urgent… have you got time for preoptimisation?
- Further history and examination
- Investigations
- Preoperative risk stratification and optimisation
- Premedication

Intraoperative
- Preparation
- Senior help
- Monitoring – invasive
- Emergency drugs and equipment
- Induction
- Maintenance
- Emergence
- Analgesia – regional technique
- Antiemesis
- Fluids
- Temperature
- Positioning

Postoperative
- Destination HDU/ITU
- Oxygen
- Analgesia
- Antiemesis
- Fluids
- DVT prophylaxis

Third section of the clinical long case viva is about a critical incident whilst in theatre or recovery – hypoxia, confusion, agitation etc.

Short cases

A mix of obstetric, general, intensive care, and chronic pain cases for just over 20 minutes… and you are done with the clinical viva!

Anatomy

In a 7-minute anatomy viva, 2-3 minutes are given to pure anatomy questions… remember this is Final FRCA, hence what is important is the application and implications related to anaesthesia.

The chosen strategy for being successful on applied anatomy is to learn it, one topic a day and to recite it the next day to someone who will listen.
'It does not matter how slowly you go so long as you do not stop'

Have a set format to answer some kinds of question. For example – factors affecting blood flow of any organ the following classification always works.
- Factors inherent to the circulation
- Pressure or myogenic autoregulation
- Chemical/metabolic factors
- Neural factors
- Humoral factors
- Others

Determinants of cerebral blood flow are
1. Autoregulation by the myogenic mechanism
2. Chemical/metabolic – O_2 and CO_2 and local metabolites like prostanoids
3. Neurohumoral – ineffective
4. Others – blood viscosity and temperature

I have jotted down the anatomy questions in the order of recurrence. It is wise to look at the rarities too as *'the cautious seldom err'*.

Most common/regular questions
Circulation
Coronary circulation and myocardial ischaemia/ECG changes
Spinal cord circulation and aortic cross clamping
Spinal cord anatomy and central neuraxial blockade
Cerebral circulation and head injury management
Blood supply of the hand and arterial line placement
Femoral triangle – CVC insertion/femoral nerve blocks
Structures
Trachea – trauma to neck and AFOI
Larynx and nerve damage
Diaphragm and hernia
Sacrum – caudal
Eye – blocks and periop injury to eye
Pleura – pressures and injury
Nerves
Cranial nerves –5, 7, and 10
Sympathetic – stellate and coeliac plexus
Intercostal block and VATS surgery
Phrenic nerve
Brachial plexus and injury/blocks
Femoral nerve
Ankle block
Sciatic nerve

<u>Fairly common</u>
Pituitary – hormonal/pressure effects and transsphenoidal surgery
Cervical plexus
Paravertebral space
Liver anatomy – blood supply
Bowel circulation and abdominal compartment syndrome

<u>Occasional popups</u>
Bone – for IO circulation
Foetal circulation
Spleen
T10 cross section
Mediastinum
Coeliac plexus

Physiology, Pharmacology, Physics, and Clinical Measurement
Same principles apply in answering these questions too. Try and classify to make your answer interesting and complete. You should have a general idea about every topic so you have a good start.
It is better to ask a question than to remain ignorant. So if you did not understand please request the examiner to rephrase it.

Behind every successful candidate there is a lot of hard work.
I hear and I forget. I see and I remember. I do and I understand….
So Practice! Practice! Practice!

section **01**

CLINICAL
VIVA

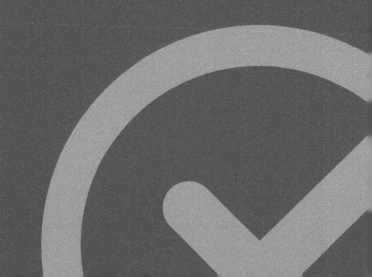

01.1 LONG CASE: EPILEPSY AND LEARNING DIFFICULTIES

HISTORY *You have been asked to review a 36-year-old man who has fallen against a radiator and sustained a penetrating injury to his right eye.*

He has a past medical history of learning difficulties and poorly controlled epilepsy with one to two fits per week, on average. He has also recently been referred to a sleep studies clinic.

He is conscious in A&E and responding to questions appropriately, despite being clearly distressed. The caregiver who is with him did not witness the fall but says that other than his eye injury, he appears to be otherwise acting normally.

STEPS	KEY POINTS	
Current medication	Carbamazepine	600 mg tds
	Levetiracetam	1.5 g bd
	Vigabatrin	1g bd
	Quetiapine	300 mg od
	Lorazepam	2–4 mg PRN
Clinical examination	Weight	135 kg
	Height	175 cm
	BMI	44 kg/m^2
	Heart rate	80/min
	Respiratory rate	16/min
	BP	165/90 mmHg
	Temperature	36.5 °C
	He is overweight with a large jaw and thick beard. Airway examination reveals poor dentition, a large tongue, and a Mallampati score of 3.	
Blood investigations	Awaited	

STEPS	KEY POINTS	
Arterial blood gas	pH	7.38
	pO_2	8.69 kPa
	pCO_2	6.98 kPa
	BE	+4.8
	HCO_3	32 mmol/L
	Hb	17 g/dl

Chest X-ray
done two months ago

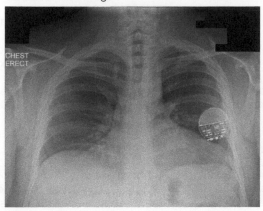

Fig. 1.1

Sleep studies
done two months ago

The polysomnogram demonstrated an apnoea-hypopnoea index (AHI) of 15 events/hr and a nadir oxygen saturation of 78%; supine AHI was 44 events/hr. Definitive obstructive events were not observed in the non-supine position. The total sleep time was 337 minutes, with a sleep time in the supine position of 113 minutes. A 2-minute epoch from the patient's polysomnogram is shown in Figure 1.2.

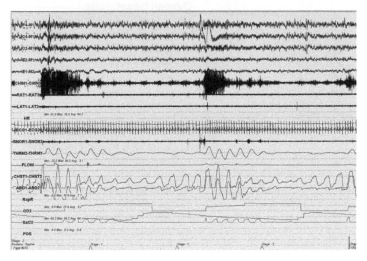

Fig. 1.2

STEPS	KEY POINTS
Summarise the case.	• 36-year-old man with penetrating eye injury • Poorly controlled epilepsy and learning difficulties • Untreated obstructive sleep apnea (OSA) • Obese with potentially difficult airway • Potential liver and renal function impairment due to antiepileptic drugs
Comment on the chest X-ray.	Obvious abnormality is the presence of a vagal nerve stimulator • Reduced lung volumes • Lung fields otherwise clear except haziness in left lower border • Normal heart borders, borderline cardio thoracic ratio
How does a vagal nerve stimulator work?	• Pulse generator/stimulator that sends regular, mild electrical stimuli to the vagus nerve • Used in drug-resistant epilepsy, particularly partial seizures and treatment-resistant depression • Often not immediately effective and rarely prevents seizures entirely • Battery-powered so requires changing every 5–10 years
What are the anaesthetic implications for patients with epilepsy?	• Increased incidence of seizures perioperatively—multifactorial • Continue anti-epileptic drugs (AEDs) with minimal fasting period (or use parenteral alternative) • Caution regarding AEDs—hepatic enzyme metabolism and other drug interactions
Correlate and comment on the ABG and sleep studies result.	• Hypoxaemia, hypercapnia, and polycythemia, related to OSA • Metabolic compensation (chronic disease) • Apnea/hypopnea index indicates severe OSA
What is AHI? How can you classify the severity of OSA?	**AHI** AHI is the number of apneas or hypopneas recorded during the study per hour of sleep. It is generally expressed as the number of events per hour. Based on the AHI, the severity of OSA is classified as follows: • None: < 5 per hour • Mild: 5–14 per hour • Moderate: 15–29 per hour • Severe: ≥ 30 per hour **Oxygen Desaturation** Desaturations are recorded during polysomnography. Although there are no generally accepted classifications for severity of oxygen desaturation, reductions to not less than 90% usually are considered mild. Dips into the 80%–89% range can be considered moderate, and those below 80% are severe.
What symptoms suggest a diagnosis of OSA?	• Snoring • Daytime somnolence • Early morning headaches • Dry or sore throat upon waking • Poor concentration and irritability
What scoring systems are used for screening for OSA?	**STOP BANG questionnaire** • **S**noring • **T**ired—daytime tiredness or fatigue • **O**bserved apnoea during sleep • **P**ressure (blood)—treatment for hypertension • **B**MI more than 35 kg/m^2 • **A**ge over 50 years • **N**eck circumference greater than 40 cm • **G**ender—high prevalence in male gender

STEPS	KEY POINTS

Epworth Sleepiness Scale
- The questionnaire looks at the chance of falling asleep on a scale of increasing probability from 0 to 3 for eight regular activities during their daily lives.
- The scores for the eight questions are added together to obtain a single number.
- Normal: 0–9; mild to moderate sleep apnea: 11–15; severe sleep apnea: 16 and above

Berlin questionnaire
- Patients can be classified into high or low risk based on their responses to similar questions.

What are the risk factors for OSA?
- Obesity
- Male gender
- Age > 40 years
- Neck circumference > 17 inches
- Family history of OSA

What are the complications or associations of OSA?

Cardiac
- Treatment-resistant hypertension
- Congestive heart failure
- Ischaemic heart disease
- Atrial fibrillation
- Dysrhythmias

Respiratory
- Asthma
- Pulmonary hypertension

GI
- Gastro-oesophageal reflux

Neurological
- Stroke

Metabolic
- Type II Diabetes Mellitus
- Hypothyroidism
- Morbid obesity

What are the anaesthetic implications for patients with OSA?

Sedative premedication
- Avoid sedating premedication
- Alpha-2 adrenergic agonist (clonidine, dexmedetomidine) may reduce intraoperative anaesthetic requirements and have an opioid-sparing effect

Difficult airway
- Ramp from scapula to head as patient is obese
- Adequate preoxygenation
- Associated gastro-oesophageal reflux disease—consider proton pump inhibitors, antacids, rapid sequence induction with cricoid pressure

Analgesia
- Minimise use of opioids for the fear of respiratory depression
- Use short-acting agents (remifentanil)
- Regional and multimodal analgesia (NSAIDs, acetaminophen, tramadol, ketamine, gabapentin, pregabalin, dexamethasone)

STEPS	KEY POINTS

Anaesthetic technique
- Carry-over sedation effects from longer-acting intravenous sedatives and inhaled anaesthetic agents
- Use propofol/remifentanil for maintenance of anaesthesia
- Use insoluble potent anaesthetic agents (desflurane, sevoflurane)
- Use regional blocks as a sole anaesthetic technique (not in this case!)

Monitoring
- Use intraoperative capnography for monitoring of respiration (mandatory anyway!)
- Arterial line if OSA associated with cardiac dysfunction

Postoperative period
- Verification of full reversal of neuromuscular blockade
- Ensure patient fully conscious and cooperative prior to extubation
- Non-supine posture for extubation and recovery
- Resume use of positive airway pressure device with close monitoring post-operatively
- May require HDU/ITU admission

What are your concerns of anaesthetising this patient now?
- Newly diagnosed hypertension
- Urgency of surgery—discuss with surgeons but likely to be urgent rather than an emergency
- Exclude other trauma, especially neck and intracranial
- Anaesthetic technique in view of potentially difficult airway
- Control of intraocular pressure
- Post-operative care—will need HDU/ITU bed

What would be your induction technique and airway management plan for this patient?
- Ideally get help—two anaesthetists present
- Awake fibreoptic intubation unlikely to be suitable (coughing, distressed, learning difficulties)
- Allow for adequate starvation time if possible
- Preoxygenate in ramped position
- Modified rapid sequence induction with rocuronium (ensuring sugammadex available) may be most appropriate
- Use of video laryngoscopy may be ideal

The patient is now extubated and in recovery. You are called to review him because he is agitated.

What are the possible causes and how might you manage them?
- Pain: analgesia
- Inadequate reversal of muscle relaxant: check the TOF count and use reversal
- Drug-induced, e.g. atropine, opioids: review anaesthetic chart
- Hypercapnia: treatment of sedative/opioid toxicity, airway manoeuvres, and adjuncts if obstructed
- Hypoxia: O_2, airway manoeuvres, and adjuncts if obstructed
- CPAP likely to be contra-indicated due to eye injury

What is your approach to deep vein thrombosis (DVT) prophylaxis in this patient?
- High risk for DVT—obese, polycythaemic
- Mechanical prophylaxis
- Early mobilisation
- Balance risk versus benefit of anticoagulation in eye trauma—get specialist help regarding the plan

01.2 SHORT CASE: COMPLETE HEART BLOCK

HISTORY *An 80-year-old male patient presents to pre-assessment clinic for SCC removal on his forehead. He complains of dizzy spells. The pre-assessment nurse wants to know what to do. See Figure 1.3.*

Vent. rate	33	BPM	3RD DEGREE A-V BLOCK
PR interval	424	ms	LEFT VENTRICULAR HYPERTROPHY WITH REPOLARIZATION
QRS duration	100	ms	ABNORMAL ECG
QT/QTc	616/455	ms	WHEN COMPARED WITH ECG OF 25-FEB-2005 03:58, (UNCONFIRMED)
P-R-T axes	38 10 242		NO SIGNIFICANT CHANGE

Loc:44

Test ind:410.90

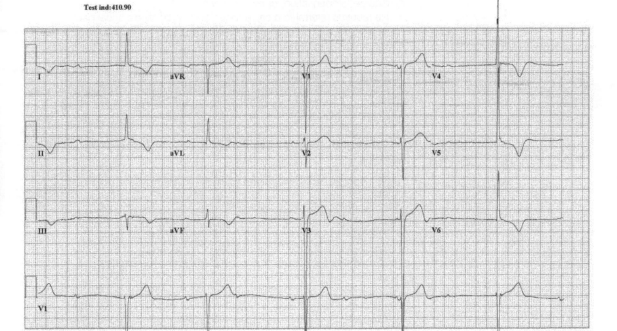

25mm/s   10mm/mV   150Hz   005D   12SL 233   CID: 1

Fig. 1.3

STEPS	KEY POINTS

What does the ECG show?

- Regular P waves and QRS complexes are seen but are unrelated to each other
- No QRS widening
- Voltage criteria for LVH
- No obvious features of coronary ischaemia

The ECG shows third-degree AV block, with a ventricular rate of 34/min.

What are the causes of complete heart block?

Congenital
- With maternal antibodies to SS-A (Ro) and SS-B (La)

Acquired
- Drugs: quinidine, procainamide, disopyramide, amiodarone, β blockers
- Infection: Lyme disease, rheumatic fever, Chagas disease
- Connective tissue disease: ankylosing spondylitis, rheumatoid arthritis, scleroderma
- Infiltrative disease: amyloidosis, sarcoidosis
- Neuromuscular disorders: muscular dystrophy
- Ischaemia: e.g. AV block associated with inferior wall MI

Iatrogenic
- AV block may be associated with aortic valve surgery, PCI

Would you anaesthetise him now?

No. Patient is at high risk of severe peri-operative bradycardia leading to cardiac decompensation, or even cardiac arrest.
- He requires referral to a cardiologist, and probably electrical pacing, ideally with a permanent pacemaker.
- Further cardiac investigations to determine the cause (e.g. angiogram) and to establish his baseline cardiac function (e.g. echocardiogram) would also be helpful.
- If the surgery is deemed too urgent to wait for further investigation and PPM implantation, other options include a temporary pacing wire, or pharmacological chronotropy via an isoprenaline infusion.

How would you manage this if it occurred intraoperatively?

Ask surgeons to stop, check correct attachment of monitoring, and feel for a pulse.

If there is no pulse palpable, start CPR and then treat the underlying problem.

Pharmacological options
- Trial of antimuscarinic drugs (e.g. atropine or glycopyrollate)
- Carefully titrated adrenaline boluses (10–100 mcg)
- Isoprenaline infusion (β-agonist): 0.02–0.2 mcg/kg/min

Electrical/mechanical options
- Percussion pacing using a clenched fist (rarely achieves electrical capture)
- Transcutaneous external pacing via defibrillator pads; increase current until electrical capture achieved. Set rate at 70–80 bpm
- If pharmacological measures fail to restore an adequate heart rate, a temporary pacing wire (inserted via a central line) will probably be necessary, but this takes time to organise (and should be done under aseptic conditions by an appropriately trained cardiologist under X-ray guidance)
- Transoesophageal pacing is also possible but similarly requires specialist equipment and expertise to set up

STEPS	KEY POINTS
	As for all emergencies, management would also require simultaneous rapid assessment/management of airway and breathing/ventilation
	- Is airway patent? Give 100% O_2, check ETT/LMA position
	- Is oxygenation/ventilation intact? Manually ventilate patient, check for bilateral chest rise, air entry on auscultation, $EtCO_2$, misting of ETT, and saturation
	- Remember to maintain anaesthesia while you sort out the new-onset complete heart block!
What are the indications for insertion of a permanent pacemaker?	• Any symptomatic bradycardia (i.e. causing collapse/syncope/presyncope) • Complete heart block • Mobitz type II block • Sick sinus syndrome • Hypersensitive carotid sinus syndrome • Symptomatic bradycardia in transplanted heart • Severe heart failure (cardiac resynchronisation therapy) • Some patients with dilated or hypertrophic cardiomyopathy
… And for temporary pacing?	All of the above indications for permanent pacemaker insertion are also indications for temporary pacing in an emergency situation (or if a permanent pacemaker is unavailable/contraindicated (e.g. systemic sepsis). • Acute myocardial infarction causing asystole/bradyarrhythmia that entails haemodynamic compromise • Drug overdose (e.g. β-blockers, calcium channel blockers, digoxin) • Surgery/general anaesthesia for patients with stable heart block not causing haemodynamic compromise but potentially at risk of worsening bradycardia/asystole • Following cardiac surgery (usually involves placement of epicardial pacing wires, rather than transvenous pacing wire, at end of surgery by surgeons)
What features are associated with a high risk of asystole?	• Pauses of >3 seconds • Previous asystolic episodes • Complete heart block with wide QRS complexes
What do you want to know before anaesthetising a patient with a PPM?	Preoperative assessment should be aimed at finding answers to the following questions: • Indication of pacemaker insertion • Check date (Does it need checking again before theatre?) • Is the patient pacing dependent? • Type of PPM (unipolar/bipolar, number of leads, biventricular/univentricular, etc) • Programmed mode Investigations/preparation • All patients should have CXR (to show PPM position and number of leads) • ECG: look for pacing spikes before each QRS to determine whether pacing-dependent • Correction of any electrolyte abnormalities (which may cause loss of capture) • Switched to fixed rate mode if necessary • PPM check if any doubts re: function/battery life/failure of capture, etc. • May need to arrange cardiac-monitored bed post-op (plus another PPM check)

STEPS	KEY POINTS
What hazards arise in theatre in patients with a PPM?	• Electromagnetic interference (mainly from monopolar diathermy) may reprogram the PPM (usually into a fixed rate back-up mode) or inhibit pacing inappropriately. To reduce the risk of PPM malfunction, use bipolar diathermy. If monopolar diathermy is unavoidable, the pad should be placed as far as possible from PPM; diathermy current should flow perpendicular to PPM current. • Patient shivering, fasciculations following suxamethonium, and sources of vibration may cause inappropriate 'sensing,' which will inhibit pacing or rate modulation (if not previously switched to fixed rate mode). • PPM may be dislodged during patient positioning or CVP line insertion. • Theoretical risk of microshock via PPM lead, which may induce arrhythmia. • All PPM-dependent patients are at risk of asystole or bradyarrhythmias if the PPM fails for any reason. Emergency drugs and pacing facilities (as discussed above) should therefore be readily available.

NAPSE/BPEG* REVISED CLASSIFICATION OF PACEMAKERS (2002)

I (chamber paced)	II (chamber paced)	III (response to sensing)	IV (rate modulation)	V (multisite pacing)
0 = none	0 = none	0 = none	0 = none	0 = none
A = atrium	A = atrium	T = triggered	R = rate modulation	A = atrium
V = ventricle	V = ventricle	I = inhibited		V = ventricle
D = dual	D = dual	D = dual		D = dual

* North American Society of Pacing and Electrophysiology/British Pacing and Electrophysiology Group

Other potential questions for this case:	Physiology of cardiac conduction Hazards associated with diathermy ICD and anaesthesia—NPSA guideline

01.3 SHORT CASE: NUTRITION IN ICU

HISTORY *Figure 1.4 shows the CXR of an ITU patient.*

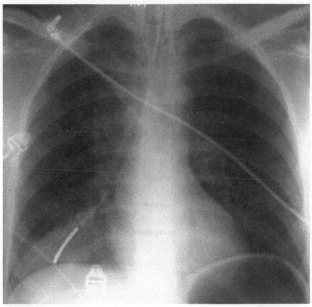

Fig. 1.4

STEPS	KEY POINTS
Comment on the most obvious finding in the film.	Nasogastric tube is above the diaphragm and follows the course of the right lower lobe bronchus.
Would you authorise the tube for enteral feeding?	No.

How can the tube position be confirmed?	**National Patient Safety Agency alert/NICE guideline**
	• Use pH paper.
	  ○ pH < 5.5 indicates gastric placement.
	  ○ If > 5.5, or no aspirate, change patient position and check in an hour.
	• X-ray is recommended only if the pH test fails.
	
	The position of all nasogastric tubes should be confirmed after placement and before each use by aspiration and pH graded paper (with X–ray if necessary) according to the NPSA guideline.

STEPS	KEY POINTS
What are the normal nutrition requirements for a healthy person?	Measuring energy use requires sophisticated equipment, so nutrition requirements are estimated using formulae.

The *Harris Benedict Equation* estimates basal metabolic rate (BMR) in kcal/day.
In men: BMR = $13.75 \times$ weight (kg) + $5 \times$ height (cm) $- 6.78 \times$ age (years) $+ 66$
For women: BMR = $9.56 \times$ weight (kg) + $1.85 \times$ height (cm) $- 4.68 \times$ age (years) $+ 655$
For an afebrile healthy individual, this is around 25 kcal/kg/day. Conditions such as fever, sepsis, surgery, and burns increase the requirements.

European Society of Parenteral and Enteral Nutrition (ESPEN)
The total energy requirements of critically ill patients are given in recent guidelines issued by the ESPEN in 2006.
- Acute initial phase of critical illness: 20–25 kcal/kg/day
- Recovery/anabolic phase: 25–30 kcal/kg/day
- **Protein** around 1.5 g/kg/day (2g/kg/day in severely catabolic patients).
- **Lipid** should be limited to 40% of total calories.
- **Carbohydrate** makes up the remaining calorie requirements.

Glutamine, arginine, fish oils, and ribonucleotides; antioxidants including Vitamins C and E; selenium and other trace elements are considered useful for immunonutrition.

Sodium	1.0–2.0 mmol/kg/day
Potassium	0.7–1.0 mmol/kg/day
Calcium	0.1 mmol/kg/day
Magnesium	0.1 mmol/kg/day
Chloride	1–2 mmol/kg/day
Phosphate	0.4 mmol/kg/day

Define malnutrition.	Malnutrition is the condition that develops when the body does not get the right amount of vitamins, minerals, and other nutrients it needs to maintain healthy tissues and organ function.

Patient has been on ITU for 5 days and has not been fed.

What is he at risk of?	Malnutrition is associated with increased morbidity and mortality.

- Increased risk of infection and pulmonary oedema
- Reduced ventilatory drive
- Impaired production of surfactant
- Prolonged weaning due to muscle fatigue
- Impaired wound healing
- Delayed mobilisation resulting from weak muscles

What are the complications of enteral nutrition?

Mechanical
- Obstruction, discomfort
- Ulceration

Metabolic
- Dehydration or overhydration
- Hyperglycaemia
- Electrolyte imbalance

Gastrointestinal
- Gastric stasis/retention, nausea, vomiting, diarrhoea, bloating
- Aspiration pneumonia due to gastro-oesophageal reflux

STEPS	KEY POINTS
What is refeeding syndrome?	Group of metabolic disturbances that occur after reinstitution of nutrition in a patient who has been malnourished for a prolonged period. • Usually starts 4 days after initiating feeding • Characterised by severe hypophosphataemia and life-threatening complications such as cardiac and respiratory failure, seizures, coma, rhabdomyolysis, and haematological disturbances
What is the underlying pathology?	• Shift occurs from fat to carbohydrate metabolism • This causes sudden increase in insulin levels, which in turn increases cellular uptake of phosphate and precipitous fall in extracellular phosphate • Levels of K, Mg also fall, leading to heart failure
How do you know if the patient is absorbing feeds?	The presence of the following features suggest nonabsorption of feeds: • Increased aspirate from NG tube • Nausea and vomiting • Bloating, abdominal distension • Diarrhoea
What do you do if patient is not absorbing feeds?	• Check correct position of NG tube. • Ensure 45° head-up position. • Use prokinetics. • Institute a high-fibre diet for diarrhoea. • Start parenteral route.

Further reading

1. Campbell Edmondson W. Nutritional support in critical care: An update. *Contin Educ Anaesth Crit Care Pain*. 2007; **7** (6): 199–202.
2. Patient Safety Alert NPSA/2011/PSA002: Reducing the harm caused by misplaced nasogastric feeding tubes in adults, children and infants. March 2011.
3. Heyland DK. Nutritional support in the critically ill patient—A critical review of the evidence. *Critical Care Clinics*. 1998; **14**: 424–40.

01.4 SHORT CASE: ELECTROCONVULSIVE THERAPY

HISTORY *After your morning list, the duty anaesthetic consultant asks you to cover the afternoon Electroconvulsive Therapy (ECT) list because the usual consultant has to cover emergency theatre. You eventually locate the ECT room in the mental health unit, which you've never visited before.*

The first patient is a 63-year-old man who is undergoing his second course of ECT. No previous notes are available, apart from those from his most recent ECT last week (including the anaesthetic chart).

STEPS	KEY POINTS
What is ECT, and how does it work?	ECT, having been in clinical use since the late 1930s, is the treatment for various psychiatric disorders and involves artificially inducing a brief generalised tonic-clonic seizure. The exact mechanism is still unclear, although a common (and probably oversimplified) view is that a tonic-clonic seizure 'resets' or 'jumpstarts' neuronal transmission (in a similar way DC cardioversion does for the heart).
What are the indications for ECT?	• Depressive illness: failed medical therapy • Mania: refractory cases • Schizophrenia • Parkinson's disease • Neuroleptic malignant syndrome • Delirium
How is it performed?	In the UK, it involves induction of general anaesthesia, and usually partial muscle relaxation, before inducing a generalised tonic-clonic seizure by passing a brief current of 30–45 J between two electrodes on either side of the patient's skull (bilateral ECT), or more commonly over one side only (unilateral) over 0.5–1.5 seconds.

STEPS	KEY POINTS

What are the main anaesthetic issues?

Remote site anaesthesia
- Unfamiliar environment and staff
- Potentially old/unfamiliar equipment (which may not have been checked recently)
- Inconsistent anaesthetic support (ODP)

The overall aims of anaesthesia are
- To induce rapid onset, brief general anaesthesia, with partial muscle relaxation to reduce the risk of limb injury during convulsions
- To avoid raising the seizure threshold (which may make seizures harder to induce and/or shorter in duration, which in turn may make the ECT less effective)
- To minimise physiological effects of ECT

Look at the ECG strip provided and explain the mechanism.

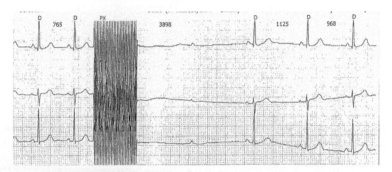

This is because of the autonomic surges that happen at the onset and maintenance of ECT, which is described below.

Only parasympathetic symptoms are shown in the ECG.

What are the main physiological effects?

Cardiac
- Initial parasympathetic discharge, lasting 10–20 seconds; bradycardia, hypotension, and asystole may occur.
- Followed by sympathetic surge, leading to increased heart rate, blood pressure, and myocardial oxygen demand.
- Potential for myocardial ischaemia or infarction, especially in those with preexisting LV impairment or coronary artery disease.

Cerebral
- Increased cerebral O_2 consumption, blood flow, and ICP
- Post-procedure cognitive deficits are common: post-ictal confusion, drowsiness, retrograde and anterograde amnesia commonly occur.

Other
- Raised intraocular and intragastric pressure are not thought to be clinically significant.
- Dental damage, tongue/lip lacerations may occur due to jaw clenching.
- Headache and myalgia.
- Fractures are rare now, due to widespread use of muscle relaxants.

STEPS	KEY POINTS
What are the key points in preoperative patient assessment?	• Often poor historians with multiple comorbidities (IHD, COPD, etc) • No absolute contraindications exist, but most anaesthetists would consider an MI or CVA within the previous 3 months, or raised ICP, to place the patient at high risk of further cardiac or cerebral events • Drug therapy may have anaesthetic implications (lithium, MAOI, etc) • Patients may not have followed fasting instructions • All patients should ideally be investigated and optimised as for any procedure; however, if ECT is deemed semi-urgent, the risks of delay must again be balanced against the benefits of optimising comorbidities
How would you conduct your anaesthetic?	**Induction** • Check patient, full monitoring, appropriate assistance and equipment as per AAGBI • Intravenous access and pre-oxygenation • Induction agent: 'minimal sleep dose', to minimise effects on raising seizure threshold. Methohexital used to be commonly employed but is no longer available; propofol is a common choice; etomidate reduces seizure threshold but affects adrenal hormone synthesis • Short-acting opioids may allow dose of induction agent to be reduced and blunt haemodynamic responses • Muscle relaxants: suxamethonium 0.5 mg/kg commonly used. If contraindicated, consider mivacurium (or rocuronium followed by sugammadex if available) **Maintenance** • Airway management: manual airway maintenance using a face mask is usually sufficient, unless specific aspiration risks warrant intubation • Bite block/mouthguard to prevent damage to the teeth or tongue • Gentle hyperventilation after induction—causing hypocapnia—helps reduce seizure threshold • Volatile not usually required, but further boluses of induction agent may be needed to maintain anaesthesia if repeated current bursts are required to induce a seizure • Have glycopyrrolate and atropine on hand to treat parasympathetic surge; consider short-acting β-blocker at induction (e.g. esmolol, labetalol) in patients at risk of myocardial ischaemia **Emergence** • Once seizure terminates, ventilation can be supported manually until anaesthesia and muscle relaxation start to wear off and spontaneous ventilation resumes • Keep oxygen applied, and transfer to recovery • Monitor standards and recovery facilities same as in a normal postoperative care unit • Anticipate post-op confusion/agitation
If severe bradycardia occurred, how would you treat it?	• Check monitoring still attached • Feel for pulse • Give atropine 3 mg stat bolus (followed by 10–20 mL flush!) • Commence CPR and put out crash call if no pulse palpable • Document on anaesthetic chart and consider prophylactic glycopyrrolate next time

STEPS	KEY POINTS
What drug therapy may influence your anaesthetic?	**Lithium** • Used mainly in bipolar disorder • Decreases the central and peripheral neurotransmitters and may prolong depolarising neuromuscular blockade • May cause nephrogenic diabetes insipidus • Has a narrow therapeutic index and signs develop at > 2.0 mmol/L. Signs of toxicity include lethargy or restlessness initially; then tremor, ataxia, weakness and muscle twitching, hypokalaemia, arrhythmias, renal failure, convulsions, and coma **SSRIs** • May cause SIADH: low [Na^+] **MAOIs** • Potential for hypertensive crisis if used with sympathomimetics (mainly indirectly acting, i.e. metaraminol, ephedrine) • Caution with opioids (unpredictable effects with pethidine; morphine and fentanyl thought to be safe) • Irreversibly inhibit MAO, so consider stopping 2 to 3 weeks pre-procedure if concerned about anaesthetic interactions
Other potential questions related to this case	Remote site anaesthesia

section 01

BASIC SCIENCE VIVA

01.5 ANATOMY: LIVER AND SPLEEN

HISTORY ...*structures at the level of T10, anatomy of the liver with blood supply, CT showing air around liver, causes of pneumoperitoneum...*

STEPS	KEY POINTS

What do you understand by the term T10?	• Vertebral level
	  Anatomical level of T10 vertebra
	
	• Dermatomal level
	  ○ Dermatome is the area of skin whose sensory innervation is derived from a single spinal nerve (dorsal root)
	  ○ Not the same as vertebral body level but refers to the cutaneous area at the level of umbilicus
	
	• Myotomal level
	  ○ Muscle distribution of a single spinal nerve (ventral root)
	  ○ T10 myotome includes the abdominal muscles
	  ○ Useful in clinical and electromyographic localisation of radicular lesion causing motor defect

Shown below is the CT of abdomen at the level of T12. Orientate yourself with the different organs at this level.	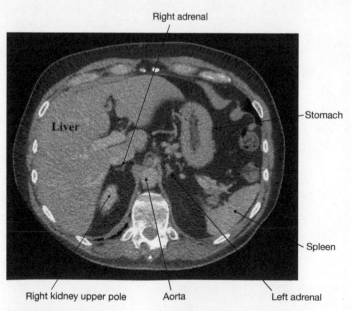

Fig. 1.5

STEPS	KEY POINTS

Look at the second CT image provided in Figure 1.6. What is your diagnosis?

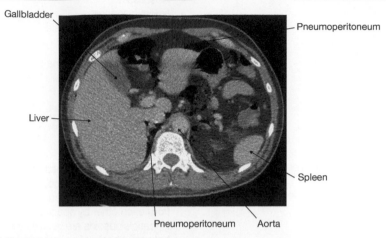

Gallbladder
Pneumoperitoneum
Liver
Spleen
Pneumoperitoneum   Aorta

Fig. 1.6

Diagnosis: Intraperitoneal and retroperitoneal free gas
Tip: Using lung windows makes free gas easier to visualise.

What are the common causes of pneumoperitoneum?

Spontaneous
- Perforated hollow viscus
- Secondary to bowel obstruction
- Secondary to peptic ulcer

Iatrogenic
- Endoscopic perforation
- Secondary to mechanical ventilation
- After laparotomy and laparoscopy

Miscellaneous
- In females, the fallopian tube acts as a conduit between the vagina and the peritoneal cavity

Look at the third CT image in Figure 1.7. Comment on the liver texture.

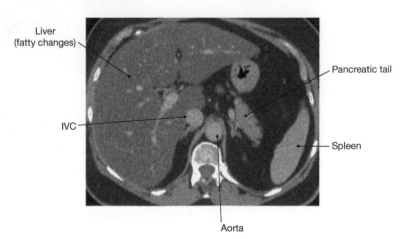

Liver (fatty changes)
Pancreatic tail
IVC
Spleen
Aorta

Fig. 1.7

Diffuse fatty liver. The liver is of low density in keeping with fatty infiltration. (Tip: Use the spleen for comparison. The liver density should be equal to or higher than the spleen.)

STEPS	KEY POINTS

What are the causes of liver lesions?

Benign lesions
- Simple cysts
- Abscesses
- Hepatic adenoma
- Focal nodular hyperplasia

Malignant lesions
- Hepatocellular carcinoma
- Cholangiocarcinoma
- Angiosarcoma

Miscellaneous
- Fatty liver
- Cirrhosis

Tell me about the liver.

The liver is the second largest organ (second to skin).
Weight is 1500 g, which accounts for 2.5% of body weight.
- Hepatocytes are polyhedral epithelial cells arranged in sheets separated from each other by spaces filled with hepatic sinusoids
- Hepatic sinusoids are vessels that arise at the portal triad and run between sheets of hepatocytes receiving blood from the portal triad to deliver to central vein

What is the significance of various types of divisions of the liver?

Anatomical division
- Divided into right and left lobes by the falciform ligament, with the caudate and quadrate lobes arising from the right lobe
- No clinical or surgical significance

Surgical divisions **(Corinaud's classification)**
- Total of eight independent segments
- Each segment has its own blood supply and biliary drainage, so they can be resected without damage to the adjacent segments

Functional classification
Liver lobule is the structural unit of liver. See Figure 1.8.

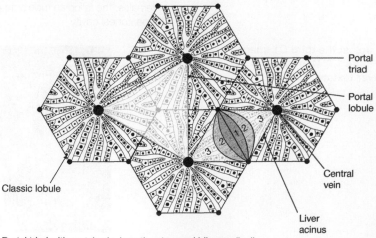

Portal triad with portal vein, hepatic artery and bile canaliculi

Fig. 1.8 Liver lobule

STEPS	KEY POINTS

- Classic lobule
  - Based on direction of blood flow
  - Hexagonal structure with the central vein in the middle and portal triad (branches of portal vein, hepatic artery, and bile duct) in the six corners. The hepatic arterial and portal venous blood flows from portal triad to the central vein

- Portal lobule
  - Based on direction of bile flow
  - The portal triad is in the middle and the central veins form the corners of the triangle

- Hepatic acinus
  - Based on changes in oxygen and nutrient content as blood flows from the portal triad to the central vein
  - It is rhomboid tissue as shown in the image, containing two triangles of adjacent classic lobule, whose apices are the central veins
  - Hepatocytes in the acinus are divided into three zones
  - **Zone 1 or periportal zone,** where the blood supply is the highest. This zone is susceptible to damage by blood-borne toxins and infection
  - **Zone 2 or intermediate zone**
  - **Zone 3 or centrilobular zone** is closer to the central vein. This area is higher in CYP 450 levels but gets the least blood supply and is susceptible to ischaemia

What is special about the blood supply of the liver?

Liver has a dual blood supply.
Total liver blood flow = 1200–1400 mls/min
$\qquad\qquad\qquad$ = 25% of cardiac output
It contains 10%–15% of the total blood volume, thereby acting as a powerful reservoir.

Hepatic artery
- High-pressure/high-resistance system
- Branch of the coeliac trunk (branch of abdominal aorta)
- Carries oxygenated blood
- 20%–30% of total blood supply
- 40%–50% of total oxygen supply

Portal vein
- Low pressure/low resistance
- Formed by the union of superior mesenteric vein and splenic vein
- Carries oxygen-poor but nutrient-rich blood from the abdominal viscera
- 70%–80% of total blood supply
- 50%–60% of total oxygen supply

Deoxygenated, detoxified blood exits the liver via hepatic veins to join the inferior vena cava.

STEPS	KEY POINTS
What are the factors that determine the hepatic blood flow?	Like any other 'factors affecting blood flow' question, have a general classification of factors. (I have listed here the factors in no order of importance.)

Myogenic autoregulation
- Applicable only to the hepatic arterial system in metabolically active liver

Metabolic/chemical control
- CO_2, O_2, and pH changes can alter the hepatic blood flow
- Postprandial hyperosmolarity increases the hepatic arterial and portal venous blood flow

Neural control
- Autonomic nervous system via the vagus and splanchnic nerves also control the hepatic blood flow
- An important example is the stimulation of the sympathetic system in haemorrhage resulting in constriction of arterioles and expulsion of blood into the general circulation, thus acting as a major reservoir of blood

Humoral control
- Adrenaline, angiotensin II, and vasopressin are the main constrictors of the arterial and venous system

Hepatic arterial buffer response (HABR)
- Phenomenon where decrease in portal venous blood flow increases the hepatic arterial blood flow and vice versa so that a constant oxygen supply and total blood flow is maintained
- The mechanism of HABR is unknown, but the local production of adenosine is predicted to be one of the causative factors

What are the functions of the spleen?
- Immune responses: formation of plasma cells and lymphocytes
- Phagocytosis
- Haematopoiesis: in foetus
- Lymphopoiesis: throughout
- Storage of red cells: 8% of the circulating red cells are present in spleen

What are the causes of splenomegaly?
- Infection: malaria, infectious mononucleosis
- Malignancy: lymphomas, leukaemia
- Portal hypertension
- Sickle cell disease
- Collagen vascular diseases
- Polycythemia

Indications for splenectomy
- Trauma
  - Commonest organ injured in blunt abdominal trauma
  - Associated with lower rib fractures

- Hypersplenism
  - Hereditary spherocytosis
  - Idiopathic thrombocytopenic purpura

- Tumour
  - Lymphoma or leukaemia

- Surgical
  - Along with gastrectomy, pancreatectomy, etc.

- Others
  - Splenic cysts and abscess
  - Hydatid cysts

STEPS	KEY POINTS
What do you understand by OPSI?	Overwhelming post-splenectomy infections (OPSI)

- Infection due to encapsulated bacteria: 50% mortality
- Organisms
  - *Strep. Pneumoniae*
  - *Haemophilus influenza*
  - *Neisseria meningitides*

- Occurs post-splenectomy in 4% patients without prophylaxis

Prevention of OPSI
- Antibiotic prophylaxis
  - Penicillin (amoxicillin)
  - Lifelong
  - Prophylaxis required in children up to 16 years

- Immunisation
  - Pneumococcal, haemophilus, and meningococcal
  - Perform 2 weeks prior to planned operation
  - Immediately post-op for emergency cases
  - Repeat every 5 to 10 years

01.6 PHYSIOLOGY: BRAINSTEM DEATH

STEPS	KEY POINTS
What are the physiological changes seen after brainstem death?	The reasons for the altered pathophysiology of the heart-beating brainstem dead person can be due to • Primary pathology suffered by the patient • Complications of ITU treatment (mainly the resuscitation of the injured brain) • Specific physiological changes and a systemic inflammatory response caused by the brainstem death **Cardiovascular changes** • Initial changes: The first change to occur is the increase in intracranial pressure (ICP). Mean arterial pressure increases to maintain cerebral perfusion in parallel with the increasing ICP. Later brain herniation causes ischaemic changes in brainstem and a hyper-adrenergic state. This in turn increases both pulmonary and systemic vascular resistance. Episodes of **'sympathetic storm'** of variable duration occur with tachycardia, vasoconstriction, and hypertension, which can lead to myocardial ischaemia. Hypertension and bradycardia (Cushing's reflex) occur in some patients secondary to reflex baroreceptor activation and activation of the parasympathetic nervous system • Subsequent changes: Cerebral herniation leads to loss of spinal cord sympathetic activity, reducing vasomotor tone, preload, and cardiac output. This is more consistent and called **'syndrome with marked vasodilation and relative hypovolaemia'.** Myocardial perfusion can be affected due to low aortic diastolic pressure **Other changes** • Ischaemia to pituitary causes diabetes insipidus, fluid and electrolyte loss, leading to further cardiovascular instability • Reduced metabolic rate, loss of hypothalamic control and vasodilatation results in heat loss and hypothermia • Coagulation abnormalities can occur due to original pathology and release of coagulation activators from the necrotic brain tissue and hypothermia • Posterior pituitary function is lost, but anterior pituitary function is preserved. There is reduction in T3 levels with normal TSH levels

STEPS	KEY POINTS

What are the contraindications of organ donation?

In order to ensure that donations are as safe as possible, the donor's medical and behavioural history is reviewed to reduce the risk of transmitting disease to a patient. There are many absolute contraindications for various tissue donations, but there are only two absolute contraindications for organ donation along with organ specific contraindications.

Absolute contraindications for organ donation
- Known or suspected new variant CJD and other neurodegenerative diseases
- Known HIV disease, not HIV infection alone

Relative contraindications for organ donation
- Disseminated malignancy
- Treated malignancy within 3 years (except non-melanoma skin cancer)
- Age >70 years
- Known active TB
- Untreated bacterial sepsis

Organ and tissue specific contraindications

Lungs
- Donor age >65
- Previous intra-thoracic malignancy
- Significant, chronic destructive or suppurative lung disease
- Chest X-ray evidence of major pulmonary consolidation

Liver
- Acute hepatitis (AST >1000 IU/L)
- Cirrhosis
- Portal vein thrombosis

Kidney
- Chronic kidney disease (CKD stage 3B and below; eGFR <45)
- Long-term dialysis
- Renal malignancy
- Previous kidney transplant (> 6 months previously)

Pancreas
- Insulin-dependent diabetes (excluding ICU-associated insulin requirement)
- History of pancreatic malignancy

Heart
- Age >65
- Documented coronary artery disease
- Median sternotomy for cardiac surgery
- LVEF ≤ 30% on more than one occasion
- Massive inotropic or vasopressor support

STEPS	KEY POINTS
You have confirmed brainstem death. How would you proceed with organ donation?	**Referral:** Early referral and communication with Donor Team (Specialist Nurse for Organ Donation – SN-OD) should be done once decision is made to test for brainstem death. Each acute trust in the UK has a nominated SN-OD. If out of hours, the on-call SN-OD can be contacted.

Patient/relatives: Once notified, the SN-OD will collect all the information about the patient and his or her relatives. The specialist nurse will do a detailed assessment of the patient for suitability of organ donation. Decision is made on this assessment and after considering factors such as coroner and relatives' views.

Transplant centre: A check on organ donation is then made by contacting the NHS Blood and Transplant Duty Office.

ITU: Once decision is made, optimal organ support is continued in the ITU and specific therapies are initiated to enhance the likelihood of successful transplantation.

What do you do to preserve organ function while waiting for organ retrieval?

General care
Care should always take place in critical care environment. Once the brain death had been confirmed, the care is mainly organ centred rather than patient centred, as patient is legally dead. Hence, in the brain-dead donor, it is appropriate to insert new lines for invasive monitoring if indicated for organ optimisation.

Continue all the basic critical care management including enteral feeding, essential drugs and antimicrobial therapy, correction of electrolytes, glucose control with insulin, prevention of hypothermia, and blood product transfusion to correct significant anaemia and coagulopathy.

Organ specific management
Cardiovascular system:
Restoration of circulating volume without overload is essential. Short-acting drugs are used during the periods of Cushing's reflux and sympathetic storm such as esmolol, GTN, and sodium nitroprusside infusions.

Vasopressin is preferred to noradrenaline as this treats diabetes insipidus and minimises catecholamine requirements. T3 replacement can improve cardiac function.

Haemodynamic targets include HR of 60–120/min, MAP of > 70 but < 95 mmHg, CVP of 10–15 mmHg, cardiac index of > 2.1 L/min/m^2, and mixed venous saturation $> 60\%$.

Respiratory system:
Methyl prednisolone 15 mg/kg given intravenously at the earliest opportunity as this is proven to reduce extra pulmonary lung water.

Use lung protective ventilation with low tidal volumes of 6–8 mL/kg, inspiratory pressures limited to < 30 cmsH$_2$O, use of PEEP and recruitment manoeuvres on regular intervals.

FiO$_2$ is adjusted to maintain SpO$_2$ of $> 90\%$ or a PaO$_2$ > 8.0 kPa.

Endocrine management:
T3 supplementation is part of many protocols but it is beneficial only in patients with poor cardiac performance after fluid loading and vasopressin.

Desmopressin is also used if diabetes insipidus persisted.

Insulin may be useful as anti-inflammatory and reduces cytokines in addition to glycaemic control.

STEPS	KEY POINTS
	Renal and fluid management: Early assessment of overall fluid status is vital as hypervolemia is associated with poor liver graft function. Fluid overload and pulmonary congestion causes poor oxygenation, which makes the lung unsuitable for transplantation. Polyuria is common due to diabetes insipidus, diuretics use, and hypothermia. Nephrotoxic drugs should be stopped and blood pressure should be maintained to ensure adequate renal perfusion.
What do you know about donation after circulatory death (DCD)?	**DBD—Donation after Brainstem Death** **DCD—Donation after Cardiac Death** DCD refers to the retrieval of organs and tissues for the purposes of transplantation after death that is confirmed using 'traditional' cardio-respiratory criteria. This pathway refers exclusively to 'controlled' DCD; that is, donation which follows a cardiac death that is the result of the withdrawal or nonescalation of cardio-respiratory support. Controlled DCD is where retrieval of organs is planned before death occurs. In uncontrolled DCD, decision for organ donation is made only after death. The main difference is in the duration of warm ischaemia time (WIT). Warm ischaemia starts when perfusion and oxygenation are inadequate after cardiac arrest or withdrawal of treatment. This period continues until cold ischaemia starts during organ retrieval. Cold perfusion slows down metabolism and ischaemic injury to the organs. This can be started earlier to reduce ischaemic injury.
What organs are available for DCD?	Kidneys, liver, pancreas, lung, and tissues such as cornea, bone, skin, and heart valves. Renal donors are the major group with a WIT of up to 2 hours or sometimes longer. Liver and pancreas are increasingly used, but WIT is only 30 min. Lung is an ideal organ as it can tolerate lack of circulation for longer times if oxygenation is provided.

Further reading

1. Organ donation.nhs.uk
2. Gordon JK, McKinlay J. Physiological changes after brain stem death and management of the heart-beating donor. *Continuing Education in Anaesthesia, Critical Care & Pain*. 2012; **12**(5).

01.7 PHARMACOLOGY: ANAESTHESIA IN PARKINSON'S DISEASE

STEPS	KEY POINTS
How is dopamine formed?	Dopamine is a neurotransmitter of the catecholamine family and is formed by removing a carboxyl group from a molecule of L–DOPA.

Phenylalanine

↓   Phenylalanine hydroxylase

L-Tyrosine

↓   Tyrosine hydroxylase (rate limiting step)

L-DOPA

↓   DOPA decarboxylase

Dopamine

↓   Dopamine β-hydroxylase

Noradrenaline

↓   PNMT (Phenylethanolamine N-methyltransferase)

Adrenaline

How is dopamine broken down?	Dopamine is converted to noradrenaline and adrenaline, which are in turn metabolised by Catechol-O-methyltransferase (COMT) and Monoamine Oxidase (MAOs).
What is Parkinsonism?	Parkinsonism is characterised by the triad of tremor, rigidity, and bradykinesia. It has multiple causes, of which 85% is Parkinson's disease.

Other causes of Parkinsonism
Pharmacological:
- Drugs affecting dopamine synthesis, storage, and release; e.g. reserpine
- Drugs blocking dopamine receptor; e.g. prochlorperazine

STEPS	KEY POINTS
	Vascular: e.g. arteriosclerosis, multi-infarct disease
	Infection: e.g. post-encephalitis
	Structural lesion: e.g. tumour, trauma (repeated head injury), normal pressure hydrocephalus
	Metabolic: e.g. hypoparathyroidism, Wilson's disease
	Post–trauma: e.g. repeated head injury
What is Parkinson's disease?	Parkinson's disease is an idiopathic neurological disease involving the extrapyramidal system. It has a prevalence of 1% in the population of >65 years old.
	It is caused by the degeneration of dopaminergic neurons in the substantia nigra of the basal ganglia.
What drugs are used to treat Parkinsons's disease?	1) Dopamine precursors with peripheral dopa decarboxylase inhibitor (DDI) Dopamine precursors (e.g. Levodopa) undergo conversion peripherally and within the CNS. DDI (e.g. benserazide) is administered together to reduce peripheral dopaminergic side effects (tachycardia, nausea, vomiting, dysrhythmias).
	2) Dopamine agonists Examples: Ropinirole, Apomorphine. They mimic actions of dopamine at the dopamine receptors.
	3) MAO-B inhibitors Example: Selegiline. Prevents breakdown of dopamine in CNS by MAO-B.
	4) COMT inhibitors Example: Entacapone. Used with Levodopa and DDI in combination to smooth out end-of-dose 'off' periods where symptoms return only a few hours after the last dose.
	5) Anticholinergics Example: Orphenadrine. Antagonises the unopposed excitatory effects of cholinergic pathways.
	6) Atypical agents Example: Amantadine. Mechanism of action not fully understood. May be useful as monotherapy in early Parkinson's disease.
When should Parkinson's disease drugs be stopped preoperatively and restarted postoperatively?	In general, it is advisable for patients to stop their drugs as late as possible preoperatively and restart it as soon as possible in the postoperative period. This is not always possible in patients who are unable to swallow or maintain enteral feeding (post major abdominal surgery). Levodopa can be administered via nasogastric or nasojejunal tubes.
	Patients can be commenced on apomorphine intravenous infusion and continue it throughout the operative period. The bolus dose of apomorphine can be determined by an apomorphine challenge—dose required to abolish the symptoms and to check that no severe adverse effects occur (e.g. profound hypotension).

STEPS	KEY POINTS
Which drugs are unsafe in this group of patients?	• Pethidine should be avoided as it can cause hypertension and muscle rigidity in patients on selegiline • Antiemetics are of importance as nausea/vomiting can hinder restarting enteral Parkinson's disease drugs. Metoclopramide, droperidol, and prochlorperazine are unsafe as they will worsen the symptoms and cause extra pyramidal effects. The antiemetic of choice is domperidone as it does not cross the blood brain barrier and therefore does not cause extra pyramidal effects • Antidepressants: tricyclic antidepressants may potentiate Levodopa-induced arrhythmias • Antipsychotics (e.g. phenothiazines, butyrophenones, piperazine derivatives) may worsen symptoms. It is best to use atypical antipsychotics (e.g. sulpiride, clozapine) • Antihypertensives may cause severe hypotension (due to postural hypotension, hypovolaemia) • Centrally acting anticholinergic drugs can precipitate central anticholinergic syndrome. Glycopyrrolate is the anticholinergic of choice

01.8 PHYSICS: MAGNETIC RESONANCE IMAGING

STEPS	KEY POINTS
What is the principle behind the working of MRI? See Figure 1.9.	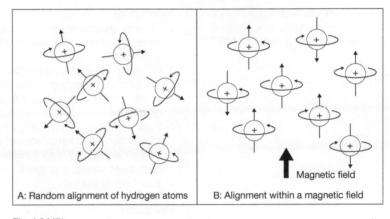

Fig. 1.9 MRI

- Unpaired protons in the body (mostly H^+ atom in water—abundant) align randomly and act as bar magnets
- When placed in an external static magnetic field (A), the protons align
- When another magnetic field (B) is applied, the protons are turned out of alignment
- When this magnetic field is intermittently turned off and on, the radiofrequency energy taken up by the protons are released before the realignment takes place. Also there is some 'Precession'—a wobbling motion that occurs when a spinning object is subject to an external force.
- This energy released is measured by a set of 3-dimensional orthogonal gradient coils in the MRI machine
- The energy released by protons in different tissues is different, and hence a 3-dimensional image with varying intensity is formed

STEPS	KEY POINTS

Some numbers
- Earth's magnetic field = 0.5–1.0 Gauss
- 10,000 Gauss = 1 Tesla
- MRI requires magnetic fields between 0.2–3 Tesla (30,000 times the earth's magnetic field)
- MRI Safe zone < 5 Gauss
- > 5 Gauss—pacemakers will malfunction and all personnel need screening
- MRI Conditional zone—50 Gauss
- > 50 gauss—ferro magnetic objects become projectiles and monitors malfunction

What do you understand by T1 and T2 weighted images?
- 'T' is the relaxation time constant.
- T1 weighted (early image)—few milliseconds after the electro magnetic field is removed
- T2 weighted (later image)—later than T1
- Protons in hydrogen take a long time to decay to original position, so fluid will appear dark (minimal signal) in T1 but white (better signal) in T2

Can you list the problems posed to the anaesthetists when taking an anaesthetised patient to MRI?
- Patient factors
  - Patients needing anaesthesia are usually ITU patients, paediatric patients, patients with learning difficulties, seizures, or movement disorders
  - Pregnancy: Currently recommended that pregnant women should ideally not be scanned during the first trimester of pregnancy due to magnetic field problems, noise, and also unscavenged anaesthetic gas issues
  - Patients with implants: Pacemakers, cochlear implants, intraocular foreign body, and ferromagnetic aneurysm clips are absolute contraindications. Modern implants such as joint prosthesis, surgical clips, heart valves, and sternal wires are deemed safe. All patients and staff need screening

- MRI factors
  - Presence of strong magnetic field
    - Exert large forces on any ferromagnetic materials in the proximity
    - Induce currents in metallic objects and cause local heating
    - Interfere with monitoring
    - Magnetic field in the vicinity can also derange the quality of images produced
    - < 5 Gauss is the safe zone
  - Noise such as that due to the gradient coils switching on and off
    - > 85 dB (above safe level)
    - Patient and staff should be protected
    - Can mask the monitor alarms
  - Heat: That produced by the radiofrequency radiation is absorbed by patient.

- Anaesthetic equipment factors
  - MRI safe: Equipment will not pose a danger to patients and staff but does not guarantee that it will function correctly
  - MRI compatible: Equipment is both safe to enter the MR examination room and will operate normally without interference to the MR scanner
  - Anaesthetic machines, cylinders, circuits, ventilators, vapourisers and scavenging are now available as MRI-compatible
  - Infusion pumps fail if field strength is > 50 Gauss

STEPS	KEY POINTS
	• Anaesthetic monitoring factors

• Anaesthetic monitoring factors
  ○ MRI-compatible short (15 cms) braided ECG leads and insulated pulse oximetry cables are necessary
  ○ NIBP—plastic connectors; IBP—pressure transducer cabling is passed through the wave guides or use MRI-compatible pressure transducers
  ○ Capnography and airway pressure monitoring requires longer sample lines with a 20-second delay
  ○ Monitoring screens should be in the control room and carbon fibre cables passed via the wave guide port

• Location factors
  ○ Usually remote
  ○ Difficult to access in case of emergency

What is Faraday's cage?

Faraday's cage is a radiofrequency shield built into the fabric of the MR room. To allow infusion lines or monitoring cables to enter the MR room, a hollow brass tube or 'waveguide' is built into the Faraday cage passing through into the control room.

Mechanism: An external static electrical field causes the electric charges within the cage's conducting material to be distributed such that they cancel the field's effect in the cage's interior.

Examples: Microwave oven, MR room.

What is quenching?

The coils used in MR magnets need to be kept cold (liquid helium) in order to maintain superconductivity.

Quenching is a process involving the rapid boil-off of the cryogen that causes an immediate loss of superconductivity. This can happen spontaneously, due to error or installation, or deliberately such as in order to switch the scanner off. This produces a large volume of helium gas, which is vented to the outside atmosphere through a quench pipe. In the event of damage to the quench pipe, the buildup of helium could potentially lead to asphyxiation.

section 02

CLINICAL
VIVA

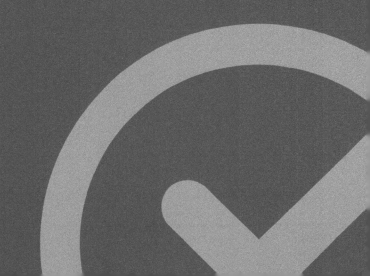

02.1 LONG CASE: FOREIGN BODY ASPIRATION IN A CHILD

HISTORY *You are called to see a 17-month-old male child who is currently in the children's ward.*

He was brought into Accident and Emergency by his mother due to grunting and looking red in the face. Two hours earlier he was eating 'Bombay mix' when he had an episode of coughing and went blue. Shortly afterwards he recovered and was well enough to eat a banana and chocolate biscuit.

STEPS	KEY POINTS
Past Medical History	Full-term normal delivery Vaccinations up-to-date No previous anaesthetics
On examination	Playing in the ward Temperature: 37°C SpO$_2$: 94% on air Respiratory rate: 22/min On auscultation: harsh breath sounds on the left with some basal crepitations
Investigations	Chest X-rays provided 1. On inspiration. See Figure 2.1.

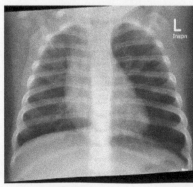

Fig. 2.1 Inspiration

STEPS	KEY POINTS

2. On expiration. See Figure 2.2.

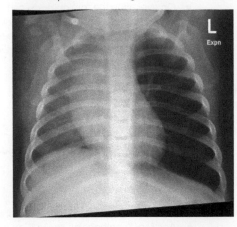

Fig. 2.2 Expiration

Summarise the case.

- Inhaled foreign body
- Some hypoxia on air
- Stable, not compromised

What are the anaesthetic concerns?

- Paediatric case
- Risk of aspiration (Wait until fasted—not urgent)
- Possible chemical pneumonia

What are the signs of respiratory distress in children?

Tachypnoea	• <1 year: 30–40/min • 1–2 years: 25–35/min • 2–5 years: 25–30/min • 5–12 years: 20–25/min • >12 years: 15–20/min • Bradypnoea suggests imminent respiratory arrest.
Tripodding or anchoring	Child may sit forward and grasp their feet or hold on to the side of the bed.
Intercostal and sternal recession	Significant if seen in a child over 6–7 years of age
Nasal flaring	Particularly seen in infants
Use of accessory muscles	Look for head bobbing in infants
Inspiratory/expiratory noises	_Stridor_: high-pitched inspiratory noise, a sign of upper airway obstruction. _Wheezing_: louder on expiration, a sign of smaller-calibre lower airway obstruction _Grunting_: exhalation against a partially closed glottis, a sign of severe respiratory distress in infants

Explain the CXRs.

X-ray on inspiration
- Minimal hyperinflation seen on the left lung
- No foreign body (FB) seen

X-ray on expiration
- Hyperinflation of the left lung.
- In both inspiration and expiration images the diaphragms have not moved.
- FB—not seen on the X-ray.

STEPS	KEY POINTS
Explain pathophysiology of hyperinflation (ball-valve mechanism).	• On inspiration both lungs will tend to appear similar in terms of their degree of aeration. The reason for this is that the trachea and bronchi normally widen on inspiration, allowing passage of air into the affected lung past the foreign body. • On expiration the foreign body can obstruct the bronchi as the diameter of the bronchi decreases slightly on expiration. The greatest difference in lung aeration will therefore be seen on the expiration image as air is exhaled from the normal lung (right lung) but not from the affected lung (left lung).
It was planned to take this child to theatre for EUA for removal of foreign body. Would you use any premedication in this child? If yes, what would you prescribe?	**Antisialogouges** Atropine/Glycopyrollate • Atropine dose 20–40 mcg/kg PO; <u>max dose 500 mcg</u> Pros: reduce secretions, so reduces suctioning during bronchoscopy, vagolytic Cons: thickening of mucus **EMLA/Ametop** • EMLA: 2.5% lidocaine and 2.5% prilocaine (leave it on for 45–60 minutes) • Ametop: Amethocaine (leave it on for 30–45 minutes); causes vasodilatation
What is the particular issue with peanuts as a foreign body?	These biological substances fragment and cause irritation and chemical pneumonia.
Explain the anaesthetic management.	• Preoperative assessment—anaesthetic and medical history, allergy and starvation status • A, B, C • Explain conduct of anaesthesia and consent parents • Bronchoscopy should be postponed because child is not compromised. **Inform** Trained assistant, senior anaesthetist **Check** • Anaesthetic equipment, airway equipment • Anaesthetic and emergency drugs **Anaesthetic plan** • Inhalational induction with spontaneous ventilation (sevoflurane + oxygen) • Avoid N_2O (because of hyperinflated lung) • Prior to bronchoscopy spraying of pharynx and vocal cords with 10% lignocaine (Max. 3 mg/kg, 1 puff = 10 mg) • Can intubate as it gives surgeon an idea of the size of scope and avoids unnecessary trauma • The correct size of scope is one which allows an audible leak of 20 cm H_2O • Maintain spontaneous breathing with a T piece attached to a side piece in the bronchoscope • A small dose of neuromuscular blocking agent or propofol to aid extraction of the foreign body through the cords • Once the procedure is finished, a tracheal tube can be inserted if a full stomach is considered a problem, and the patient woken up and extubated once protective reflexes have returned. • Analgesia not usually required as the procedure is not painful. Paracetamol can be given as required.

STEPS	KEY POINTS
What are the different types of bronchoscopes?	• Rigid: STORZ ventilating bronchoscope, Venturi scopes • Flexible: Fibreoptic scope (Dormia basket can be used to extract foreign body)
What are the complications of bronchoscopy, particularly with rigid bronchoscopes?	• Trauma to lips, teeth, base of tongue, epiglottis, and larynx. • Damage to the tracheobronchial tree is rare but causes pneumothorax, pneumomediastinum, and surgical emphysema. • Haemorrhage is usually minor and settles spontaneously. The child is in recovery. The nurse is concerned as he is tachycardic and in respiratory distress.
What are the differential diagnoses?	• Residual anaesthetic • Hypothermia • Hypovolemia • Hypercarbia • Laryngospasm • Aspiration • Anaphylaxis • Barotrauma
An X-ray is done in recovery. See Figure 2.3. What is your diagnosis?	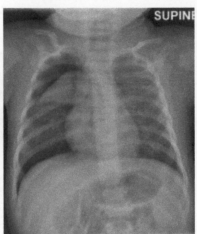 **Fig. 2.3** Pneumomediastinum Barotrauma and right-sided pneumothorax with mediastinal shift.
What are the clinical signs you would expect in a child with pneumothorax?	• Hypoxic • May be shocked • Decreased air entry and hyper resonance on affected side • Distended neck veins • Later, trachea deviates away from affected side
How would you manage?	• High flow oxygen via reservoir mask • Immediate needle thoracocentesis to relieve tension • Chest drain urgently to prevent recurrence
After he recovers, he is thirsty. Would you give him fluids?	No. It can be given after the lignocaine wears off; wait at least 1 hour.

02.2 SHORT CASE: ANAESTHESIA FOR LUNG RESECTION

HISTORY *A 78-year-old female is booked for bunion operation. She complains of chest pain on her right side, cough, and weight loss.*

STEPS	KEY POINTS
What is the most obvious finding on the CXR in Figure 2.4?	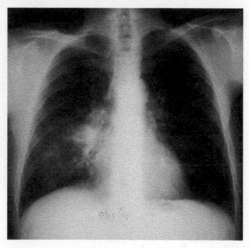 Fig. 2.4
What are the differential diagnoses?	**Infection** • Tuberculosis, abscess **Inflammation** • Lymphadenopathy **Neoplasm** • Primary bronchogenic carcinoma • Metastatic neoplasm • Lymphoma **Other** • Pulmonary artery aneurysm
How would you decide what it is?	History, examination, bloods, CT, bronchoscopy, and biopsy *It is diagnosed as a nonsmall cell carcinoma, and she is now posted for a lung resection.*

STEPS	KEY POINTS
How do you preassess her?	**History** • Anaesthetic history, paying particular attention to cardiac and respiratory function • Smoking history **Examination** • Signs of weight loss and cachexia • Cardiovascular and respiratory examination **Investigations** • Routine bloods, cross matching • Arterial blood gas • Lung Spirometry, diffusion capacity (DLCO), predicted postoperative FEV1 • Cardiopulmonary exercise testing (CPET)
What is DLCO, and how do you measure it?	DLCO is the diffusion capacity and is calculated by measurement of carbon monoxide taken up by patient in unit time. It is a gross estimate of alveolar/capillary function.
How do you predict postoperative FEV1?	The predicted or estimated postoperative (epo) values of FEV1, FVC, and diffusion capacity can be obtained by consideration of the lung volume removed at surgery. For lobectomy, the simple calculation uses the number of bronchopulmonary segments removed compared with the total number (19) in both lungs. Example: Consider a patient with a preoperative FEV1 of 1.6 litre, which is 80% of predicted normal. For right middle lobectomy (two segments), $$\text{epo-FEV1} = 1.6 \times 17/19 = 1.43 \text{ litre}$$ $$\text{ppo-FEV1\%} = 80\% \times 17/19 = 71\%$$ Often a V/Q scan is used to measure how much the lung that will not be operated on contributes to lung function and then combine with a formula to calculate postoperative FEV1.
What values of the lung function tests would you accept before proceeding to surgery?	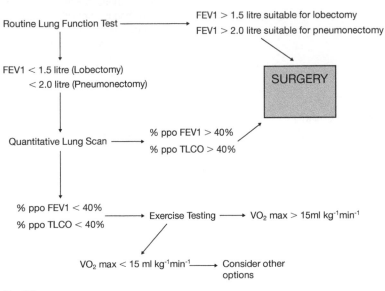

Fig. 2.5

STEPS	KEY POINTS

The flow chart in Figure 2.5 is an amalgamation of the British Thoracic Society and American College of Chest Physicians' guidelines.

The initial screening tool is of preoperative measured FEV1 with >2 litre required for pneumonectomy and >1.5 litre for lobectomy. If there is no diffuse lung disease and no comorbidity, achievement of the appropriate lung volume is sufficient.

When these threshold lung volumes are not present, full respiratory function testing allows calculation of the predicted postoperative FEV1 and DLCO. If both are >40% and the oxygen saturation is >90% on air, the patient is in an average risk group. If either (or both) the predicted postoperative FEV1 or DLCO are <40%, the patient should undergo formal CPET. The threshold VO_2 max of 15 ml/kg/min delineates between high- and medium-risk patients.

This patient is undergoing a thoracotomy and lung resection.

What are your airway options?

For thoracotomy, one lung ventilation is desired and hence you can use a double lumen tube (DLT) or bronchial blocker.

How would you choose and insert a DLT?

- Commonly used tube is left-sided Mallinckrodt. Size 39–41 for male and 37 for female.
- Insert with stylet, pass vocal cords, then remove stylet, and rotate the tube to 90 degrees and advance. Once resistance is felt, inflate tracheal cuff and check both lungs.
- Then inflate bronchial cuff and clamp off tracheal lumen. Confirm single lung ventilation. Repeat on opposite side.
- Gold standard: Check with fibreoptic scope before and after positioning. On the left side, blue bronchial cuff should just be visible below carina; on the right side, also check that right upper lobe corresponds to opening "slit" in distal bronchial lumen.

What are the pain relief options postop?

- Systemic
- Paracetamol, NSAIDs, IV opioids
- Neuraxial
  - Epidural—Gold standard but failure rate and hypotension from bilateral sympathetic blockade.
  - Intrathecal—Not often used.
  - Paravertebral—Getting more popular, can be placed by surgeon by direct vision or anaesthetist. Single-side blockade makes for less incidence of hypotension.
  - Intercostal and intrapleural—Can be used but the limited effectiveness makes its use not as popular.

Further reading

1. Gould G, Adrian P. Assessment of suitability for lung resection. *Continuing Education in Anaesthesia, Critical Care & Pain.* 2006; | **6**(3).

02.3 SHORT CASE: AMNIOTIC FLUID EMBOLISM

HISTORY *A 37-year-old female who is 30 minute postpartum with an epidural suddenly becomes short of breath and is worsening.*

STEPS	KEY POINTS
What are the causes of shortness of breath in pregnancy?	**Patient factors** • Asthma • Pulmonary Infection • Anaemia **Obstetric factors** • Preeclampsia • Amniotic fluid embolism (AFE) • Pulmonary embolism • Ergometrine use • Cardiomyopathy **Anaesthetic factors** • High block assuming that the epidural is still being used in this case Another way to classify the differential diagnoses is to take the obstetric versus nonobstetric approach.
What is the pathophysiology of AFE?	First described by Steiner in 1941, it is a diagnosis of elimination after other causes of cardiovascular instability and collapse have been rejected. Difficult diagnosis is reflected by a wide ranging incidence of 1:8000 to 1:80 000 deliveries **Pathogenesis** • Embolic: due to an emboli caused by entry of amniotic fluid or fetal cells in the circulation • Immunological: similar to anaphylaxis as fetal cells are not always present **Presentation** • Occurs usually during labour and delivery (including LSCS) but can occur up to 48 hours post delivery, typically in two phases • Phase 1: characterised by acute shortness of breath and hypotension followed by cardiac failure, cardiac arrest, pulmonary oedema, acute lung injury, convulsions. and loss of consciousness. The maternal mortality rate is 26%–60%. • Phase 2: 40% of women who survived the first stage will go on to develop the haemorrhagic phase due to DIC.

STEPS	KEY POINTS
What are the risk factors for AFE?	No proven risk factors, but the following may be associated with a higher risk of developing AFE:
	Advanced maternal age, multiparity, meconium stained liquor, intrauterine fetal death, polyhydramnios, strong frequent or tetanic uterine contractions, microsomia, chorioamnionitis, uterine rupture, and placenta accreta.

What systemic changes occur during AFE?

Haemodynamic changes
- Increase in systemic and pulmonary vascular resistance, resulting in acute pulmonary hypertension, left ventricular dysfunction and pulmonary oedema.
- Myocardial dysfunction results from ischaemia and as a direct depressant effect of endothelin and humoral factors.

Pulmonary
- Vasospasm and ventricular dysfunction lead to hypoxia.
- Survivors develop an ARDS-like picture.

Coagulation
- DIC
- Amniotic fluid contains activated coagulation factors II, VII, and X. It induces platelet aggregation, releases platelet factor III, and has a thromboplastin-like effect.
- The clinical picture is one of massive haemorrhage and haemodynamic collapse.

What is the management of AFE?

The management is mainly supportive, invasive monitoring, and transfer to ITU.

Management goals in the operating theatre are
- Maintaining oxygenation—use of PEEP.
- Haemodynamic stability—inotropes are usually required.
- Maintenance of uterine tone.
- Management of DIC—Liaise with haematologist. FFP, cryoprecipitate, and platelets are usually required. Recombinant factor VII has been used in massive haemorrhage.

02.4 SHORT CASE: POSTOPERATIVE EYE PAIN

HISTORY *A 66-year-old previously fit and well male patient had a total hip replacement under a general anaesthetic. In recovery, he is complaining of unilateral eye pain.*

STEPS	KEY POINTS	
What is your differential diagnosis?	**Ocular causes** Conjunctivitis Corneal abrasion Corneal ulceration Foreign body Trauma	**Orbital causes** Glaucoma Iritis Optic neuritis Migraine Trauma
What are the most common/ likely causes?	• Corneal abrasion due to mask, eye tape, and decreased tear production • Chemical injury from antiseptic solutions and drugs • External pressure resulting in optic neuropathy • Retinal ischaemia • Exacerbation of glaucoma	

What are the factors that make a patient high risk to attaining an eye injury?	• Position
	   ◦ Lateral: abrasion/trauma
	   ◦ Prone: optic nerve pressure/conjunctival oedema
	• Pre-existing eye disease
	• History of diabetes and hypertension
	• Prolonged surgery	

What is glaucoma?	Glaucoma is the condition where the free flow of aqueous humour is hindered, which can increase the intraocular pressure (IOP). • Closed angle • Open angle • Normal tension glaucoma In all types of glaucoma the loss of vision is due to optic nerve damage.	
What is open- and closed-angle glaucoma?	Open-angle glaucoma (chronic glaucoma) is the condition in which aqueous fluid drains very slowly due to clogging of the trabecular mesh. Closed-angle glaucoma, also called acute glaucoma, is an ophthalmologic emergency. This occurs when the iris completely blocks fluid access to the trabecular meshwork. The pressure builds up, causing the patient excruciating eye pain, and vision is lost quickly. In normal tension glaucoma optic nerve damage is present but with normal IOP. The cause is mainly familial and history of systemic heart disease such as irregular heart rhythm.	

STEPS	KEY POINTS
What are the determinants of IOP? What are the normal values?	IOP is dependent on • Contents, such as volume of aqueous, vitreous, and blood • Scleral compliance • Tone of extra ocular muscles • Drainage of aqueous, which depends on venous pressure Normal IOP = 16+/− 5 mmHg; >25 mmHg is pathological.
Can the IOP be normal in glaucoma?	Yes. In open-angle and normal tension types, the IOP can be normal. The sclera adapts to increased volume, and hence IOP is normal.
Explain the pathophysiology of closed-angle glaucoma.	Normally the aqueous humour produced by the ciliary body is drained to the veins through the Canal of Schlemm. If the angle between iris and cornea is acute/blocked, then the drainage is affected, resulting in increased intraocular pressure. • Pain and loss of sight in extreme conditions; "silent thief of sight" Avoid drugs that dilate the pupils as this also can close the angle. See Figure 2.6.

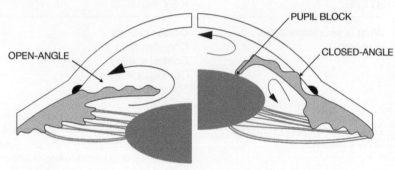

Fig. 2.6 Glaucoma

What is the effect of anaesthesia on IOP?	Consider IOP equivalent to ICP and structure your answers similarly. Any increase in volume and pressure intraocularly and obstruction to venous drainage would cause an increase in IOP. • IV induction drugs: decrease IOP except ketamine. • Muscle relaxants: suxamethonium increases IOP up to 10 mmHg due to extraocular muscle twitching. This can be overcome by giving adequate dose of IV induction agents. Nondepolarising muscle relaxants decrease IOP. • Hypoxia, hypercarbia, neck ties/coughing: increase IOP.
How would you decrease the IOP in an acute setting?	**General** • Head up tilt • Avoid neck ties/coughing/vomiting, etc. • Maintain oxygenation, and avoid hypercarbia and hypotension. **Drugs** • Acetazolamide • Mannitol • Propofol

STEPS	KEY POINTS
Can you tell me the pathway of the light and corneal reflexes?	**Pupillary (light) reflex** Afferent—Optic nerve, which terminates in the pretectal area of midbrain. Axons from here then radiate bilaterally to terminate in the Edinger-Westphal nucleus ➤ Ciliary ganglion ➤ parasympathetic postganglionic axons travel in the short ciliary nerve and end on the iris sphincter. Efferent—Oculomotor nerve Ganglion—Ciliary ganglion Central mediator—Occipital lobe of brain **Corneal reflex** Afferent—Ophthalmic or nasociliary division of trigeminal nerve ➤ trigeminal nerve ➤ trigeminal ganglion ➤ spinal trigeminal tract ➤ spinal trigeminal nucleus Efferent—Facial motor neurons ➤ facial nerve branch to orbicularis oculi Ganglion—Trigeminal ganglion Central mediator—Pons

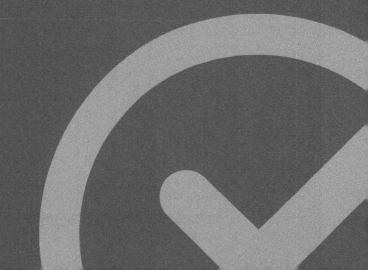

section 02

BASIC SCIENCE VIVA

02.5 ANATOMY: SPINAL CORD BLOOD SUPPLY

HISTORY

STEPS	KEY POINTS
Describe the blood supply of the spinal cord.	The spinal cord derives its blood supply from a single anterior spinal artery (ASA), paired posterior spinal arteries (PSA), and by the communicating segmental arteries and the pial plexus.

ASA

Single artery formed at the foramen magnum by the union of each vertebral artery. Blood flows centrifugally supplying the anterior two-thirds of the spinal cord in front of the posterior grey column.

PSA

Derived from the posterior inferior cerebellar artery (PICA) or vertebral artery, with blood flowing centripetally in this arterial system. The arteries lie along the postero lateral surface of the spinal cord medial to the posterior nerve roots.

Pial arterial plexus

Surface vessels branch from the ASA and PSA forming an anastomosing network that penetrates and supplies the outer portion of the spinal cord.

Segmental branches

Segmental or radicular branches arise from various arteries—vertebral, deep cervical, costo cervical, aorta, and the pelvic vessels.

Arteria radicularis magna, or the artery of Adamkiewicz

Arises from the thoracolumbar part of the aorta, usually on the left, and enters the spinal cord at the level of L1.

Various regions of spinal cord are vascularised unevenly. The cervical and lumbosacral parts are well vascularised whereas the thoracic part of the spinal cord, especially the anterior region, derives the branches from intercostal and iliac arteries, which vary in location and numbers making it prone to ischaemic damage. See Figures 2.7 and 2.8.

STEPS

KEY POINTS

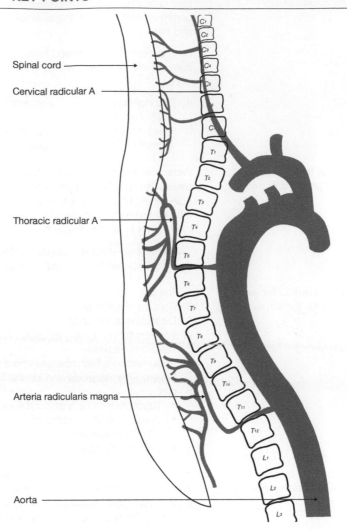

Spinal cord

Cervical radicular A

Thoracic radicular A

Arteria radicularis magna

Aorta

C₁
C₂
C₃
C₄
C₅
C₆
C₇
T₁
T₂
T₃
T₄
T₅
T₆
T₇
T₈
T₉
T₁₀
T₁₁
T₁₂
L₁
L₂
L₃

Fig. 2.7 Spinal cord blood supply

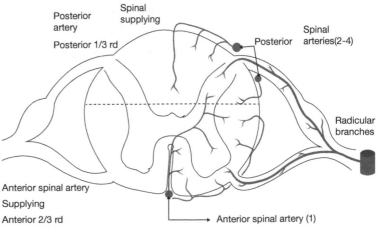

Posterior artery

Posterior 1/3 rd

Spinal supplying

Posterior

Spinal arteries(2-4)

Radicular branches

Anterior spinal artery
Supplying
Anterior 2/3 rd

Anterior spinal artery (1)

Fig. 2.8 Spinal cord blood supply

STEPS	KEY POINTS
Describe the venous drainage. What is its importance?	Radicular and spinal veins drain into the internal vertebral venous plexus and later drain into the azygos system and the superior vena cava. The plexus communicates with the basilar sinus in the brain and with the pelvic veins and inferior vena cava.
	So in patients with increased intra-abdominal pressure, blood is diverted from the inferior vena cava to the plexus, leading to engorgement of epidural veins.
	a. This increases the risk of accidental venous puncture during the conduct of epidural anaesthesia.
	b. It also decreases the effective epidural space volume, thereby requiring a smaller volume of local anaesthetic.
Which part of the spinal cord acts as a watershed zone?	Watershed effect occurs when two streams of blood flowing in opposite directions meet. This happens where the radicular artery unites with the ASA, where blood courses upward and downward from the entry point, thus leaving a watershed region between the adjacent radicular areas where blood flows in neither direction.
	The watershed effect is maximum in the mid-thoracic area due to the greater distance between the radicular arteries.
What are the causes for poor blood supply to the cord?	1. Trauma
	2. Rupture of aortic aneurysm
	3. Dissection of the aorta
	4. Inflammation of aorta—vasculitis, collagen disorders
	5. Venous hypertension
	6. Degenerative spinal diseases and disc herniation
	7. Severe atherosclerosis and luminal narrowing
	8. Iatrogenic
	• Vasoconstrictors in epidural space
	• Surgical cross clamping of the aorta
	• Coeliac plexus block
	• Deliberate/accidental hypotension
What are the risk factors for spinal cord ischaemia during aortic surgery?	According to recent statistics, incidence of spinal cord ischaemia following thoracoabdominal aortic aneurysm repair is 3% –18% despite improved surgical technique, transfusion, and perfusion technology. The factors that determine the neurological outcome after aortic cross clamping are:
	1. Presence of predisposing factors, such as atherosclerosis, diabetes, and renal disease
	2. Extent of aneurysm
	3. Duration of cross clamp
	4. Surgical difficulty
	5. Previous aortic surgery
	6. Severity of perioperative hypotension
What are the different spinal cord protection strategies undertaken during thoracoabdominal aneurysm repair?	1. Mild systemic hypothermia (32°–34°C): The most reliable protective adjunct and helps by decreasing metabolic demands and attenuating inflammatory response to ischaemia.
	2. Maintaining spinal cord perfusion pressure (SCPP) depends on the mean arterial pressure and cerebrospinal fluid pressure (CSFP).
	$$SCPP = MAP - CSFP$$
	Cross-clamping leads to proximal hypertension and increased cerebrospinal fluid pressure. So controlling the arterial pressure with vasopressors or decreasing CSFP via lumbar drains plays a significant role in maintaining SCPP.

STEPS	KEY POINTS

3. Distal aortic shunting through femorofemoral bypass and left heart bypass increases the blood flow to the distal aorta.
4. Pharmacological neuroprotection: Agents such as free radical scavengers, barbiturates, steroids, opiate antagonists, etc., have been evaluated in decreasing the risk of ischaemic damage of the cord.
5. Monitoring spinal cord function with MEPs/SSEPs have proved effective in preventing damage by avoiding important radicular arteries.

What is ASA syndrome? What are the findings?

ASA syndrome—problems in the anterior spinal artery territory resulting in critical ischaemia of the anterior part of the spinal cord.
The characteristic findings are

Motor
Loss of motor function bilaterally below the level of lesion due to the involvement of corticospinal tracts

Sensory
Loss of spinothalamic tracts resulting in bilateral thermoanaesthesia
But intact light touch, vibration, and proprioception due to preservation of posterior columns

Autonomic
Sexual dysfunction; loss of bladder and bowel function due to the effect on descending autonomic tract
See Figure 2.9.

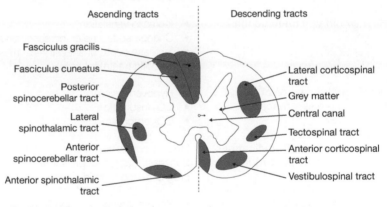

Ascending tracts   Descending tracts

Fasciculus gracilis
Fasciculus cuneatus
Posterior spinocerebellar tract
Lateral spinothalamic tract
Anterior spinocerebellar tract
Anterior spinothalamic tract

Lateral corticospinal tract
Grey matter
Central canal
Tectospinal tract
Anterior corticospinal tract
Vestibulospinal tract

Fig. 2.9 Blood supply to spinal cord

02.6 PHYSIOLOGY: PNEUMOPERITONEUM

HISTORY

STEPS	KEY POINTS
What are the causes of increased CO_2 intra-operatively?	• Hypoventilation • Rebreathing • Sepsis • Malignant hyperpyrexia (MH) • Skeletal muscle activity/hypermetabolism • CO_2 insufflation
How would you manage this?	• Increase ventilation • Change soda lime or increase flows • Increase depth of anaesthesia, muscle relaxants • Specific treatment of MH
What are the causes of raised CO_2 during a laparoscopic procedure?	• Hypoventilation • CO_2 insufflation • CO_2 embolism
Are there any contraindications for laparoscopic procedure?	Medical contraindications to laparoscopic surgery are always relative. Successful laparoscopic surgery has been performed on anticoagulated, pregnant, and morbidly obese patients.
What are the specific anaesthetic issues for laparoscopic procedures?	• Pneumoperitoneum and its effects • Positioning: extreme head up or head down • Surgical issues: trauma of a viscus, vascular trauma

What are the problems with gas insufflation?	• Cardiovascular
	  ◦ ↓cardiac index: ↓venous return due to compression of IVC and Trendelenburg position
	  ◦ ↑SVR: Aortic and splanchnic compression
	  ◦ ↑MAP
	  ◦ Ischaemia: alteration in supply and demand
	  ◦ Arrhythmia: Vagally mediated and ventricular due to high CO_2
	  ◦ Cardiac failure
	
	• Respiratory
	  ◦ ↓FRC
	    - Diaphragmatic splinting and cephalad displacement
	    - Atelectasis
	    - Pulmonary shunting
	    - Hypoxaemia

STEPS	KEY POINTS
	○ ↑Airway pressures: barotrauma or pneumothorax ○ ↑CO_2: Rises by 1 kPa—needs 25% increase in minute volume ○ Endobronchial intubation ○ Gas embolism: Rare and CO_2 is safe • Renal effect: ↓Renal blood flow and GFR • Acid aspiration
At what pressures is a healthy patient at risk of cardiovascular compromise?	>20 mmHg >30 mmHg, Cardiac index might fall by 50%
What are the issues with positioning?	• Head up: Hypotension and cerebral hypoperfusion • Head down: Cerebral oedema, retinal detachment (long operations) • Soft tissue damage due to pressure; e.g. Brachial plexus injury with pressure on the shoulder and neck if used with harness to prevent the patient from slipping down with extreme head down.
What are advantages and disadvantages of laparoscopic surgery?	**Pros:** • Pulmonary function better preserved following laparoscopic surgery; FVC↓ 27% after laparoscopic surgery and by 48% after open surgery • Less painful, earlier discharge from hospital • Cosmetic appealing surgical scars **Cons:** • Postoperative nausea and vomiting—50% of patients require antiemetics, so prophylactic antiemetics may be given routinely • Pain following laparoscopic surgery consists of early transient vagal abdominal and shoulder discomfort due to peritoneal irritation by residual carbon dioxide
What are the factors that determine the morbidity in gas/air embolism?	• Volume of gas entrainment: The closer the vein of entrainment is to the right heart, the smaller the lethal volume. As little as 0.5 mL in Lt anterior descending artery or 2 mL in cerebral circulation is fatal. Traditional estimation is 5 mL/kg • Rate of accumulation: > 0.30 mL/kg/min • Patient's position at the time of the event
What is the pathophysiology of gas embolism?	• Pressure effect: Air entering the systemic venous circulation puts a substantial strain on the right ventricle, and rise in pulmonary artery pressures. This increase in PA pressure can lead to right ventricular outflow obstruction and decrease pulmonary venous return to the left heart, which in turn would lead to resultant decreased cardiac output and eventual systemic cardiovascular collapse. • Inflammatory effect: The air embolism effects on the pulmonary vasculature can lead to serious inflammatory changes in the pulmonary vessels such as direct endothelial damage and accumulation of platelets, fibrin, neutrophils, and lipid droplets. Secondary injury as a result of the activation of complement and the release of mediators and free radicals can lead to capillary leakage and eventual noncardiogenic pulmonary edema. • V/Q mismatch: Alteration in the resistance of the lung vessels and ventilation-perfusion mismatching can lead to intra-pulmonary right-to-left shunting and increased alveolar dead space with subsequent arterial hypoxia and hypercapnia.

02.7 PHARMACOLOGY: DRUGS USED IN MALIGNANCY

HISTORY

STEPS	KEY POINTS
What drugs are used in the treatment of malignancy?	*This is one of the difficult questions but keeps reappearing at the FRCA.*
	Control of disease progression
	• Cytotoxics
	Immunosuppressants
	• Immunoglobins, anti-lymphocytes such as cyclosporine and tacrolimus
	Control of symptoms
	• Analgesics
	• Antiemetics
	• Anxiolytics
	• Antisialogogues
	Prevent/treat metastasis
	• Bone-modifying drugs (e.g., Alendronic acid)
Classify cytotoxic drugs.	• Alkylating agents Act by chemically altering DNA by adding alkyl groups to the electronegative groups of cancer cells. (e.g. Cisplatin, Carboplatin, Chlorambucil, Cyclophosphamide)
	• Anti-metabolites The anti-metabolites function as the building blocks of DNA by imitating the role of purine or pyrimidine and stop cell division. (e.g. Methotrexate, cytarabine)
	• Plant alkaloids They block cell division by inhibiting microtubule function. (e.g. vinca alkaloids)
	• Topoisomerase inhibitors Topoisomerases are enzymes that are essential to maintain the topology of the DNA. Interfering with these enzymes prevents the normal functions of the DNA, such as transcription, replication, and repair. (e.g. amasacrine and etoposide)

STEPS	KEY POINTS

- Antitumour antibiotics
  (e.g. Dactinomycin, daunorubicin, doxorubicin)

- Hormones
  Prednisone and dexamethasone in high doses can damage lymphoma cells.
  Tamoxifen is a selective oestrogen receptor modulator.
  Finasteride is a 5 alpha reductase inhibitor.

- Monoclonal antibodies
  Monoclonal antibodies attach themselves to tumour-specific antigens,
  thereby increasing immune response to tumour cell. (e.g. rituximab,
  cetuximab, trastuzumab)

What are the common side effects of chemotherapy drugs?

Pulmonary toxicity
- Infection due to neutropenic myelosuppression
- Pneumonitis: methotrexate and cyclophosphamide
- Pulmonary fibrosis: bleomycin

Cardiac toxicity
- Arrhythmias, myocardial infarction, congestive cardiac failure,
  cardiomyopathy, myocarditis, and pericarditis: cyclophosphamide
- Torsades de Pointes: cisplatin and anthracyclines

Renal toxicity
- Acute and chronic renal failure: cisplatin and carboplatin

Hepatotoxicity
- Fatty change, cholestasis, and hepatocellular necrosis: methotrexate and
  cyclophosphamide

Neurotoxicity
- Peripheral and cranial neuropathy, autonomic dysfunction, and seizures:
  Vinca alkaloids and methotrexate

Haematological toxicity
- Myelodepression and neutropenic sepsis: most agents

What specific problems arise with the use of steroids?

Water and sodium retention, hypokalaemia, hypertension, hyperglycaemia,
diabetes, osteoporosis, proximal myopathy, dyspepsia, peptic ulcer,
euphoria, depression, infection, poor wound healing, Cushing's, etc.

What are the problems in methotrexate?

Increased infection, abnormal LFTs, thrombocytopenia, photosensitivity

What is tumour lysis syndrome (TLS)?

It is a group of metabolic complications that can occur after treatment
of cancer, usually lymphomas and leukaemias. Precipitating medication
includes combination chemotherapy or steroids, and it sometimes
occurs without any treatment and is known as 'spontaneous tumour lysis
syndrome'.

What are the pathophysiological changes in TLS?

Hyperkalaemia
High turnover of tumour cells leads to spill of potassium into the blood.
- Cardiac conduction abnormalities (can be fatal)
- Severe muscle weakness or paralysis

Hyperphosphataemia
Causes acute renal failure because of deposition of calcium phosphate
crystals in the renal parenchyma

STEPS	KEY POINTS
	Hypocalcaemia Calcium precipitates with phosphate to form calcium phosphate, leading to hypocalcaemia. • Tetany • Seizures • Emotional instability/agitation/anxiety • Myopathy ***Hyperuricaemia*** Acute uric acid nephropathy (AUAN)
How can TLS be prevented?	• Adequate IV hydration • Alkalinisation of urine • Prophylactic oral or IV allopurinol • Rasburicase as an alternative to allopurinol
Describe the analgesia in cancer patients.	Simple analgesics: Paracetamol and nonsteroidal agents Weak opioids: tramadol and codeine Strong opioids: morphine, diamorphine in oral, parenteral, transdermal and neuraxial routes Special drugs: gabapentin, pregabalin Nerve blocks
What is breakthrough pain?	Breakthrough pain is defined as pain of moderate or severe intensity occurring against a background of controlled chronic pain. It could be spontaneous, incidental, or procedural. As with any cancer pain, treatment relies on detailed assessment and formulation of a multidisciplinary therapy plan. Rapid acting opioids have been successfully used to treat breakthrough pain, but it remains a difficult therapeutic problem.

02.8
PHYSICS: SODALIME

HISTORY

STEPS	KEY POINTS
Name the compounds used to absorb carbon dioxide in the breathing system.	• Soda lime Commonly used, it has been proven that presence of sodium hydroxide, at any level, provides the basis for anaesthetic agent dehalogenation, which can lead to formation of compound A and carbon monoxide. • Baralyme or barium lime It is made of 80% calcium hydroxide and 20% barium hydroxide. This is less efficient than soda lime and also produces compound A more quickly. • Litholyme or lithium lime Also an effective carbon dioxide absorbent, litholyme is free of the strong bases (NaOH, KOH) and does not produce compound A or carbon monoxide. Lithium chloride acts as the catalyst to accelerate the formation of calcium carbonate. • Amsorb Contains calcium hydroxide and calcium chloride and is not associated with the formation of carbon monoxide or compound A. • Amsorb Plus It is a new generation carbon dioxide absorbent, free from strong alkali metal hydroxides. It utilizes calcium hydroxide as the active base with minor constituents that promote speed and capacity of absorption. Amsorb Plus is specifically designed for low and minimal flow anaesthesia. • Dragersorb and Medisorb These are produced by Drager and GE healthcare, respectively, with varying proportions of constituents.
Describe soda lime in detail.	Soda lime consists of 94% calcium hydroxide, 5% sodium hydroxide, and a small amount of potassium hydroxide (0.1%) and silica to prevent disintegration. A dye or colour indicator such as ethyl violet is also added, which changes the colour when the soda lime is exhausted. This happens at pH < 10. pH 13.5 Moisture content 14%–19% 1 kg absorbs 120 L of carbon dioxide

STEPS	KEY POINTS
	When exhaled gases reach the canister, carbon dioxide absorption takes place and heat and water are produced. The warmed and humidified gas rejoins the fresh gas flow (FGF).
	In a patient with tidal ventilation of 6 L/min and CO_2 production of 250 ml/min, the soda lime will be exhausted in 6 hours at FGF of 1 L/min and in 8 hours if the FGF is 3 L/min.

What is the chemical reaction during the absorption of CO_2 by soda lime?

$CO_2 + H_2O \longrightarrow H_2CO_3$

then

$H_2CO_3 + 2\,KOH \longrightarrow K_2CO_3 + 2\,H_2O + Energy$

then

$K_2CO_3 + Ca(OH)_2 \longrightarrow CaCO_3 + 2KOH$

OR

$CO_2 + 2NaOH \longrightarrow Na_2CO_3 + H_2O + heat$

then

$Na_2CO_3 + Ca(OH)_2 \longrightarrow CaCO_3 + 2NaOH$

Each mole of CO_2 (44 g) reacted produces one mole of water (18 g). The overall reaction is

$Ca(OH)_2 + CO_2 \longrightarrow CaCO_3 + H_2O + heat$

What are the harmful products that are formed when using soda lime?

Compound A
- Is a fluoro methyl ether produced when sevoflurane is used with soda lime due to dehydrohalogenation in the presence of KOH.
- Factors that increase the production of compound A are
  - High sevoflurane
  - Increasing temperature
  - Low FGF
  - Use of baralyme

Carbon monoxide
- Occurs when inhalational agents with CHF_2 moiety such as desflurane, enflurane, and isoflurane are used with desiccated soda lime granules. This happens when the system is left unused for a long time. This can lead to formation of carboxyhaemoglobin and can be significant in smokers especially when very low flows are used.
- Factors increasing the production of CO include
  - Type of inhaled anaesthetic agent (magnitude of CO production from greatest to least is desflurane > enflurane > isoflurane > sevoflurane)
  - High absorbent dryness
  - Type of absorbent (at a given water content, baralyme produces more CO than soda lime)
  - Increased temperature
  - Higher anaesthetic concentration
- Other insignificant substances like methane, acetone, ethanol, etc.

What is the size of the soda lime granules? How does this affect its performance?

The typical size is expressed as between 4–8 mesh. It means the granules will pass through a mesh with 4–8 strands per inch in each axis. The uniformity in size is necessary to provide a smooth flow. They should provide larger surface area but lesser resistance to flow. Bigger molecules would cause gas channelling, and smaller granules can increase the resistance to gas flow.

STEPS	KEY POINTS
What are the uses and advantages of using soda lime?	• Anaesthetic use • Non anaesthetic use—in submarines and recompression chambers • Metabolic monitoring—in alkaline fuel cells to extract carbon dioxide as it affects the measurement **Advantages** • Permits low flows without rebreathing carbon dioxide, making the system cost effective • Less waste and pollution • Humidification of inspired gases due to the inherent exothermic reaction
Is the colour indicator always accurate and represent the usage of soda lime?	No. The decrease in pH causes the indicator to change colour, so any product that causes a decrease in pH can mimic an exhausted soda lime. In partial exhaustion, the carbonic acid levels increase and cause the change in colour of the indicator. If the soda lime is unused, then the free hydroxyl ions from the depth of the canister migrate to the surface and neutralise the acid, reverting the colour change. As a result, the soda lime appears fresh although it is partially exhausted.
What are the clinical signs of soda lime exhaustion?	• Increased spontaneous respiratory rate in the absence of muscle relaxant • Increase in sympathetic drive • Respiratory acidosis • Increased surgical bleeding due to hypertension and coagulopathy
What are the pros and cons of using a circle system?	**Advantages** • Economy of anaesthetic consumption • Warming and humidification of the inspired gases • Reduced atmospheric pollution **Disadvantages** • Unstable if closed-system is used • Slow changes in the inspired anaesthetic concentration with low flows and out-of-circuit vaporiser
What are the components of a circle system and rough dimensions of tubing?	• CO_2 absorber canister • Breathing bag • Unidirectional inspiratory and expiratory valves • Fresh gas supply • Pressure-relief valve • Corrugated hoses and a Y-piece The body of the absorber is connected to the patient by means of inspiratory and expiratory tubes and a Y-piece the size of which is important when anaesthetising paediatric patients as very small tidal volumes may not generate enough pressure to open the valves effectively. The effective dead space of the Y-piece is larger than it appears, and so there can be rebreathing of exhaled gas. These difficulties are overcome by the use of purpose-built infant absorbers and paediatric tubing and Y-pieces.

Further reading

1. Leslie RA, Johnson EK, Goodwin APL. Dr Podcast Scripts for the Primary FRCA.
2. Al-Shaikh B, Stacey S. *Essentials of Anaesthetic Equipment*. 4th Revised edition.

CLINICAL VIVA

03.1 LONG CASE: PREGNANT WOMAN WITH DIABETIC KETOACIDOSIS

HISTORY *You are asked to see a 20-year-old female who is 30/40 pregnant. Her past medical history consists of Insulin Dependent Diabetes Mellitus (Type I DM) and asthma.*

She has been admitted with an infected hand and a short history of abdominal pain.

Her current medications are salbutamol inhaler prn, insulin glargine (Lantus) 20 U nocte and actrapid 6–8units TDS with meals.

STEPS	KEY POINTS	
On examination	Weight	80 kg
	Height	165 cm
	BMI	25
	Heart rate	80/min
	Respiratory rate	20/min
	BP	140/80 mmHg
	Temperature	36°C
Investigations	Hb	10.0 g/L
	WCC	16.9×10^9/L
	Neutrophils	10×10^9/L
	Platelets	400×10^9/L
	Urea	12.0 mmol/L
	Creatinine	140 mmol/L
	Na	134 mmol/L
	K	5.9 mmol/L
Arterial Blood Gas	FiO_2	0.3
	pH	6.89
	PaO_2	17.0 kPa
	$PaCO_2$	2.48 kPa
	HCO_3	4.7 mmol/L
	BE	−29.2 mmol/L
	Blood glucose	30 mmol/L

STEPS	KEY POINTS
Urine dipstix	White cells + Proteins ++ Ketones +++ Glucose +
Summarise the case.	A 20-year-old woman with known Type I DM presenting with an infected hand requiring surgical debridement complicated by the fact that she is 30 weeks pregnant and showing signs of diabetic ketoacidosis (raised blood sugar, compensated metabolic acidosis, and abdominal pain).
Can you explain the blood results? Which are consistent with pregnancy?	• Most striking abnormality is metabolic acidosis on blood gas with raised blood glucose and ketones in urine consistent with diabetic ketoacidosis (DKA) • Raised urea consistent with dehydration, bordering on acute renal failure when taken in context with creatinine (GFR is usually much increased in pregnancy ~ 50% at term; therefore, although creatinine is in range, it is much higher than would be expected for the increase urea and creatinine clearance than one would expect at this stage of pregnancy) • Raised white cell count with neutrophilia consistent with bacterial infection (infected hand) • Mild anaemia consistent with physiological anaemia of pregnancy (plasma volume increases by up to 45% with only a 20%–30% increase in red cell mass, hence a 'physiological' anaemia)

Discuss the management of DKA.	*The answer is based on diabetes.org.uk guideline.*
	
	General management
	• Managed in HDU setting
	• Joint care with obstetricians and medical team
	
	DKA consists of the biochemical triad of ketonaemia, hyperglycaemia, and acidaemia. Therefore, management is directed at correcting these key issues.
	• Full clinical history and examination
	• Rapid ABC assessment including a full set of observations and Glasgow coma score
	• Large-bore IV access (or central access if this is not possible)
	• Consider precipitating causes and treat appropriately
	• All patients with DKA need specialist diabetic team input within 24 hours of admission
	
	Initial investigations
	• Blood: blood glucose, urea and electrolytes, full blood count, blood cultures, blood gas
	• ECG to look for arrhythmias due to associated electrolyte abnormalities
	• Chest radiograph if clinically indicated
	• Urinalysis and culture to rule out infection
	
	Specific Treatment
	• Drugs
	   o Establish usual medication for diabetes
	   o Commence a fixed rate insulin infusion (FRII), if weight not available from patient estimate weight in kg (in pregnancy you should use patients current weight)

STEPS	KEY POINTS
	• Fluids
	○ Restore circulating volume with boluses of 500 mL–1000 mL 0.9% sodium chloride if systolic blood pressure is < 90 mmHg (may need more depending on response and may need to consider use of vasopressors to maintain BP)

	○ The suggested regime in a previously healthy 70 kg adult would be:
	    - 1L 0.9% sodium chloride over first hour
	    - 1L 0.9% sodium chloride with potassium chloride over next 2 hours
	    - 1L 0.9% sodium chloride with potassium chloride over next 2 hours
	    - 1L 0.9% sodium chloride with potassium chloride over next 4 hours
	    - 1L 0.9% sodium chloride with potassium chloride over next 4 hours
	    - 1L 0.9% sodium chloride with potassium chloride over next 6 hours
	    - Mandatory reassessment of cardiovascular status at 12 hours

	○ Once blood glucose is less than 14 mmol/L, then 10% dextrose should be commenced at 125 mL/hr and ran with the normal saline
	• Electrolyte replacement
	○ If potassium is > 5.5 mmol/L, no potassium replacement is given in fluid infusions
	○ If 3.5–5.5 mmol/L, 40 mmol per litre of saline should be given
	○ Below 3.5 mmol/L requires senior ITU input as more potassium will need to be given with extra monitoring
	• Goals
	○ Aim is to reduce blood ketones and suppress ketogenesis
	○ Achieve a fall of ketones of at least 0.5 mmol/L/hr
	○ Get resolution within 12–24 hours
	• The precipitating cause needs to be treated (in this case, the infected hand)
How do you make a sliding scale insulin or Variable Rate Intravenous Insulin Infusion (VRIII)?	• The latest guidelines for the management of DKA no longer recommend the use of a sliding scale insulin • A fixed rate insulin infusion is made by drawing up 50 units of human soluble insulin (e.g. actrapid) and making it up to 50 mL with 0.9% sodium chloride. This is then run at 0.1 units/kg/hr until the ketone level is less than 0.6 mmol/L

Which fluids would you give her and why?	• There are several mechanisms responsible for fluid depletion in DKA
	  ○ Osmotic diuresis due to hyperglycaemia
	  ○ Vomiting—commonly associated with DKA
	  ○ Inability to take in fluid due to a diminished level of consciousness
	
	• Electrolyte shifts and depletion are in part related to the osmotic diuresis
	• Hyperkalaemia and hypokalaemia need particular attention
	
	I would follow the fluid regime above and tailor it to the specific needs of the patient. I would use 0.9% sodium chloride with potassium chloride as required as it is compliant with NPSA safety regulations, but I would be aware of the risk of hyperchloraemic acidosis.

The surgeons are keen to debride her hand. Describe how you would anaesthetise her.	At this stage I wouldn't anaesthetise her; she needs her DKA treated and her fluid status optimised prior to receiving an anaesthetic, be that regional or general

STEPS	KEY POINTS
You arrange a bed for her on the high-dependency unit, and 18 hours later her DKA has corrected but her hand still requires surgical debridement. What is your anaesthetic choice?	Regional vs. general anaesthesia.

Regional vs. general anaesthesia.
- My preferred method would be regional in view of recent metabolic derangement and pregnancy.

Axillary brachial plexus block is the choice for forearm and hand surgery.
- If GA is planned, then this would need to be a rapid sequence induction. There is a risk of difficult airway and a need for left lateral tilt.
- Ensure well-balanced anaesthetic avoiding hypoxia, hypercarbia, and hypothermia.
- Fetus would require CTG monitoring.

Describe the technique for performing an axillary brachial plexus block.

General
- Full anaesthetic history and examination
- Informed consent of the patient
- Trained assistant
- Full monitoring as per AAGBI guidelines
- Ultrasound machine
- IV access

Conduct of block
- Aseptic technique
- Ultrasound probe positioned with short axis to arm just distal to pectoralis major insertion
- Aim to achieve local anaesthetic spread around the axillary artery covering median, ulnar, and radial nerve and a separate injection to cover the musculocutaneous nerve
- Total volume of local anaesthetic 20–25 mls of 0.25% L – Bupivacaine (5–7 mL around each nerve)

Look at the ultrasound image in Figure 3.1a and name the structures.

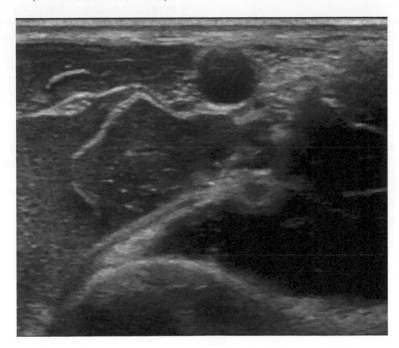

Fig. 3.1a

STEPS	KEY POINTS

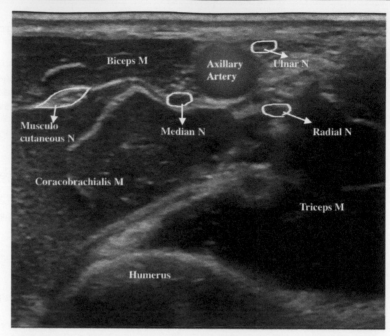

Fig. 3.1b

Median, ulnar, and radial nerves are seen scattered around the axillary artery with the tissue sheath. The musculocutaneous nerve is seen between the biceps and coracobrachialis away from the rest of the brachial plexus. The axillary vein is compressed leading to the possibility of accidental intravascular injection of local anaesthetic

As you inject the local anaesthetic for your block, the woman begins to have a seizure. What is your differential diagnosis?	• Non-pregnancy-related: local anaesthetic toxicity, hypoxia, hypoglycaemia, epilepsy, metabolic derangement (e.g. cerebral oedema from DKA) • Pregnancy-related: Eclampsia
Describe how you would manage the seizures.	• Call for help. • Give 100% oxygen. • Maintain an airway, with intubation if necessary. • Establish IV access. • Give IV benzodiazepine in incremental doses to terminate the seizure. • Ensure left lateral position. • Treat the cause.

STEPS	KEY POINTS

Describe the specific management of seizures related to local anaesthetic toxicity.	• **Recognise:** change in mental status, severe agitation or loss of consciousness with or without seizures, and cardiovascular collapse.
	
	• **Immediate management:**
	  ○ Stop injecting local anaesthetic.
	  ○ Call for help.
	  ○ ABC: Maintain airway (secure with ETT if necessary), give 100% oxygen, confirm and establish IV access.
	  ○ Control seizures with incremental doses of benzodiazepine, propofol or thiopental, assess cardiovascular status throughout. Conventional therapies to treat hypotension, bradycardia, and tachyarrhythmia.
	
	• **Intralipid:**
	  ○ Initial bolus: 20% lipid emulsion 1.5 ml/kg over 1 min and start an infusion at 15 ml/kg/hr. After 5 min, if cardiovascular stability not restored, give further two boluses. Continue infusion at same rate, but if she remains unstable after 5 min, increase to 30 ml/kg/hr.

Further reading

1. Diabetes in Pregnancy. *NICE Clinical Guideline July 2008*. Available at http://www.nice.org.uk/nicemedia/live/11946/41320/41320.pdf
2. The Management of Diabetic Ketoacidosis in Adults. *Joint Diabetes Societies Inpatient Care Group*. Second Edition. September 2013.
3. Ultrasound guided brachial plexus block. The New York School of Regional Anaesthesia.
4. *AAGBI Safety Guideline: Management of Severe Local Anaesthetic Toxicity.* The Association of Anaesthetists of Great Britain & Ireland 2010.

03.2 SHORT CASE: ICU WEAKNESS

HISTORY *A 62-year-old patient ventilated on ICU with pneumonia is now experiencing difficulty in weaning.*

STEPS	KEY POINTS
What may be the causes for difficult weaning?	**Respiratory causes** • Insufficiently treated pulmonary disease • Auto-PEEP and hyperinflation **Cardiac causes** • Concomitant cardiac disease **Others** • Poor nutrition • Electrolyte imbalance • Critical illness neuropathy/ICU weakness • Poor technique—inadequate rest following an exhausting spontaneous breathing trial
You mentioned ICU weakness. How can you define it?	ICU-acquired weakness (ICUAW) is 'clinically detected weakness in critically ill patients in whom there is no plausible aetiology other than critical illness'. The criteria for diagnosing ICUAW are the presence of most of the following factors: • Weakness developing after the onset of critical illness • Weakness being generalised, symmetrical, flaccid, and generally sparing the cranial nerves (e.g. facial grimace is intact) • Muscle power assessed by the Medical Research Council (MRC) score of < 48 (or a mean score of < 4 in all testable muscle groups) noted on > 2 occasions separated by > 24 hours • Dependence on mechanical ventilation • Other causes of weakness having been excluded
Can you list the differential diagnosis for ICUAW?	• Spinal cord dysfunction • Critical illness myopathy • Guillain-Barre syndrome • Motor neuron disease • Preexisting neuropathy • Myasthenia
What can cause ICU weakness?	ICUAW can be classified into those with critical illness polyneuropathy (CIP), critical illness myopathy (CIM), or critical illness neuromyopathy (CINM). The causes are unknown, though they are thought to be a possible neurological manifestation of systemic inflammatory response syndrome.

STEPS	KEY POINTS
	Risk factors for CIP, CIM and CINM include:
	• Severe sepsis/septic shock with multi-organ failure
	• Prolonged mechanical ventilation
	• Prolonged bed rest
	• Glucose and electrolyte abnormalities
	• Use of parenteral nutrition, renal replacement therapy, steroids, muscle relaxants, vasopressors, and aminoglycosides
What is the difference between CIP and CIM?	• Similar symptoms and presentations • Often distinguished largely on the basis of specialised electrophysiological testing or muscle and nerve biopsy
Can you tell me the details of the electrophysiological investigations required for diagnosis?	• Nerve conduction studies to determine nerve conduction velocities and stimulated amplitudes [compound motor action potentials (CMAPs) and sensory nerve action potentials (SNAPs)] • Electromyography to look at muscle electrical activity [motor unit potential (MUP) amplitudes, durations, and fibre recruitment patterns] both at rest and during activity
How may it be treated?	• No intervention has been shown in prospective study to improve the outcome • Focus on prevention • Optimise rehabilitation
	Prevention of ICUAW • Minimisation of the risk factors (as above) • Intensive insulin therapy
Can you mention a few care bundles you are aware of in the intensive care unit?	**Ventilator Care Bundle** • Elevation of the head of the bed • Peptic ulcer disease prophylaxis • Deep venous thrombosis prophylaxis • Daily oral care with Chlorhexidine
	Central Line Bundle • Appropriate hand hygiene • Chlorhexidine skin prep • Maximal barriers for central line insertion • Subclavian vein placement is preferred site • Review lines daily and remove unnecessary catheters
	Sepsis Care Bundle Three-hour bundle • Measure lactate level • Obtain blood cultures prior to administration of antibiotics • Administer broad spectrum antibiotics • Administer 30 mL/kg crystalloid for hypotension or lactate $\geq$ 4 mmol/L

STEPS	KEY POINTS
	Six-hour bundle • Apply vasopressors (for hypotension that does not respond to initial fluid resuscitation) to maintain a mean arterial pressure (MAP) $\geq$ 65 mm Hg • Measure central venous pressure (CVP) and central venous oxygen saturation (ScvO$_2$) in refractory hypotension • Remeasure lactate if initial lactate was elevated

Further reading

1. Appleton R, Kinsella J. Intensive care unit-acquired weakness. *Contin Educ Anaesth Crit Care Pain.* 2012; doi: 10.1093/bjaceaccp/mkr057v.
2. Dellinger RP, Levy MM, Rhodes A, et al. Surviving Sepsis Campaign: International Guidelines for Management of Severe Sepsis and Septic Shock: 2012. *Crit Care Med.* 2013; **41**: 580–637.

03.3 SHORT CASE: CONSENT ISSUES

HISTORY *A 16-year-old girl with learning difficulties is put on the operation list for dental corrective surgery (surgery due to last 1 to 2 hours). You are asked to preassess this patient.*

STEPS	KEY POINTS
What are the causes of learning difficulties?	The underlying problems in these children may include neurological disability, developmental delay, behavioural disorders, autism, and mental health or personality problems.
What are the issues with this case?	• Poor dental hygiene. • Uncooperative and communication may be challenging. • Higher risk of infection like hepatitis B, especially in institutionalised individuals. • Other medical conditions and physical abnormalities may co-exist, such as epilepsy, reflux, and cardiac anomalies. • Consent issues.
What is capacity? How will you assess capacity in this patient?	A capable (or competent) person is one who has reached 18 years of age and who has the capacity to make decisions on their own behalf regarding treatment. In England and Wales competent young people of 16 or 17 years of age can give consent for any surgical, medical, or dental treatment; it is not necessary to obtain separate consent from the parent or guardian. *The Mental Capacity Act 2005 governs the treating of an incapable person.* Occasionally in some cases the Act permits medical treatment to be given without the patient's consent, as long as it is in their best interests and has not been refused in a valid and applicable advance directive (living will) or advance decision. **In adult:** Every adult is assumed to be capable. The default position, therefore, is that all adults have capacity until they are proven otherwise. No other person can consent to treatment on behalf of any adult, including incompetent adults. Any treatment, investigation, or physical contact with the patient undertaken without consent may amount to assault. But treatment may be given if it is in their best interests, as long as the requirements of the Mental Capacity Act 2005 are adhered to.

STEPS	KEY POINTS

In children:
Only people with 'parental responsibility' are entitled to give consent on behalf of their children.

Parental responsibility is defined in the Children Act (1989) as "All the rights, duties, powers, responsibilities, and authority which by law a parent of a child has in relation to a child and his property" (Children Act 1989, section 3).

What are the consent and parent-guardian issues in adolescents?

'Consent' is a patient's agreement for a health professional to provide care. Patients may indicate consent nonverbally, orally, or in writing.

Parent-guardian:
The mother has an automatic right to parental responsibility. The father has an automatic right only if he was married to the mother at the time of birth, although he can acquire parental responsibility by court order or by agreement.

In some circumstances, another person may have acquired parental responsibility (e.g. a legal guardian, adoptive parent, or a social worker).

Age:
- If a person under 18 years of age refuses treatment that is deemed essential, then the patient can be made a ward of the Court and the Court may order that an operation may be carried out lawfully.
- If a young person of 16 or 17 years of age is not competent to give consent, then the consent of a parent should be sought, unless immediate treatment is required to prevent death or permanent injury.
- If a child under the age of 16 years achieves a sufficient understanding of what is proposed, he or she may consent to treatment. The child must be Gillick competent.

What is Gillick competence?

This term is used in medical law to decide whether a child (16 years or younger) who has achieved sufficient understanding of what is being proposed is able to consent to his or her own medical treatment, without the need for parental permission or knowledge. However, in cases where a competent child has refused or resisted medical treatment, the courts have upheld the right of the parents to consent for the child's treatment up to the age of 18 years.

Lord Scarman's test is generally considered to be the test of 'Gillick competency'. He required that a child could consent if he or she fully understood the medical treatment that was being proposed.

Fraser guidelines are concerned only with contraception and focus on the desirability of parental involvement and the risks of unprotected sex in children younger than 16.

Who are IMCAs?

The IMCA service is provided for any person aged 16 years or older, who has no one able to support and represent them, and who lacks capacity to make a decision about either:
1. a long-term care move
2. a serious medical treatment
3. adult protection procedures
4. a care review

What are the different types of consent forms you have come across?

Form 1: For adults or competent children
Form 2: For parental consent for a child or young person
Form 3: For cases where the patient will remain alert throughout the procedure and no anaesthetist will be involved in their care
Form 4: For adults who are unable to consent to investigation or treatment

STEPS	KEY POINTS
What problems might you encounter while anaesthetising her in the anaesthetic room?	Difficult rapport and aggressive and combative behaviour at induction requiring sedation. Premedicants like midazolam reduce anxiety at induction of anaesthesia and reduce postoperative behavioural disturbances.
	Parent-guardian presence at induction and in the recovery area is necassary to eliminate separation anxiety.
	Starvation status may not be adequately followed by the patients.
What are criteria for offering GA in a day-care dentistry?	The General Dental Council and the Royal College of Anaesthetists guidelines state that general anaesthesia for dentistry should only be administered for:
	• Situations in which it would be impossible to achieve adequate local anaesthesia and complete treatment without pain
	• Patients who, because of problems related to age/maturity or physical/learning disability, are unlikely to allow safe completion of treatment
	• Patients in whom long-term dental phobia will be induced or prolonged

Further reading

1. NHS Choices. *Consent to Treatment.*
2. UKCEN. UK Clinical Ethics Network.
3. General Medical Council (GMC). *Consent guidance: patients and doctors making decisions together.*

03.4 SHORT CASE: WPW SYNDROME

HISTORY *You are preassessing a 22-year-old female patient for Functional Endoscopic Sinus Surgery (FESS). She gives a history of palpitations for which she was admitted to A&E a year ago.*

STEPS	KEY POINTS
What are the causes of palpitations?	• Anxiety • Exercise • Panic attacks • Caffeine, alcohol • Drugs: Thyroxine, cocaine, beta 2 agonists • Cardiac: MI, arrthymias, ectopics, AF, flutter, VT, reentry tachyarrhythmia • Endocrine: hyperthyroidism, hypoglycaemia, phaeochromocytoma
Why do arrthymias occur?	• Reentry circuits • Enhanced automaticity • Triggered activity
What investigations would you like her to have?	• History and examination is paramount • ECG: 12-lead, 24-hour, ambulatory • Cardiac electrophysiological study • Bloods, to rule out endocrine causes
Figure 3.2 illustrates her ECG. Comment on the positive findings. What is the diagnosis?	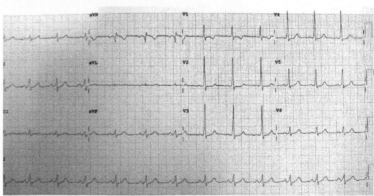

Fig. 3.2

STEPS	KEY POINTS
	Rate: 75/min Sinus rhythm Normal axis PR interval: 3–4 small squares (not very short) Initial slow upstroke of QRS but later becomes normal complexes Presence of delta waves
Explain to me what Wolff–Parkinson-White (WPW) syndrome is.	• Presence of faster accessory pathway (bundle of Kent) between atrium and ventricle (accessory AV pathway) • This pathway conducts impulses faster than the normal AV node • Electrical signals traveling down this abnormal pathway may stimulate the ventricles to contract prematurely, resulting in a unique type of supraventricular tachycardia
What are the characteristics of ECG in WPW?	• Sinus, normal axis, short PR interval • Presence of delta waves
What is a delta wave?	• Accessory pathway conducts impulse faster than AV node, resulting in short PR interval • The initial depolarization takes place in ventricular muscle; hence, the slow and slurred delta wave • Later, when the impulse arrives at the AV node, bundle of His and Purkinje carries the impulse, which is normal and faster than ventricular wave; hence, the rest of the QRS is normal
What are the treatment options for patients with WPW syndrome?	• Risk stratification to exclude patients who are at risk of sudden death. This is done with the presenting symptoms of syncope, etc., and with invasive electrophysiological studies • Pharmacological therapy for stable tachyarrhythmias and cardioversion for decompensated patients • Drugs: Commonly used drugs are amiodarone and procainamide. Drugs such as adenosine, diltiazem, verapamil, and beta blockers are avoided due to the risk of slowing the heart's normal conduction and favouring accessory conduction leading to unstable dysrhythmias • Ablation: Definitive treatment is by radiofrequency ablation of the accessory pathway
What are the implications of WPW for anaesthesia?	There is a tendency to paroxysmal supraventricular tachycardia in the perioperative period and there may be associated congenital cardiac abnormality. Unmasking of WPW syndrome under either general or regional anaesthesia has been reported, which means the patient was asymptomatic with normal ECG preoperatively and under anaesthesia re-entrant arrhythmia gets unmasked with clinical symptoms. Anaesthetic drugs tend to change the physiology of AV conduction. If the patient is asymptomatic, then risk of perioperative arrhythmias is much less. • General anaesthesia Avoid light planes of anaesthesia and drugs that can precipitate tachycardia (like atropine, glycopyrrolate, ketamine) resulting in paroxysmal supraventricular tachycardia or atrial fibrillation. Opioids, such as fentanyl, and benzodiazepines, including midazolam, have been found to have no effect on the accessory pathway.

STEPS	KEY POINTS
	There are references showing disappearance of delta waves after propofol administration, making it the drug of choice for induction. Isoflurane and sevoflurane have been found to have no effect on AV node conduction, making these agents preferable for maintenance of cardiostability. Short acting nondepolarizing muscle relaxant without histamine release would be an acceptable choice as reversal of neuromuscular blockade using neostigmine and glycopyrrolate is not required.

• Regional anaesthesia
  There is significant advantage over general anaesthesia as multidrug administration, laryngoscopic stimulation, intubation, and light planes leading to sympathetic stimulation are avoided.

What are the common types of tachyarrhythmias that can develop in the perioperative period?

There are two common life-threatening arrhythmias that occur in patients with WPW.
• Atrial fibrillation leading to ventricular fibrillation
• Circus re-entrant tachycardia causing ventricular or paroxysmal supraventricular tachycardias. Ventricular tachycardias are very difficult to treat and may even be life threatening

How would you manage intraoperative tachyarrthymias?

After taking all precautions, if arrhythmias develop, the patient is treated after a careful ABC assessment.

Atrial fibrillation
• The treatment principle is to prolong the anterograde refractory period of the accessory pathway relative to the AV node. This slows the rate of impulse transmission through the accessory pathway and, thus, the ventricular rate. This is in direct contradiction to the goal of treatment of non-WPW atrial fibrillation, which is to slow the refractory period of the AV node

Paroxysmal supraventricular tachycardia
• Vagal manoeuvres initially
• Haemodynamically stable: Lignocaine, adenosine, disopyramide, and procainamide can be used. These drugs block transmission via the accessory pathway by blocking fast sodium channel
• Haemodynamically unstable: Synchronized DC cardioversion at 25–50 J may be needed for atrial fibrillation. Digitalis and verapamil are strictly contraindicated in patients with pre-excited atrial fibrillation or flutter with rapid conduction over an accessory pathway

Treat possible triggers: hypoxia, hypercarbia, acidosis, and electrolyte imbalance

section 03

BASIC SCIENCE
VIVA

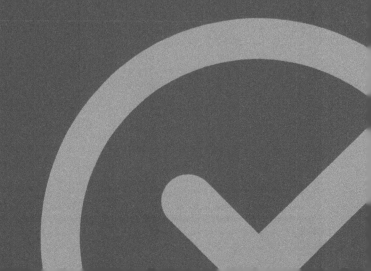

03.5 ANATOMY: CRANIAL NERVE MONITORING

Your knowledge of cranial nerves can be tested in different ways.

...Diagnostic features of chronic pain, pathogenesis, features, medical, radiological and surgical treatment of trigeminal neuralgia and management, anatomy of trigeminal nerve, Gasserian ganglion block.

...How would you assess the degree of neuromuscular blockade, mechanism of work, various modalities, which nerves are commonly used, facial nerve anatomy, surgeries where it can be damaged?

...Reasons for assessing cranial nerves, criteria for brainstem death, brainstem death testing—how each CN is tested, the afferent and efferent pathways.

...When would you monitor vagus nerve intraoperatively, why and how it is done, anatomy of vagus, causes and features of injury—general and laryngeal.

STEPS	KEY POINTS
When would you monitor cranial nerves (CN)?	**Surgical** • Intraoperatively during a surgical procedure to identify the nerve, preserve function, and prevent intraoperative injury. Several neurosurgical procedures warrant routine monitoring of cranial nerves depending on the position and extent of surgery. All cranial nerves except CN I can be monitored. As most cranial nerves are motor, placing the EMG electrodes on muscles supplied by the nerve tests their function. CN VIII, being a sensory nerve, is tested by brainstem evoked auditory potential (BAEP). CN II is rarely monitored. • III, IV, and VI: removal of tumours at clivus or skull base • V: microvascular decompression for trigeminal neuralgia • VII: acoustic neuroma and parotid gland surgery • VIII: cerebello pontine angle tumours • IX: radical neck dissection • X: thyroid or vocal cord surgery • XI and XII: skull base (jugular glomus tumour) surgery

STEPS	KEY POINTS

Neurophysiological
- Intraoperative nerve monitoring to assess the degree of neuromuscular block (commonly used technique is the **T**rain **o**f **F**our (TOF)). Peripheral branches of the facial nerve are used due to their ability to cause visible muscular contractions and their proximity to the skin.
- Brainstem testing in ITU: to confirm brainstem death.

What are the anaesthetic implications of using CN monitoring for neurosurgery?

(The question is not about anaesthetic implications of neurosurgery but of CN monitoring.)
- Choice of anaesthetic—use of inhalational agents and muscle relaxants
- Physiological factors that influence evoked potentials—temperature, acid-base, blood pressure, haematocrit, etc.
- Electrical artefacts—electrical interference can be a problem as SSEP is believed to simulate pacemaker spikes on ECG tracing

Neurophysiological monitoring	Muscle relaxant	Volatile agent
EMG: Electromyogram	<<	<->
MEP: Motor-evoked potential	<<	<<
BAEP: Brainstem-evoked auditory potential	<->	<->
SSEP: Somatosensory-evoked potential	<->	<<

The degree of muscle relaxation is the only anaesthetic factor for concern when myogenic (EMG) activity is used for monitoring purposes. Special anaesthetic consideration is not required with BAEP.
- If MEP is monitored, then use of TIVA with Propofol and Remifentanil with no muscle relaxation is the anaesthetic of choice (as volatile limited to ≤ 0.5 MAC)
- With SSEP, a similar technique is used but without the need to restrict the use of neuromuscular blocker

Choose a cranial nerve and tell me about its origin and course.

Choose the nerve with a less confusing anatomy. (…There is no such nerve!) I would personally choose Trigeminal nerve. It is just that it has a fairly succinct origin and course and it can lead to further questioning on trigeminal neuralgia, which is a treat! Vagus nerve has a complex course, and it seems there is nothing special about Facial nerve.

Trigeminal nerve is the largest cranial nerve.

Function
- Motor: to the muscles of mastication
- Sensory: to the face, orbit, tongue, nose and anterior scalp

Nuclei of origin
- One motor: upper pons below the floor of IV ventricle
- Three sensory
  - Mesencephalic nucleus (proprioception): midbrain
  - Principal sensory nucleus (touch): upper pons
  - Nucleus of spinal tract (pain and temperature): pons to spinal cord

STEPS	KEY POINTS

Course
- The sensory fibres decussate and emerge at the upper pons as a larger sensory and smaller motor root
- Gasserian (trigeminal or semilunar) ganglion is crescent-shaped swelling formed by the sensory fibres situated at the apex of the petrous temporal bone. The ganglion is surrounded superiorly by the temporal lobe, medially by the internal carotid artery and cavernous sinus, and inferiorly lies the motor root
- The motor fibres bypass the ganglion and join the mandibular division

Division and distribution
- Ophthalmic (V_1): sensory only
  - Emerges *via superior orbital fissure*
  - Frontal, lacrimal and nasociliary nerves

- Maxillary (V_2): sensory only
  - Leaves the base of skull via *foramen rotundum*
  - Gives off branches to supply the pterygopalatine fossa and the face before it exits through the infraorbital foramen as the infraorbital nerve

- Mandibular (V_3): sensory and motor
  - Via *Foramen ovale*
  - Sensory: auriculotemporal, buccal, lingual, and inferior alveolar nerves

- Motor: muscles of mastication

How is trigeminal nerve tested to confirm brainstem death?

It is tested by the interrogation of brainstem-mediated V and VII cranial nerve reflexes.
- Corneal reflex
  - Cornea is touched with a wisp of cotton wool. Blinking of the eyelids is the normal response
  - No response should be elicited in brainstem death
  - Reflex: Afferent fibres via ophthalmic branch of CN V and efferent pathway via CN VII

- Deep central somatic stimulation
  - Apply deep supraorbital pressure and look for a central motor response in the distribution of the facial nerve (grimace)
  - Reflex: afferent via CN V and efferent via CN VII

What are the causes of trigeminal nerve injury?

Mainly surgical; during neurosurgical decompression of trigeminal ganglion, maxillofacial procedures, and dental injections.

When can facial nerve be damaged?

Anaesthetic: compression from facemasks and endotracheal tube ties, stretching of the nerve because of faulty positioning, direct injury due to nerve blocks.

Surgical: direct surgical trauma.

The risk factors associated with incidence of nerve injury are diabetes, intraoperative hypotension, hypoxia, hypothermia, and electrolyte imbalance.

03.6 PHYSIOLOGY: APNOEA PHYSIOLOGY

STEPS	KEY POINTS
What are the preconditions for brainstem testing?	• Identifiable pathology causing irremediable brain damage • Coma with exclusion of hypothermia, depressant drugs, reversible circulatory, metabolic and endocrine disturbances • Apnoea, needing mechanical ventilation
What is the basic neurological principle of apnoea test component of brainstem death testing?	The intact respiratory centre will initiate breathing if the threshold $PaCO_2$ is reached, which is usually 6.65 kPa. In brainstem death the respiratory centre is destroyed and apnoea persists above this threshold.
How is oxygenation maintained during the apnoea test?	By apnoeic mass transfer of oxygen.
Can you explain the physiology of apnoeic oxygenation?	The oxygen consumption (VO_2) remains fairly constant at ~250 mL/min. This is delivered to the tissues by haemoglobin, whose oxygen is then replenished, on return to the pulmonary circulation. In an apnoeic patient, approximately 250 mL/minute of oxygen will move from the alveoli into the bloodstream; only 8 to 20 mL/minute of carbon dioxide moves into the alveoli, with the remainder being buffered in the bloodstream. The end result is that the net pressure in the alveoli becomes slightly subatmospheric, generating a mass flow of gas from pharynx to alveoli. This process where the alveoli continue to take up oxygen even without diaphragmatic movements or lung expansion is called the mass transfer of oxygen or apnoeic oxygenation. In healthy people under ideal circumstances, PaO_2 can be maintained at > 100 mm Hg for up to 100 minutes without a single breath, although the lack of ventilation will eventually cause marked hypercapnia and significant acidosis. Apneic oxygenation with nasal cannulae works because the pharynx is filled with high FiO_2 gas and functions as an oxygen reservoir. The discrepancy between the 10 mL CO_2 entering the alveolar space and the 250 mL O_2 leaving it causes an influx of gas from the airway above the alveolar space. If it is open and filled with 100% O_2 (pre-oxygenation and catheter with O_2), then 240 mL is drawn into alveolar space. This is only 10 mL O_2 less than requirement; therefore, PaO_2 falls at 0.5 kPa/min.

STEPS	KEY POINTS

What are the various factors that significantly influence the time period from the onset of apnoea to critical hypoxia?	• Functional residual capacity (FRC)
	  o Conditions where there is a decreased FRC such as obesity, lung disease, kyphoscoliosis, pregnancy, and children, critical hypoxia is reached more rapidly
	
	• Preoxygenation
	  o Denitrogenation due to preoxygenation greatly increases the time for hypoxia after apnoea
	
	• Maintenance of patent airway
	  o Closed airway: In closed airway, apnoea commences with an intrathoracic pressure equal to ambient pressure. The extraction of oxygen results in subatmospheric intrathoracic pressure and alveolar collapse almost immediately, thereby dangerously reducing the alveolar partial pressure of oxygen
	  o Patent airway: An open airway will allow oxygen to diffuse into the apnoeic lung, which has been shown in animal and simulated human studies to maintain oxygen saturation for up to 100 min
	
	• Haemoglobin level
	  o Anaemia will cause a small reduction in the time to critical hypoxia, although this effect will be more noticeable in patients who also have a reduced FRC
	
	• Basic metabolic demand (VO_2)
	
	The more the demand, the quicker the hypoxia
	(This question tests a core knowledge and is fairly difficult to explain well even if the candidate has read up on it. The values are not important but the principle is.)

Further reading
1. Sirian R, Wills J. Physiology of apnoea and the benefits of preoxygenation. *Contin Educ Anaesth Crit Care Pain.* 2009; **9**(4): 105–108.

03.7 PHARMACOLOGY: COMPARING VOLATILE AGENTS

STEPS	KEY POINTS
What is the volatile agent you use for inhalational induction and why?	Sevoflurane Nonirritant, sweet smelling, and has optimal oil:gas and blood:gas coefficients.

Properties	Isoflurane	Sevoflurane	Desflurane
Physical	Irritant Coughing and breath holding	Nonirritant Sweet smelling	Laryngospasm Excessive secretions
Pharmacokinetic	B:G—1.4 O:G—98 MAC—1.1	B:G—0.7 O:G—80 MAC—1.8	B:G—0.45 O:G—29 MAC—6.6
Pharmacodynamic	0.2% metabolised	3%–5%	Resistant to metabolism

Compare and contrast the three commonly used volatiles: Isoflurane, Sevoflurane, and Desflurane.

What is Blood:Gas solubility coefficient? What does it explain? Can you draw a graph to explain? See Figure 3.3.

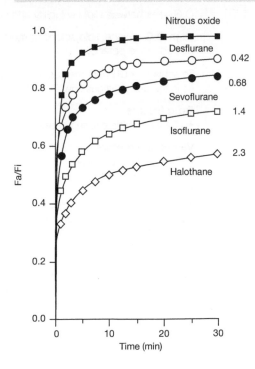

Fig. 3.3 Blood:Gas solubility

STEPS	KEY POINTS

Ratio of the amount of anaesthetic in blood and gas when the two phases are of equal volumes and pressure and in equilibrium at 37°C.

High B:G—The gas is more soluble in the blood, so low partial pressure in blood leading to low partial pressure in brain; slow onset.
And vice versa

What do you understand by Oil:Gas partition coefficient? Again, draw a graph to show its importance. See Figure 3.4.

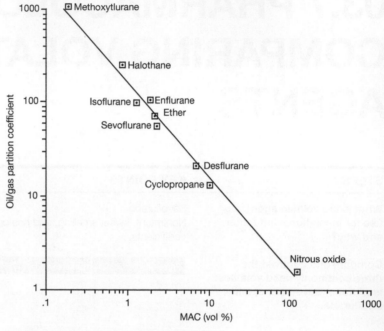

Fig. 3.4 Meyer Overton hypothesis relating to O:G

O:G—link between lipid solubility and potency.

High O:G—Higher lipid solubility; more gas reaches brain. Hence, the drug has got good potency.

What factors influence the speed at which inhaled agents attain equilibrium?

To achieve equilibrium the gas must be at the same concentration in the brain as in the delivered gas flow. The rate at which this occurs depends upon:

Drug factors
- Dilution within existing gases

Ventilation factors
- Inhaled concentration
- Alveolar ventilation
- Diffusion
- Blood/gas partition coefficient. A low b/g partition coefficient indicates low solubility so equilibrium will be reached with relatively small transfers of gas, and therefore will be rapid
- Pulmonary blood flow
- V/Q matching
- Concentration effect: More of the gas means greater concentration which equates to a quicker attainment of equilibrium
- Second gas effect: As nitrous is absorbed it increases the concentration of the volatile

Circulation factors
- Cardiac output
- Distribution to other tissues: Uptake in tissues is related to their blood flow, solubility and arterio-venous difference

03.8 PHYSICS: INTRACRANIAL PRESSURE MONITORING

STEPS	KEY POINTS
What are the clinical features of raised intracranial pressure (ICP)?	• Headache • Nausea and vomiting • Confusion • Personality or behavioural changes • Visual disturbances due to papilloedema Headache is worse in the morning as cerebral oedema is worse in the lying position and there is a relative increase in hypoxia of the brain due to hypoventilation during sleep. It is also worse when bending down, coughing, and sneezing. Acute severe increase in ICP leads to a decrease in GCS, Cushing's reflex; as ICP continues to rise, it leads to fixed and dilated pupils, Cheyne Stokes breathing pattern, and eventually hypotension and death.
What are the causes of increased intracranial pressure?	Raised ICP may be due to an increase in the blood, tissue, or CSF components of the brain. • Blood—Increased blood flow or impaired venous drainage (e.g. venous sinus thrombosis) • Tissue—Tumour, brain abscess, haematoma, and cerebral oedema • CSF—Hydrocephalus or increase in CSF production, which happens in meningitis or choroid plexus tumour
What is the Monroe-Kellie theory?	The cranial cavity is a rigid closed container; thus, any change in intracranial blood volume is accompanied by the opposite change in CSF volume if ICP is maintained.

STEPS	KEY POINTS

Can you draw the ICP elastance curve? See Figure 3.5.

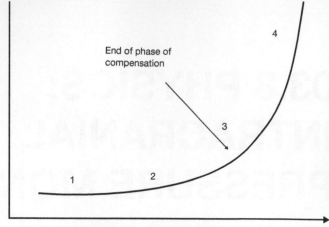

Fig. 3.5 ICP elastance curve *(change in pressure per unit change in volume)*

Stage 1/2 = compensation phase. As the volume of one of the intracranial constituents increases, the other two constituents decrease in volume in order to keep the intracranial pressure constant.

Stage 3/4 = decompensated phase. When compensatory mechanisms are exhausted, small increases in the volumes of intracranial constituents cause large increases in ICP.

The slope of the curve is dependent on which intracranial constituent is increasing. The curve is steeper with blood and CSF as they are incompressible and less steep with brain tissue as it is compressible.

What is the Cushing's reflex?

A hypothalamic response to brain ischaemia wherein the sympathetic nervous system is activated, which causes increased peripheral vascular resistance with a subsequent increase in blood pressure. The increased BP then activates the parasympathetic nervous system via carotid artery baroreceptors, resulting in vagal-induced bradycardia.

The brain ischaemia that leads to Cushing's reflex is usually due to the poor perfusion that results from increased ICP due to haematomas or mass lesions.

Cushing's reflex leads to the clinical manifestation of Cushing's triad: hypertension, bradycardia, and irregular respirations (Cheyne-Stokes breathing).

How do you manage raised ICP?

This can be described as a reduction in blood, tissue, and CSF.

Blood
- Ventilation
  Both hypoxia and hypercapnia can increase cerebral blood flow, and hypoxia of the brain can increase lactic acid, which further causes vasodilatation. Hence, to prevent this, mechanical ventilation is preferred. Hyperventilation can be employed as a method to decrease the PCO_2, and this in turn causes vasoconstriction. This can be used in an acute setting, but its efficacy is limited. If controlled ventilation is used, adequate muscle relaxation and sedation should be used.

STEPS	KEY POINTS

- Positioning: Patients should be nursed in the head-up position, and jugular compression should be avoided to encourage venous drainage

Hypothermia and barbiturate therapy may be used to decrease cerebral blood flow.

Tissue
- Surgical decompression or removal of tumour and haematoma
- Cerebral oedema can be treated with mannitol/frusemide or hypertonic saline
- Corticosteroids may be used for oedema secondary to mass lesions

CSF
Shunts via the lateral ventricle to drain CSF in hydrocephalus.

How do you measure ICP?

Noninvasive
- From history and symptoms of headache, nausea/vomiting, confusion, and behavioural changes
- Papilloedema on eye examination
- CT scan or MRI of the head

Invasive
- External ventricular drain placement: catheter is placed in the lateral ventricle at the level of foramen of Munro
- Intraparenchymal fibre optic catheter placement: monitor is placed in the prefrontal area

How do you interpret the ICP waveforms? See Figures 3.6 and 3.7.

There are four kinds of waves.
1. *Normal*
   - Normal waves have a systolic upstroke (P1) and a diastolic downstroke (P3) with a dicrotic notch (P2)

2. *A waves*
   - Lundberg A waves, 'or plateau waves', are steep increases in ICP lasting for 5 to 10 minutes. They are always pathological and represent reduced intracranial hypertension indicative of early brain herniation

3. *B waves*
   - Lundberg B waves are oscillations of ICP at a frequency of 0.5 to 2 waves/min and are associated with an unstable ICP. Lundberg B waves are possibly the result of cerebral vasospasm

4. *C waves*
   - Lundberg C waves are oscillations with a frequency of 4–8 waves/min and are probably caused by interaction between the cardiac and respiratory cycles

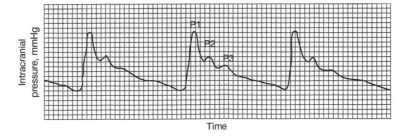

Fig. 3.6 Normal

STEPS   **KEY POINTS**

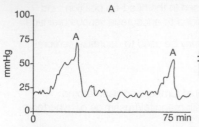

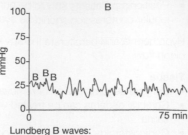

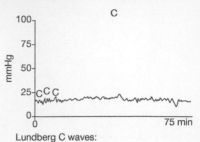

Lundberg A waves:

- Steep ramp up to 50–80 mmHg, over 2–15 minutes

- Peak is followed by an abrupt fall to baseline

- Reflect extreme compromise of intracranial compliance

Fig. 3.7 Lundberg waves

Lundberg B waves:

- Pressure pulses of 10–20 mmHg, over 0.5 to waves per minute

- Also reflect intracranial non–compliance but to a lesser degree

Lundberg C waves:

- These waves represent diminished compliance in a qualitative fashion

CLINICAL VIVA

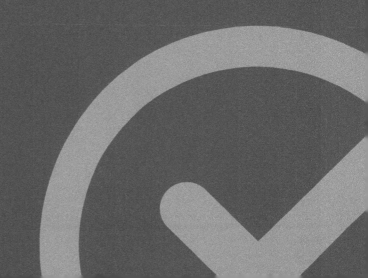

04.1 LONG CASE: GUILLAIN BARRE SYNDROME

HISTORY *You are asked to review a 13-year-old male by the paediatric team. He has been an inpatient for 10 days and was admitted with lethargy, unsteady feet, slurred speech, and general unwellness. Over the past 24 hours he has developed weakness in all four limbs and has started to drool saliva. His parents are Jehovah's Witnesses.*

STEPS	KEY POINTS		
On Examination	Facial weakness is present		
	Absent tendon reflexes		
Investigations	Haemoglobin	11.7 g/dL	(13.0−17.0)
	RBC	$4.2 \times 1012/L$	(3.80−5.50)
	Haematocrit	0.29	(0.38−0.56)
	MCV	84 fL	(80.0−100.0)
	WBC	$5.1 \times 10^9/L$	(4.0−11.0)
	Platelet Count	$434 \times 10^9/L$	(140−400)
	INR	1.0 Ratio	(0.8−1.2)
	Sodium	137 mmol/L	(137−145)
	Potassium	3.4 mmol/L	(3.6−5.0)
	Urea	4.4 mmol/L	(1.7−8.3)
	Creatinine	74 umol/L	(62−124)
	Glucose	6.0 mmol/L	(3.5−6.0)
	Magnesium	0.56 mmol/L	(0.76−0.96)
	Calcium	2.24 mmol/L	(2.10−2.60)
Arterial Blood Gas	FiO_2	0.21	
	pH	7.35	
	PCO_2	6.2	
	PaO_2	11	
	BE	+5	
	HCO_3	28	
	Anion Gap	21	
CSF Analysis	Protein	3	
	White cells	< 3	
	No organisms seen		

STEPS	KEY POINTS
Summarise the case.	• Complex critically ill paediatric patient • Severe neurological pathology with threatened airway and failure of ventilation needing urgent multidisciplinary input from senior clinicians • Parents are Jehovah's Witnesses
What abnormality do you note in the blood results?	• Normocytic anaemia • Platelets are high, depicting inflammation • Low magnesium
What are the causes of normocytic anaemia?	• Decreased production of normal-sized red blood cells (e.g. anaemia of chronic disease, aplastic anaemia) • Increased production of HbS as seen in sickle cell disease • Increased destruction or loss of red blood cells (e.g. haemolysis, post-haemorrhagic anaemia) • An uncompensated increase in plasma volume (e.g. pregnancy, fluid overload) • B2 (riboflavin) and B6 (pyridoxine) deficiency

What are the causes of hypomagnesaemia?	• Decreased magnesium intake
	  ○ Starvation
	  ○ Alcohol dependence
	  ○ Total parenteral nutrition
	• Redistribution of magnesium from extracellular to intracellular space
	  ○ Treatment of diabetic ketoacidosis
	  ○ Alcohol withdrawal syndrome
	  ○ Refeeding syndrome
	  ○ Acute pancreatitis
	• Gastrointestinal magnesium loss
	  ○ Diarrhoea, vomiting, and nasogastric suction
	  ○ Hypomagnesaemia with secondary hypocalcaemia (HSH)
	• Renal magnesium loss
	  ○ Renal tubular defects

Interpret the arterial blood gas.	• Compensated respiratory acidosis • Type 2 respiratory failure • Normal glucose and lactate • Anion gap 21

What is anion gap? How do you calculate it?	• Anion gap is the difference in the measured cations and the anions in serum.
	  ○ Measured cations: Na^+, K^+, Ca^{2+}, and Mg^{2+}
	  ○ Unmeasured cations: serum proteins (normal) and paraproteins (abnormal)
	  ○ Measured anions: Cl^-, $H_2PO_4^-$, HCO_3^-
	  ○ Unmeasured anions: sulphates and some serum proteins
	• Used to determine the cause of metabolic acidosis
	• Expressed as mEq/L
	• Anion gap $= (Na + K) - (Cl + HCO_3)$

STEPS	KEY POINTS
What are the reasons for an increased anion gap?	• Lactic acidosis/ketoacidosis/alcohol abuse • Toxins: methanol/aspirin/cyanide • Renal failure causes high anion gap acidosis by decreased acid excretion and decreased HCO_3^- reabsorption. Accumulation of sulphates, phosphates, urate, and hippurate accounts for the high anion gap.
What is the significance of a high anion gap?	• The anion gap is affected by changes in unmeasured ions. A high anion gap indicates acidosis (e.g. in uncontrolled diabetes, there is an increase in ketoacids i.e. an increase in unmeasured anions) and a resulting increase in the anion gap. • Bicarbonate concentrations decrease in response to the need to buffer the increased presence of acids (as a result of the underlying condition). The bicarbonate is consumed by the unmeasured anion (via its action as a buffer), resulting in a high anion gap.
Comment on the CSF analysis.	Increase protein in the absence of organisms is called albumino cytological dissociation
Why is there increase in CSF protein?	The increase in CSF protein is due to widespread inflammation of the nerve roots.
What would you expect the CSF glucose to be?	Normal—i.e. approx. 2/3 of plasma glucose
What is the differential diagnosis?	• Guillain Barre Syndrome (GBS) • Myasthenia Gravis • Multiple Sclerosis • Transverse myelitis • Encephalitis • Meningitis • Space-occupying lesion • Sepsis
What is the likely diagnosis? What is the pathogenesis?	My diagnosis is Guillain Barre Syndrome. The history of prodromal infection and the course of presentation favour my diagnosis. There is often history of campylobacter or cytomegalovirus infections or vaccinations (influenza, polio, rabies, and rubella). It is postulated that the immune responses directed towards the infecting organisms cross-react with neural tissues resulting in widespread segmental demyelination of peripheral nerves.
How will you differentiate this from myasthenia gravis?	Differences in Myasthenia (the following are features of myasthenia): • Early involvement of muscle groups including extra-ocular, levator, pharyngeal jaw, neck, and respiratory muscles. Sometimes presents without limb weakness • Excessive fatigability and variation of symptoms and signs throughout the day are common • Reflexes are preserved and sensory features, dysautonomia, and bladder dysfunction are absent • Electrophysiological study shows normal nerve conduction and presence of decremental response to repetitive nerve stimulation • EMG shows abnormal jitter and blocking • Edrophonium test is normally positive

STEPS	KEY POINTS
How will you manage this case?	**General—ICU care** • ABC approach: 30% cases require ventilation • Temperature control • VTE prophylaxis • Pain relief • Feeding **Specific** • Steroids • Immunoglobulin G (IgG) • Plasma exchange • CSF filtration
Discuss autonomic dysfunction in these patients.	• Autonomic dysfunction is a major cause of morbidity and mortality, particularly in ventilated patients • May cause refractory orthostatic hypotension, paroxysmal hypertension, bradycardia, ventricular tachyarrhythmias, ileus and urinary retention • Autonomic dysfunction is of particular importance at the induction of anaesthesia. Careful consideration should be given to the use of suxamethonium and inotropic and vasopressor agents may produce markedly atypical responses in heart rate and blood pressure. Even tracheal suction may lead to significant cardiovascular instability
How do you decide when to intubate this patient?	• Intubation should be performed on patients who develop any degree of respiratory failure • Clinical indicators for intubation include hypoxia, rapidly declining respiratory function, poor or weak cough, and suspected aspiration • Typically, intubation is indicated when the FVC is less than 15 mL/kg
How would you intubate this child?	• Avoid suxamethonium • Size 7 cuffed tube (Age/2 +12 cm at lips)
What are the specific treatment options?	• Plasma exchange: removes auto antibodies, immune complexes, etc., and has shown to halve the recovery time • Immunoglobulins: easier and safer than, and equally effective as plasma exchange. Useful in unstable patients • Steroids: ineffective as monotherapy • Complement inhibitors: e.g. Eculizumab has been trialed. • CSF filtration
What is the problem with IgG use in this patient?	• Jehovah's parents may refuse this.
How do you deal with this situation?	• Assess the child's capacity—Gillick competence. • Involve hospitals Jehovah liaison group/legal service/social services. *This child is now transferred to ICU.*

STEPS	KEY POINTS

What are the problems encountered during his stay?

This condition needs long-term care and ventilatory support. This makes way for the usual and common ICU-related problems on top of the pathology-related complications.

Non-pathology-related
- Infections—lines, chest, UTI, septicaemia, etc.
- DVT, pressure sores, and contractures
- Nutritional deficits
- Psychological

Pathology-related
- Autonomic neuropathy
- Pain

The ICU team has tried to do an early percutaneous tracheostomy, which was unsuccessful due to technical reasons. An X-ray is done after the procedure. See Figure 4.1.

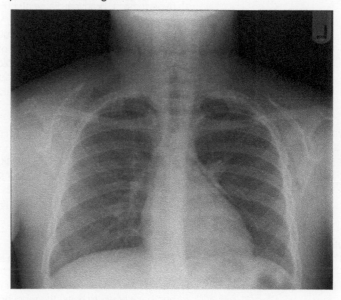

Fig. 4.1

Comment on the chest X-ray.

- Pneumomediastinum

Cause of pneumomediastinum: Traumatic intubation or tracheostomy/NG insertion as children have fragile soft tissue in trachea and oesophagus

Should a percutaneous tracheostomy procedure be followed by X-ray to look for complications?

Immediate CXR after uncomplicated percutaneous tracheostomy performed under bronchoscopic guidance rarely reveals unexpected radiological abnormalities. The role of CXR appears to be restricted to those patients undergoing technically difficult and complicated procedures.

04.2 SHORT CASE: INTRAUTERINE FETAL DEATH

HISTORY *You are the anaesthetic registrar on call in the labour ward. You are asked to review a 29-year-old female who is 28 weeks pregnant, gravida 4, para 3. She has presented to the labour ward with decreased fetal movement for the past 5 days. Subsequently after doing an ultrasound, the obstetricians have confirmed intrauterine fetal death. She is about to be induced. The midwives ask you to see patient and offer advice on subsequent pain management.*

STEPS	KEY POINTS
What would you do?	<ul><li>Full history and examination, especially looking for associated problems (e.g. preeclampsia, haemorrhage, abruption, chorioamnionitis, DIC)</li><li>Sensitive approach as likely to be upset</li><li>Plan analgesia in a stepwise fashion with multi-modal approach<ul><li>Regular paracetamol +/− codeine, progressing to opiates if required.</li><li>PCA analgesia (diamorphine/morphine preferable to pethidine), some units also have protocols for remifentanil PCAs.</li><li>Epidural analgesia: Good analgesia but risk of clotting abnormality (DIC), increasing risk of epidural haematoma and subarachnoid haemorrhage. Also increased risk of epidural abscess if raised temperature, signs of sepsis especially in intrauterine fetal death.</li></ul></li></ul>
What investigations will you do and why?	<ul><li>FBC (may be anaemic if had antepartum haemorrhage, may have raised WCC associated with sepsis)</li><li>U&E (may have multi-organ failure associated with haemorrhage or infection)</li><li>Coagulation profile (risk of DIC)</li><li>Blood cultures (maternal sepsis possible cause of fetal death)</li><li>Group and save (as at risk of haemorrhage)</li><li>12-lead ECG (risk of arrhythmias with metabolic disturbance)</li></ul>

STEPS	KEY POINTS

Your examination and investigations yield the following:

Alert and talking patient

Heart rate	100 bpm
BP	90/60 mmHg
Temp	38.9°C
Hb	9.0 g/dL
WCC	22×10^9/L
Platelets	100×10^9/L
INR	1.7
Urea	12 mmol/L
Creatinine	90 µmol/L

What is your immediate management?

- Sepsis management as per surviving sepsis campaign (fluid resuscitation with crystalloid, early antibiotics, lactate measurement, close monitoring)
- Haematology involvement with regards to DIC and correction with blood products as necessary
- Nurse in obstetric HDU

Which antibiotic would you choose to give this patient and why?

Broad-spectrum antibiotics (including anti-chlamydial) like clindamycin. This is decided after discussion with the microbiologist.

What do you think of a creatinine of 90 µmol/L in a pregnant woman?

It falls within the normal range of creatinine for women, but creatinine is generally very low in pregnancy. Therefore, taken in context of this case, it could represent early renal dysfunction secondary to sepsis.

What is the incidence of intrauterine fetal death?

CMACE define intrauterine death as those babies with no signs of life in utero. (Stillbirth: baby born with no signs of life after 24/40.)
One in 200 babies are born dead, and the overall adjusted stillbirth rate is 3.9 per 1000.

What are the causes of intrauterine fetal death?

No specific cause is found in 50% of stillbirths.
The causes can be multiple and are as follows:

Maternal causes
- Preeclampsia
- Chrioamnionitis
- Placental abruption
- Antepartum haemorrhage
- Maternal disease (e.g. Diabetes Mellitus)

Fetal causes
- Cord prolapse
- Idiopathic hypoxia-acidosis
- Congenital malformations
- Congenital fetal infections

Further reading

1. Green-top Guideline No. 55. *Late Intrauterine Fetal Death and Stillbirth*. October 2010. Royal College of Obstetricians and Gynaecologists.

04.3 SHORT CASE: EISENMENGER'S SYNDROME

HISTORY *A 50-year-old man is admitted for urgent fixation of fracture neck of femur following an accidental fall. He is known to have Down's syndrome, VSD at birth with occasional 'blue spells'.*

STEPS	KEY POINTS
What is the association of VSD with 'blue spells'?	VSD is an acyanotic heart disease, but in the presence of increased right heart pressures causes a right-to-left shunt leading to cyanotic spells. This is called Eisenmenger's syndrome.
What is Eisenmenger's syndrome?	Eisenmenger's syndrome (after German physician Dr Viktor Eisenmenger, 1897) is an untreated congenital heart defect with intracardiac communication that causes pulmonary hypertension, reversal of flow, and cyanosis. The initial cardiac defects could be VSD, PDA, or less commonly, ASD. Other causes include AV septal defect, double-outlet right ventricle, tetralogy of Fallot, transposition of great vessels, and truncus arteriosus. (Eisenmenger's syndrome secondary to VSD is called Eisenmenger's Complex.)
What are cyanotic heart diseases? How is Eisenmenger's syndrome different from them?	Cyanotic heart diseases are congenital cardiac defects where deoxygenated blood is shunted to systemic circulation. Examples are: • Tetralogy of Fallot • Total anomalous pulmonary venous connection • Hypoplastic left heart syndrome • Transposition of great vessels • Truncus arteriosus • Tricuspid atresia Eisenmenger's syndrome causes cyanosis at a later age. The congenital cardiac defect is not cyanotic, but secondary to the development of pulmonary hypertension the previous left-to-right shunt is converted to a right-to-left shunt.

STEPS	KEY POINTS

What is the pathophysiology of Eisenmenger's syndrome?

Systemic to pulmonary connection

↓

Left-to-right shunting

↓

Increased pulmonary flow

↓

Irreversible pulmonary vascular injury

↓

Increased pulmonary vascular resistance

↓

Right-to-left shunting

↓

Hypoxia and erythrocytosis

Initially the communication between right and left sides of chambers allows blood flow from left to right, as SVR (1000 dynes.sec/cm^5) is much higher than PVR (150 dynes.sec/cm^5). Increased blood flow in the right heart increases blood flow through the pulmonary artery and produces shear forces in pulmonary microvasculature. This with volume overload causes increase in PVR. Gradually PVR becomes equal or higher than SVR over years. Thus the shunt becomes bidirectional, and later, when reversal occurs, deoxygenated blood flows from right to left causing cyanosis and chronic hypoxaemia. This stage with right-to-left shunt and cyanosis is termed Eisenmenger's syndrome.

What are the signs and symptoms?

Eisenmenger's syndrome is an insidious disease process. In patients with left-to-right shunt, only 11% develop reversal of shunt and Eisenmenger's syndrome.

Main symptoms include dyspnoea on exertion, palpitations, syncope, fatigue, angina, and haemoptysis. Important signs are cyanosis, clubbing of fingers, dysrhythmias on ECG, polycythaemia, signs of congestive cardiac failure, hyperviscosity, and endocarditis. It also causes cholelithiasis, renal dysfunction, gout, and haematological abnormalities.

The quality of life is poor, and exercise tolerance is limited.

What are the implications of anaesthetising this patient?

• Anaesthesia in patients with Down's syndrome is not discussed here.

The theoretical risks of anaesthesia in these patients are considerable. The cornerstone of safe anaesthesia in such patients is maintenance of preoperative levels of systemic vascular resistance and to reduce the amount of right-to-left shunt during the perioperative period.

Avoid any increase in PVR: By reducing anxiety with premedication, good analgesia, avoiding acidosis, hypoxia, and hypercarbia.
Avoid any reduction in SVR: Titration of induction and inhalational agents, avoiding regional techniques, and use of alpha agonists to maintain SVR.

• Careful premedication with a benzodiazepine may be useful.
• For IV access, it is crucial to avoid any small air bubbles entering the circulation as this can cross to the arterial side and cause stroke and ischaemia to vital organs (paradoxical air embolus).

STEPS	KEY POINTS

- General anaesthesia is better tolerated than spinal anaesthesia. Ketamine maintains SVR, while the other agents reduce it. Inhalational agents also reduce SVR, but their dose-dependent reduction in PVR might be useful.
- Controlled ventilation is recommended. Hyperoxemia and low CO_2 reduce PVR and shunt.
- Adequate analgesia is vital as pain causes increase in PVR, SVR, and cardiac oxygen requirements.
- Invasive monitoring is recommended and postoperative HDU or ITU care might be needed.

In general, avoid
- Increase in PVR
- Decrease in SVR
- Air in IV line
- Hypoxia and hypercarbia

Will you consider regional anaesthesia in this case?

Advantages of regional technique
- Avoidance of cardiac effects of anaesthetic agents
- Avoidance of the need for airway management (possibly difficult in Down's syndrome)
- Good postoperative analgesia

Disadvantages
- Significant and uncontrolled drop in SVR caused by spinal can be detrimental.
- Also in a patient with learning difficulties, an awake procedure can be challenging and sedation can cause CO_2 retention and worsening of right-to-left shunt.
- Epidural and incremental spinal (with spinal catheter) with invasive monitoring and use of fluids and vasopressors to avoid fall in SVR have been described in the literature.

04.4 SHORT CASE: MYOTONIC DYSTROPHY

HISTORY *You are asked to preassess a 32-year-old man with myotonic dystrophy, booked for wisdom tooth removal.*

STEPS	KEY POINTS
What is the definition of myotonic dystrophy?	Progressive, hereditary neuromuscular disorder characterised by • Myotonia (prolonged contraction/delayed relaxation of the skeletal muscles after voluntary stimulation) • Dystrophy (progressive weakness and muscular atrophy) Autosomal dominant disorder with an incidence of 2.4–5.5 cases per 100 000 in the UK.
What is the pathophysiology of myotonic dystrophy?	Locus for myotonic dystrophy is found on chromosome 19. The underlying pathophysiology is related to abnormal sodium or chloride channels, which results in the muscle being in an abnormal hyperexcitable state. This leads to repetitive action potentials and sustained muscle contraction, manifesting in the inability to relax.
What are the complications and system manifestations of this disease?	**Facial feature** • Frontal balding, muscle wasting, ptosis, cataracts **Cardiac** • Conduction defects (heart block, bundle branch block, wide QRS, increased QTc, PR intervals) • Heart failure • Cardiomyopathy • Mitral valve prolapse **Respiratory** • Respiratory muscle weakness • OSA • Decreased hypercapnic drive, hypoxaemia, cor pulmonale • Mucus/sputum retention, poor cough, risk of respiratory infection **Neurological** • Bulbar palsy, dysphagia • Intellectual impairment **Endocrine** • Hypothyroidism • Diabetes **GI** • Delayed gastric emptying, constipation • Aspiration

STEPS	KEY POINTS
How could you preoptimise him?	He would require a thorough preoperative assessment including a full history and examination looking for the multisystem involvement as listed above, with special mention of:

He would require a thorough preoperative assessment including a full history and examination looking for the multisystem involvement as listed above, with special mention of:

- Bulbar problems: dysphagia, slurred speech (aspiration risk)
- Cardiac abnormalities: conduction defects (may need pacing)
- Respiratory muscle fatigue: poor cough (risk of chest infection), OSA (need for NIV/overnight ventilation)
- Endocrine: presence of diabetes/hypothyroidism

Investigations
- 12-lead ECG (check for conduction abnormalities and consider need for pacing intraoperatively)
- FBC, U&Es, Blood glucose (may have anaemia of chronic disease, polycythaemia associated with lung disease, hyperkalaemia due to muscle dysfunction, raised blood glucose secondary to associated diabetes mellitus)
- Pulmonary function tests (to look for restrictive lung disease)
- ABGs (may have chronic hypoxaemia)
- CXR (may have evidence of aspiration pneumonitis, evidence of cardiac failure)
- Echocardiogram (to exclude structural abnormality, e.g. mitral valve prolapse)

Precounseling
- Local versus general anaesthesia (see below)
- Discussion regarding factors that precipitate myotonia
- Risk of deterioration of disease with anaesthesia and need for overnight stay

He states that anything in his mouth precipitates his myotonia and that he might bite the surgeon's fingers off (if done under local anaesthesia).

How could you prevent this?

- Sedation may be an option but has a risk of inducing severe respiratory depression
- Local anaesthetic infiltration of the masseter has been shown to reduce myotonia

He refuses the option of local anaesthetic.

How would you proceed with regard to giving a general anaesthetic?

Preoperative
- Ensure preoperative optimisation (as above), take a good history, and explain potential complications
- Premedication: Avoid respiratory depressants and give antacids

Intraoperative
- Full monitoring as per AAGBI guidelines, consider invasive monitoring if history of cardiomyopathy or arrhythmias. Have pacing capability available
- Avoid precipitation of myotonias: hypothermia, shivering, mechanical and electrical stimulation. Use warming blankets, warm fluid, monitor temperature
- Induction: Etomidate, thiopentone, and propofol have all been shown to be safe, though propofol is associated with less postoperative ventilation

STEPS	KEY POINTS

- Muscle relaxation: Depolarizing neuromuscular blocking agents (suxamethonium) may induce generalized muscular contractures and are therefore not recommended. Non depolarizing neuromuscular blocking agents are not associated with myotonia, but the use of anticholinesterases may precipitate contractures, due to increased sensitivity of acetylcholine
- Maintenance: Avoid volatiles as they may induce shivering, and therefore myotonia, at high concentrations. Propofol and remifentanil total intravenous anaesthesia has been shown to be very effective and avoids the need for muscle relaxation
- Airway: Will require intubation as significant risk of aspiration and possibly nasal route to facilitate surgical access
- Emergence: Avoid anticholinesterase agents (precipitate myotonia), extubated with care to prevent aspiration

Postoperative
- Consider need for prolonged ventilation, at high risk of delayed onset apnoea and should have ECG and oxygen saturations monitored for 24 hours postop
- Consider need for ICU/HDU. Try to avoid depressant analgesics. May require chest physiotherapy postoperatively depending on prior lung function

What other muscular dystrophies are you aware of and how do they differ?

Duchene Muscular Dystrophy
It is most common in childhood affecting males and is inherited as X linked recessive disorder. It is characterized by proximal muscle wasting and weakness associated with contractures, scoliosis, restrictive lung disease, and cardiomyopathy. Death occurs usually in second or third decade from cardiorespiratory failure. The causative factor is shown to be the lack of dystrophin (protein that anchors muscle to extracellular matrix).

Becker's Muscular Dystrophy
It is a milder form of muscular dystrophy affecting 1 in 30,000 men. In this condition, dystrophin is only partially absent. It presents in teenage years and has a protracted course, and death happens at fourth or fifth decade from cardiorespiratory failure.

Further reading
1. Baust J. *Myotonic Dystrophy: Decision Making in Anaesthesiology*. 4th Edition. 2007, P160–163.
2. Marsh S, Pittard A. Neuromuscular disorders and anaesthesia. Part 2: Specific neuromuscular disorders. *CEACCP*. 2011; **4**: 119–23.
3. Campbell N et al. Practical suggestions for the anesthetic management of a myotonic dystrophy patient. *Myotonic Dystrophy Foundation Toolkit: 2007*. 73–80. Available from http://www.myotonic.org/sites/default/files/pages/files/Anesthesia%20Guidelines.pdf

section 04

BASIC SCIENCE
VIVA

04.5 ANATOMY: MEDIASTINUM

STEPS	KEY POINTS

What is mediastinum?	• The mediastinum lies between the right and left pleurae
	• It extends from the sternum in front to the vertebral column behind, and it contains all the thoracic viscera excepting the lungs
	
	• **Superior mediastinum**
	  ○ Located above the manubriosternal angle
	  ○ Bounded posteriorly by T1-4; above it is continuous with the neck; below it is continuous with both anterior and posterior mediastina
	  <u>Organs</u>: Thymus, oesophagus, thoracic duct, trachea and bronchi
	  <u>Vessels</u>: Aorta (arch) and brachiocephalic trunk, SVC and both brachiocephalic veins, left common carotid artery, left subclavian artery
	  <u>Nerves</u>: Both phrenic nerves and vagi, left recurrent laryngeal nerve
	
	• **Anterior mediastinum**
	  ○ Between sternum anteriorly and the pericardial sac posteriorly
	  ○ Contains the sternopericardial ligament, fat, and lymph nodes
	
	• **Middle mediastinum**
	  ○ Between anterior and posterior mediastinum
	  ○ Structures include the pericardium, heart, phrenic nerves, pericardioacophrenic vessels, and origin of great vessels
	
	• **Posterior mediastinum**
	  ○ Between pericardial sac and anterior surface of the vertebral bodies
	  ○ Structures include descending aorta, oesophagus, azygous system of veins, vagus nerve, thoracic duct, lymph nodes, and thoracic splanchnic nerves

What is the nerve that traverses through the neck/chest and abdomen?	Vagus nerve

Where does it lie in the neck, chest, and abdomen?	• <u>Neck</u>: within carotid sheath along the tracheo oesophageal groove
	• Chest
	  ○ <u>Right</u>: passes behind the right brachiocephalic vein, crosses right subclavian artery, is crossed by azygos vein, and travels posterior to the hilum of right lung
	  ○ <u>Left</u>: behind left brachiocephalic vein, crosses aortic arch, and travels posterior to the hilum of left lung

STEPS	KEY POINTS

	• Abdomen
	  ○ <u>Right</u>: enters abdomen via the oesophageal hiatus of the diaphragm, right and posterior to the oesophagus, runs along left gastric artery to the coeliac plexus
	  ○ <u>Left</u>: is left and anterior to the oesophagus in the hiatus, lesser curvature of the stomach and pylorus

Where does the oesophagus start and how long is it?	• At C6 and it is 25 cm long
Why is the oesophagus important to anaesthetists?	• Mode of feeding—so placement of NG tube • Mode of monitoring—doppler/ TOE/temp • Inadvertent injury—bougie, tracheostomy • Air into stomach especially in children—regurgitation risk • Inadvertent oesophageal intubation

How would you anaesthetise for food bolus removal or ingested foreign body?	Eighty percent of ingested foreign bodies will pass without the need for intervention.
	
	Implications
	• Risks of impaction, with obstruction or perforation depending on the type of the foreign body
	• Risk of aspiration depending on the location of the foreign body
	• Usually (not necessarily) paediatric population
	• All issues relating to a shared airway
	• Underlying oesophageal motility disorder causing impaction
	
	Management
	• History, examination, and investigations to ascertain the type and location of the foreign body
	
	Timing of intervention
	• <u>Emergency</u> intervention in patients with esophageal obstruction or ingestion of sharp objects leading to perforation or batteries leading to liquefaction necrosis and perforation
	• <u>Nonurgent</u>: Coins in the esophagus may be observed for 12–24 hours in an asymptomatic patient
	
	Airway control
	• The most acceptable technique to remove a gastrointestinal foreign body remains controversial. Initial management includes assessment of the patient's ventilatory status and an airway evaluation.
	
	GA with endotracheal intubation
	  a. Patients unable to manage their secretions (high aspiration risk)
	  b. Cases of proximal oesophageal foreign body ingestion
	  c. Objects that are difficult to remove
	  d. When rigid oesophagoscopy is needed
	  e. Pediatric population
	
	Conscious sedation
	With midazolam in other patient groups

04.6 PHYSIOLOGY: CEREBRAL CIRCULATION

STEPS	KEY POINTS
During which surgeries is cerebral circulation likely to be affected?	• Surgeries performed in the head-up position; e.g. posterior fossa craniectomy, cervical laminectomy, and sometimes thyroid operations • Beach chair position; e.g. shoulder surgery • Trendelenburg position; e.g. in laparoscopic colorectal surgery, gynaecological operations • Surgery needing cardiopulmonary bypass, as aortic cannulation can lead to cerebral embolism
Describe the arterial supply.	This can be divided into the anterior and posterior cerebral circulations that are connected via the anterior and posterior communicating arteries forming the Circle of Willis. Two thirds of the cerebral arterial supply is via the internal carotid arteries and one third via the vertebral arteries. See Figure 4.2.

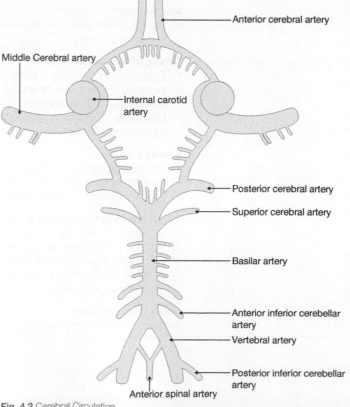

Fig. 4.2 Cerebral Circulation

STEPS	KEY POINTS
	• The anterior cerebral artery supplies the medial portion of the frontal lobe and the superior medial parietal lobe • The middle cerebral artery supplies the lateral cerebral cortex. It also supplies the anterior temporal lobe and the insular cortices • The posterior cerebral artery supplies the occipital lobe and medial side of temporal lobe
What factors affect cerebral blood flow?	• Arterial pCO_2: Hypercapnia increases blood flow whereas hypocapnia decreases it • Arterial pO_2: Does not affect it until the pO_2 reaches 6.7 kPa. The cerebral blood flow increases below this • Cerebral metabolic rate of oxygen ($CMRO_2$): There is a linear correlation between cerebral blood flow and $CMRO_2$ • Cerebral perfusion pressure: Autoregulation occurs between a MAP of 60 and 160 mmHg. The mean arterial pressure at which autoregulation occurs in hypertensive population is in a higher range and is impaired in pathology (e.g. traumatic brain injury) • Drugs used in anaesthesia: Intravenous induction agents except ketamine decrease cerebral blood flow. Inhalational anaesthetic agents and nitrous oxide increase cerebral blood flow as they cause vasodilatation. Opiates cause very little change in blood flow • Temperature: Decrease in temperature decreases cerebral blood flow
What is the mechanism of cerebral autoregulation?	The autoregulatory vessel caliber changes are mediated by interplay between myogenic, neurogenic, and metabolic mechanisms. • Metabolic control: balance between demand and supply of oxygen (i.e. between cerebral metabolism and oxygen delivery mediated by vasoactive substances such as NO, H^+, etc.) • Myogenic control: sensing mechanisms in smooth muscle of the arterioles detect changes in transmural pressure. The calibers of vessels are changed to maintain blood flow • Neurogenic control: The vascular smooth muscle resistance is controlled via autonomic innervations
What is the management of raised intracranial pressure (ICP)?	Raised ICP may be due to an increase in any compartment of the brain (i.e. blood, brain tissue, or CSF). The treatment of raised ICP involves the reduction in any of them and may be achieved in the following ways: **Blood** • The cerebral blood flow can be decreased by hyperventilation and thus a decrease in $PaCO_2$. Attention should be paid to not affect venous drainage by nursing the patient in a head-up position and avoiding compressing the jugular veins by not tying endotracheal tubes too tight. Coughing should be avoided, and adequate muscle relaxation and sedation must be used • Therapeutic hypothermia to decrease CBF • Use of barbiturate infusions (e.g. thiopentone to decrease CBF and $CMRO_2$) **Brain tissue** • Osmotic diuretics such as mannitol and hypertonic saline draw out water from the extracellular and intracellular spaces • Surgery (e.g. frontal lobectomies and removal of tumours) **CSF** • Drainage via shunts and catheters

04.7 PHARMACOLOGY: SEROTONIN

STEPS	KEY POINTS
Outline the production and metabolism of serotonin.	**Production:** Serotonin (5-Hydroxytryptamine) is produced by hydroxylation and decarboxylation of tryptophan, an essential amino acid. **Metabolism:** Reuptake and inactivation by monoamine oxidase (MAO) to produce 5-hydroxyindoleacetic acid, which is renally excreted.
Where is serotonin found?	• Platelets • Gastrointestinal tract (primarily in enterochromaffin cells) • Brain (the hypothalamus, limbic system, spinal cord, retina, and cerebellum)
What are the types of receptors you know of, and what are the functions of serotonin?	Seven families have been identified (5-HT1 through to 5-HT7). Most of the receptors are coupled to G proteins and produce an effect via adenyl cyclase or phospholipase C. The one exception is 5HT3, an ion channel. The effect of serotonin varies with each receptor. 5-HT2 receptors mediate platelet aggregation and smooth muscle contraction. 5-HT3 receptors are concentrated in the GI tract and the area postrema and are involved in vomiting. 5-HT6 and 7 receptors are involved in limbic function.
What is serotonin syndrome?	Serotonin syndrome (SS), or serotonin toxicity, was first described in the 1950s. It is a spectrum of clinical findings due to excess of serotonin in the CNS. Classical triad of symptoms • Change in mental status • Autonomic dysfunction • Neuromuscular excitability

STEPS	KEY POINTS
What are the signs and symptoms?	• Change in mental status: agitation, delirium, disorientation, anxiety, lethargy, seizures, and hallucinations • Autonomic dysfunction: diaphoresis, hypertension, hyperthermia, vomiting, tachycardia, dilated pupils, diarrhoea, and abdominal pain • Neuromuscular changes: tremors, muscle rigidity, hyperreflexia, nystagmus • Others: rhabdomyolysis, acute renal failure, disseminated intravascular coagulation, and circulatory failure Clinical features are highly variable but usually correlate with degree of toxicity, and the onset can be dramatic or insidious in nature.
How is it diagnosed?	The diagnosis is purely clinical. Most validated diagnostic criteria—*Hunter Criteria*—84% sensitive and 97% specific. The *Hunter Criteria for Serotonin syndrome* are fulfilled if the patient has taken a serotonergic agent and has a combination of one or more of the following: • Spontaneous or inducible clonus • Ocular clonus • Agitation • Diaphoresis • Tremor • Hyperreflexia • Hypertonia • Temperature > 38°C *History* should concentrate on prescription and other medications, illicit substance abuse, alternative medications, and any recent changes to medications. *Laboratory investigations* are of very little use in the diagnosis. Serum serotonin levels do not correlate with toxicity, and other findings are generally nonspecific. There may be an elevated white cell count and increased CK.
Outline the principles of treatment.	• Stopping all drugs acting on serotonin • Supportive care such as supplemental oxygen, intravenous fluids, and cardiac monitoring. • Benzodiazepines for agitation and BP control • Management of autonomic instability—can use short-acting agents such as esmolol • Controlling hyperthermia • Considering serotonin antagonists if available (Cyproheptadine is the serotonin antagonist that has been used.)

STEPS	KEY POINTS
Which drugs can precipitate the syndrome?	Co-administration of two serotonergic agents, usually monoamine oxidase inhibitors (MAOI) and selective serotonin reuptake inhibitors (SSRIs) • *Increased serotonin formation*: L-tryptophan • *Increased serotonin release*: Cocaine, ecstasy, amphetamines, alcohol • *Reduced serotonin reuptake*: SSRIs, TCAs, pethidine, tramadol, fentanyl, ondansetron, St. John's wort, etc. • *Inhibits serotonin metabolism*: MAOIs, serotonin agonists, LSD • *Increases sensitivity of receptor*: Lithium
What are the anaesthetic implications?	Serotonin syndrome is uncommon but is often undiagnosed in milder cases. Drugs that alter serotonin are given routinely in anaesthetic practice. Patients already on one drug are being prescribed a second serotonergic agent such as alcohol, tramadol, or ondansetron. Serotonin syndrome can be prevented by • Understanding individual patient's triggers, symptom patterns, and preferred therapies • Continuing preventative medication • Minimising variations in arterial blood pressure, temperature, and arterial CO_2

04.8 PHYSICS: MONITORING IN SCOLIOSIS SURGERY

HISTORY *You are asked to preassess a 14-year-old boy who is booked for thoracic scoliosis correction surgery.*

STEPS	KEY POINTS
What are the challenges presented to the anaesthetist by this patient undergoing surgical correction of scoliosis?	Scoliosis is a spinal deformity associated with lateral curvature of the spine, rotation of vertebral body, and thoracic cage deformity. The main concerns in anaesthetising this particular case are as follows: **Patient factors** • Paediatric age group • Coexisting neuromuscular disorders—muscular dystrophy, cerebral palsy, and increased incidence of malignant hyperthermia • Associated comorbidities—respiratory and cardiac compromise • Difficult airway—depending on the level of scoliosis **Surgical factors** • Difficult positioning—prone or lateral • Potential for excessive blood loss • Risks of prolonged surgery—hypothermia and thromboembolic risks • Need for intraoperative neurophysiological monitoring (IONM) • Need for insertion of double lumen tube in certain approaches
What are the two main system involvements in patients with scoliosis?	• *Respiratory system* Thoracic curvature decreases the mechanical efficiency of the chest wall causing a restrictive pulmonary picture with decreased lung volumes and compliance, but preservation of FEV1/FVC ratio. In severe cases, restricted ventilation may lead to alveolar hypoventilation, arteriovenous shunting, and V/Q mismatch. A thorough assessment of functional impairment and optimisation of any reversible cause of pulmonary dysfunction such as chest infection with antibiotics, bronchodilators, and physiotherapy. • *Cardiovascular system* Patients with high-degree spinal curvature are at risk of developing corpulmonale. Hypoxic pulmonary vasoconstriction develops in the face of arterial hypoxaemia, and the resulting pulmonary hypertension leads to right heart failure.

STEPS	KEY POINTS
What investigations would you consider necessary in this patient?	• Full blood count, urea and electrolytes, clotting screen, cross-matching of blood and blood products • Plain CXR for respiratory and cardiac assessment • 12-lead ECG to assess cardiac function • Echocardiogram in patients with long-standing and severe scoliosis • Lung function tests: Preoperative vital capacity of < 35% is associated with increased postoperative respiratory morbidity and is considered a relative contraindication for surgery • In cases where difficult airway is suspected, flexion and extension radiographs and CT/MRI of cervical spines are recommended *From this first question the viva can go to different areas:* • *One-lung anaesthesia and double lumen tubes* • *Positioning for spinal surgery* • *Spinal cord blood supply and spinal cord ischaemia* • *Monitoring of the spinal cord*
Describe the blood supply of the spinal cord. Which part of the spinal cord is most at risk of ischaemia?	The anterior spinal artery supplies the anterior two-thirds of the spinal cord, and the posterior spinal arteries supply posterior third. In addition, radicular branches from local arteries feed into the spinal arteries, including the artery of Adamkiewicz at the lower thoracic/upper lumbar level. This segmental blood supply results in the formation of watershed areas. The areas of the spinal cord, which are the most at risk of ischaemia, are T3–5 and T12–L1.
How can you monitor the neurological function during scoliosis surgery?	Given the risk of spinal cord ischaemia during surgery, methods of detection of spinal cord compromise are essential for preservation of function. IONM of evoked potentials provides information about the functional integrity of neural pathways in anaesthetised patients. The most commonly used techniques include: • **Transcranial Motor Evoked Potentials (Tc-MEPs):** Significant changes in muscle MEP during scoliosis surgery bears a strong correlation to cord injury. This involves monitoring of the descending anterior and lateral corticospinal tracts by transcranial electrical stimulation of excitable regions in the cortex producing segmental muscle contraction. • **Somato Sensory Evoked Potentials (SSEPs):** Electrical impulses are delivered to a peripheral nerve via surface electrodes, which reach the primary sensory cortex through the dorsal column; this electrical activity is recorded via scalp electrodes. Changes in the SSEP waveforms reflect loss of integrity of the dorsal column sensory pathways. • **Spontaneous and triggered electromyographic (EMG) responses:** Detects peripheral nerve injury quickly and easily. • **Stagnara wake-up test:** Despite limitations, this method still remains 'gold standard' for assessment of motor function. The test involves lessening the level of anaesthesia until the patient is able to follow commands, allowing for a gross assessment of motor function. In many studies the advantage of using multimodal monitoring has been suggested.

STEPS	KEY POINTS
How do anaesthetic drugs affect these techniques?	• **IV induction agents:** The use of bolus doses of i.v. induction agents reduces the amplitude of evoked potential responses, and in particular, cortical responses, but these effects do not prevent useful intraoperative recording of SSEPs and MEPs. • **Inhalational agents:** There is a dose-dependent reduction in SSEP and MEP amplitude. Muscle relaxants do not affect SSEPs, but MEPs are affected with moderate doses. When myogenic motor evoked responses are to be recorded, stable level of muscle relaxation as reflected by one or two twitches on train of four (TOF) should be maintained. • **Opioids:** Small effect on waveform amplitude and latency. • **Hypothermia:** Decreases nerve conduction and decreases the amplitude of SSEP waveform. • **Hypotension:** SSEPs are lost and ischaemic injury can occur when MAP < 60 mm Hg.
What problems exist with patient positioning for this procedure?	Different approaches call for different modes of positioning: knee-to-chest, prone, or lateral. Ensure optimal position to aid free excursion of chest wall to promote adequate ventilation; in the presence of restrictive pattern, this could otherwise be detrimental to the respiratory function. Also prevent increased intra-abdominal pressure to avoid engorgement of epidural venous plexus and increased surgical site bleeding.
What can you do to decrease blood loss during surgery?	Typical blood loss may exceed 50% of patient's blood volume and is related to the duration and extent of surgery, anaesthetic factors such as induced hypotension, optimal positioning, and use of antifibrinolytic agents.
What determines the need for postoperative ventilation?	**Patient factors** • Presence of pre-existing neuromuscular disorder • Severe restrictive pulmonary disease (< 35% vital capacity) • Associated cardiac involvement and right heart failure • Obesity **Surgical factors** • Duration and extent of surgery • Invasion of thoracic cavity • Blood loss > 30 mL/kg • Presence of complications such as pneumothorax and haemothorax
What are the analgesic options?	The surgery involves a large incision over several dermatomes, and significant postoperative pain can be expected. A multimodal analgesic technique involving the combination of simple analgesics, opioids, and regional blocks is chosen. Nonsteroidal anti-inflammatory drugs are generally avoided for the fear of increased bleeding and renal failure because of the high incidence of intraoperative hypotension and hypovolemia. Various regional techniques: spinal and epidural catheters inserted intraoperatively by the surgeon; paravertebral and intrapleural infusion of local anaesthetics are used variedly in the UK. **Key points** • Scoliosis surgery poses significant challenges • Preoperative lung function determines postoperative respiratory morbidity • IONM has shown to effectively predict the adverse outcomes of nerve injury • Anaesthetic technique is tailored to suit the use of IONM and to prevent blood loss

section 05

CLINICAL VIVA

05.1 LONG CASE: ABDOMINAL AORTIC ANEURYSM FOR EVAR

HISTORY *An 80-year-old gentleman presents for an elective repair of an 8 cm infrarenal abdominal aortic aneurysm. You have been asked by surgeons to review this patient in the preassessment clinic.*

STEPS	KEY POINTS
Past Medical History	His past medical history includes a left pneumonectomy and thoracoplasty for tuberculosis 40 years ago and two occasions where he had angioplasty and insertion of coronary stents 5 and 8 years ago.
Drugs	Enalapril 5 mg OD Atenolol 25 mg OD Isosorbide mononitrate 20 mg BD Paracetamol 1g PRN
Social History	Ex-smoker for over 40 years Drinks alcohol occasionally
On Examination	Heart rate 76/min Blood pressure 160/90 mmHg BMI 33 kg/m^2 Dependent ankle oedema, which he attributes to venous stasis.
Blood Investigations	Hb 13.1 g/dL (13–16) WCC 3.0 × 10^9/L (4–11) Platelets 242 × 10^9/L (140–400) PCV 0.35 (0.38–0.56) Na 138 mmol/L (137–145) K 4.3 mmol/L (3.6–5.0) Urea 12 mmol/L (1.7–8.3) Creat 170 umol/L (62–124)

STEPS	KEY POINTS
ECG (See Figure 5.1.)	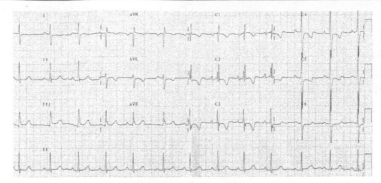

Fig. 5.1

CXR (See Figure 5.2.)	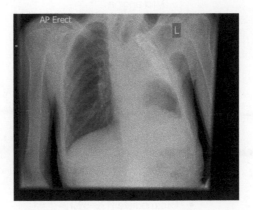

Fig. 5.2

Lung function tests	FVC (L)	1.02	48% predicted
	FEV$_1$(L)	0.8 L	51% predicted
	DLCO (ml/min/mmHg)	7.3	30% predicted

Summarise the case.

This 80-year-old patient presents as a high-risk patient with multiple comorbidities for high-risk surgery. He is elderly with significant cardiac history, poorly controlled hypertension, pre-existing moderate chronic kidney disease, and significant restrictive lung disease. The size of his aortic aneurysm and his poor physiological status puts him at increased risk of perioperative cardiac and surgical complications, bleeding, and long-term severe renal dysfunction.

I would like to take a full history, examination, and review and consider additional investigations and ensure full optimisation of his comorbidities before considering his options with both the patient and his surgeon.

Discuss assessment of risk.

Abdominal aortic aneurysms are incidental findings in two thirds of patients. Surgery is recommended when they reach 55 mm. At this stage there is less than 1% risk of spontaneous rupture. By 60 mm there is more than 17% risk of spontaneous rupture. We can see that simply the size of this gentleman's aneurysm places him at high risk from rupture without surgical intervention.

STEPS	KEY POINTS

In terms of proceeding with surgery, risk assessment should be done taking into consideration the likelihood of a perioperative cardiovascular event.

Original cardiovascular risk scoring systems include Goldman's Criteria, Detsky's, and Lee's Revised Cardiac Index. The American College of Cardiology (ACC)/American Heart Association (AHA) guidelines for Perioperative evaluation of Non-Cardiac Surgery (2003) have been developed subsequently.

Patient Risk (cardiac risk by patient comorbidities)

- Minor
  - Age > 70
  - Abnormal ECG
  - Nonsinus rhythm
  - Uncontrolled hypertension
  - Stroke

- Moderate
  - MI > 6 months
  - Mild angina
  - Compensated heart failure
  - Diabetes

- Major
  - MI < 6 months
  - Unstable angina
  - Decompensated heart failure
  - Severe valvular heart disease
  - Symptomatic arrhythmias

Surgical Risk (cardiac risk by type of surgery)

- Minor (< 1%)
  - Endoscopy/cataract surgery
  - Plastics/breast surgery

- Intermediate (1%–5%)
  - Thoracic/head and neck surgery
  - Orthopaedic/minor vascular surgery

- Major (> 5%)
  - Aortic/major vascular surgery
  - Emergency surgery
  - Prolonged surgery

From a surgical risk basis, this is aneurysm surgery in the high-risk category and independently, cardiac risk is more than 5% for undergoing surgery alone irrespective of comorbidities.

In recent times it is apparent that more comprehensive scoring systems are needed to categorise patient risk. A system known as EuroSCORE is increasingly being used.

Could you go through his investigations and positive findings?

Bloods
His blood tests reveal that he has chronic kidney disease.

ECG
- PR interval is at the upper limit of normal (200 msec)
- Tall R waves in lateral leads V5 and V6 with mild ST segment depression suggests left ventricular hypertrophy
- rSR pattern in V1 with T wave inversion in V1–V3, suggestive of right bundle branch block

STEPS	KEY POINTS

CXR

CXR reveals evidence of his previous surgery and signs within his existing lung.

It demonstrates marked volume loss of the left hemithorax with shift of the mediastinum and elevation of the hemidiaphragm. Also the pleura is calcified.

Lung function test

Lung function tests reveal severe restrictive disease and a very low DLCO. DLCO is a measurement of carbon monoxide take-up per unit time. It measures alveolar/capillary function. DLCO < 80% is associated with increased pulmonary complications, and a DLCO < 30% is associated with increased morbidity.

A full history together with an echocardiogram and baseline ABGs would help assess him further.

What methods are there for assessing his functional capacity?

Functional capacity assesses patient response to increased physical demand. I would like to ask about his exercise tolerance. This can be done by using the Duke Activity Status Index, which quantifies numbers of METs (metabolic equivalents), a measure of basal oxygen consumption (i.e. at rest). One MET equates to 3.5 ml O_2/kg/min.

7–10 METs suggests good function (e.g. carrying shopping upstairs, cycling, jogging).
4–7 METs suggests moderate function (e.g. climbing two flight of stairs without stopping).
1–4 METs suggests impaired function (e.g. basic ADLs, eating, dressing, walking on flat surface).

Tests of functional capacity

Exercise ECG (Bruce Protocol): Looking for evidence of ischaemia while walking on a treadmill which goes through intervals of walking on a flat surface to graduated inclines.

6-minute walk test: To record the furthest distance walked at own pace back and forth along a 30 m walkway in 6 minutes on a flat surface.

Incremental Shuttle walk test: Externally paced, incremental distance walked back and forth, final result measured in this is the number of shuttles, which can help predict VO_2 max.

Pharmacology-induced stress testing: Dobutamine Stress Echo, thallium scan; echocardiographic or nuclear medicine imaging changes based on drug injected to look for any regional wall motion abnormality or cold spots depending on the test. This may be useful if unable to walk due to arthritis or other conditions.

Cardiopulmonary Exercise Testing (CPET)

This is usually done on a bicycle with assessment of both ECG and analysis of gases and is valuable in considering when the aerobic metabolism crosses over to anaerobic metabolism in a patient and assessing maximal oxygen consumption at peak exercise. It provides many other parameters that can help uniquely assess cardio respiratory risk in combination.

STEPS	KEY POINTS
How is EVAR performed?	Endovascular repair of abdominal aortic aneurysms involves a joint procedure performed by a radiologist in conjunction with a vascular surgeon. An aortic stent graft is placed via femoral arteries to extend both above and below the edges of the aneurysm. One or both groins may be used. Local anaesthetic is used for the entry site, but regional or general anaesthesia may also be given, though less frequently. Arterial blood pressure monitoring is ideal. It is not suitable if there is significant peripheral vascular disease or atherosclerotic plaques.

What are the benefits of EVAR versus open surgery?

Mortality of EVAR versus open repair is quoted as 0.9% versus 4.3% according to AAAQIP report from 2009–2010.

Advantages
- Shorter, less invasive procedure
- Less associated bleeding
- Early ambulation
- Reduced hospital stay

Disadvantages
- Costly
- Technically difficult
- Reasonable incidence of poor seating of the graft and therefore leak around the graft

How will you discuss risk with the patient?

I would explain risk to the patient in terms of the patient's comorbidities and the surgery they are undergoing. I will need a full history and possible additional investigations in order to provide a more comprehensive picture. It is important to use terms that the patient can understand such as percentages or use of 'common' or 'rare'. The Royal College of Anaesthetists has produced guidance and a patient information leaflet relating to aortic surgery that I could give the patient.

In this case there is the risk of his age and comorbidities, which may lead him to a higher risk of a heart attack and chest infection around the time of his operation, the higher risk of bleeding given the size and length of operation, and the possibility of long-term dialysis. This should be balanced against his high risk of spontaneous rupture given the size of the aneurysm. It is important that all concerns are addressed before proceeding from both the anaesthetic and surgical side.

Despite his high risk, how would you anaesthetise him?

I would give him a general anaesthetic. Ensure he has taken all his regular medications except an ACE inhibitor preoperatively.

Preinduction
- Full noninvasive monitoring
- Awake mid-thoracic epidural after informed consent under aseptic technique
- Invasive arterial monitoring

Induction
- Intubation with the use of high-dose opiate and propofol intravenous induction with use of a muscle relaxant
- Central venous line for assessment of fluid status and provision of vasopressors, blood, and multiple drugs if needed
- Cardiac output monitoring would also be helpful
- Maintaining his mean arterial pressure within 15% of his baseline where possible will help reduce risk of hypoperfusion to organs
- Optimal positioning
- Fluid and body warmers and temperature monitoring
- Nasogastric tube to empty the stomach

STEPS	KEY POINTS
During the operation he has a massive bleed when the clamp is released. How will you manage this?	This will require good communication within the theatre team to avoid adverse sequelae. The clamp should be reinstated and then both medical and surgical aspects managed.
	From a surgical perspective, it is important that there is no ongoing surgical site bleeding and this should be addressed. The bleeding may have in part been related to haemodynamic changes associated with the release of the clamp. This can be minimised by giving a fluid bolus and maintaining vascular tone with vasopressors when clamp is next released. It is also important to ensure that the current bleed has been dealt with and blood and other products transfused appropriately if needed and haemodynamic parameters restored before a repeat attempt at releasing the clamp.
Define massive transfusion, products available, and transfusion triggers for each product.	Massive transfusion occurs when there is more than 50% blood volume transfused in 4 hours or 10 units in 24 hours. Products available are red cells, fresh frozen plasma, platelets, and cryoprecipitate. Adjuncts include fibrinolytics, such as tranexamic acid, aprotinin, recombinant factor 7, and prothrombin concentrate.
	The main principles are to recognise it early, maintain tissue perfusion and oxygenation by considering oxygen delivery, arrest the cause of bleeding (surgical versus coagulopathy), and use blood products appropriately and in a timely fashion. Until bleeding is controlled, it is recommended to give products in a ratio of 1:1:1 (red cells:FFP:platelets).

Transfusion triggers during ongoing bleeding

Hb	< 10
APTT	> 1.5 times normal
Platelets	< 50 or < 75 with ongoing haemorrhage
Fibrinogen	< 1.5

Other goals to achieve

Temperature	> 36 degrees
Ionised Ca^{2+}	> 1.1
pH	> 7.2

What are his options for analgesia?	In view of his poor lung function and undergoing a laparotomy, I feel that a thoracic epidural is in his best interests. I will discuss the procedure with the patient and make appropriate plans for removal later given perioperative heparin use. This should be performed awake preinduction and should facilitate postoperative deep breathing and together with regular chest physiotherapy help reduce the risk of postoperative respiratory infection.
	The alternative would be to perhaps perform transversus abdominis plane blocks and use a fentanyl/morphine PCA with regular paracetamol. It should be borne in mind that due to his age he is likely to be opiate sensitive and due to his additional risk of further renal impairment postoperatively he may have difficulty clearing opiates, which may impair his recovery and cooperation with physiotherapy.
What will decide the criteria for extubation at the end of the operation and where will he go postoperatively?	Providing he has normal acid base, temperature, reasonably corrected haematological and electrolyte parameters and is fully reversed, it would be ideal to plan for an early wakening and extubation to assess neurology and encourage early chest physiotherapy. With his comorbidities, intensive care would be necessary in the first instance until both ventilation and kidney function have been assessed as adequate.
	Preoperative cardiopulmonary exercise testing (CPET) may have helped plan postoperative care if he has undergone this.

STEPS	KEY POINTS

Can you discuss relevance of CPET in more depth with respect to elective AAA surgery?

In recent years various studies have looked at the use of CPET to help stratify risk in patients undergoing aneurysm surgery. In the UK the national vascular society has recommended the use of the AAAQIP (Abdominal Aortic Aneurysm Quality Improvement Project) preoperative care bundle (2011), which incorporates the following:

- Preoperative assessment and risk scoring
- CT angiography to aid decision making between open repair or EVAR
- Assessment by a vascular anaesthetist
- Case reviewed at an MDT meeting involving both surgeon and radiologist
- Patient to be given evidence-based written information

CPET has become a routine part of preassessment for elective aneurysm surgery and helps plan postoperative care. Some variables of significance are as follows.

VO_2 max of 15 ml/kg/min is thought to be equivalent to four METs and hence predictive of poor functional capacity below this value. A value of at least 20 ml/kg/min is desirable for abdominal aortic aneurysm surgery.

AT, or anaerobic threshold, denotes the VO_2 value when there is a switch from aerobic to anaerobic metabolism and therefore when oxygen demand is greater than supply. An AT of 11 ml/kg/min is thought to be needed to undergo significant surgery, and below this there may be a need for postoperative critical care. In addition, below this value on a case-by-case basis there may be a preference for EVAR instead of an open procedure.

A low-peak VO_2, AT, and ventilatory equivalent for CO_2 have been shown to be associated with poor outcomes after this surgery.

Further reading

1. Minto G and Biccard B. Assessment of the high-risk perioperative patient. *Contin Educ Anaesth Crit Care Pain* (2014) **14**(1): 12–17.
2. Al-Hashimi M and Thompson J. Anaesthesia for elective open abdominal aortic aneurysm repair. *Contin Educ Anaesth Crit Care Pain* (2013).
3. Nataraj V and Mortimer AJ. Endovascular abdominal aortic aneurysm repair. *Contin Educ Anaesth Crit Care Pain* (2004) **4**(3): 91–94.
4. Blood Transfusion and the Anaesthetist: Management of Massive Haemorrhage. *AAGBI Guideline.* 2011.
5. Your anaesthetic for aortic surgery. *RCOA patient information leaflet.* May 2008.
6. Abdominal Aortic Aneurysm Quality Improvement Project.
7. Agnew N. Preoperative cardiopulmonary exercise testing. *Contin Educ Anaesth Crit Care Pain* (2010) **10**(2): 33–37.

05.2 SHORT CASE: FRACTURE MANDIBLE

HISTORY *A 19-year-old male who is normally fit and well has been booked for repair of a fractured mandible. When you go to see him in the ward, you notice that his breath smells strongly of alcohol.*

STEPS	KEY POINTS
What are your concerns?	• Mode of injury • Loss of consciousness and current GCS • Airway involvement • Associated head and neck injuries • Intoxication – alcohol, drugs • Starvation status
How would you assess the airway?	Patients with facial trauma often pose the greatest airway challenges to the anaesthetist. For this patient with isolated facial trauma, preoperative airway evaluation must be detailed and thorough. • Particular attention should be focused on jaw opening, mask fit, neck mobility, maxillary protrusion, macroglossia, dental pathology, nasal patency, and the existence of any intraoral lesion or debris. • Trismus is often caused by pain and can disappear on induction of anaesthesia. However, it may persist for mechanical reasons and this needs to be discussed with the surgical team. • Preoperative imaging should be reviewed. X-ray of the mandible (AP, lateral oblique, or panoramic) and neck (AP, lateral), CT if possible.
What are the possible associated injuries?	• Cervical vertebrae fracture • Head injury • Airway: soft tissue injury with risk of oedema and obstruction, tracheal injury • Other facial fractures (i.e. nose, maxilla Le Fort fracture type I horizontal, type II pyramidal, type III transverse)

STEPS	KEY POINTS

What are Le Fort fractures?
See Figure 5.3.

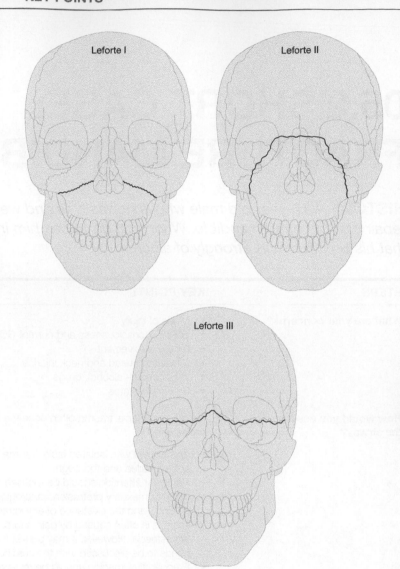

Leforte I

Leforte II

Leforte III

Fig. 5.3 Le Fort classification.

They are midfacial fractures caused by anteriorly directed force.

In Le Fort I fractures, a horizontal fracture line separates the inferior portion of the maxilla from the superior two-thirds of the face, which remain associated with the skull. The entire maxillary dental arch may be mobile or wedged in a pathologic position.

In Le Fort II fractures, the pyramidal mid-face is separated from the rest of the facial skeleton and skull base.

In Le Fort III fractures, the face is essentially separated along the base of the skull due to force directed at the level of the orbit.

When are you happy to anaesthetise this patient?

If the airway is not compromised and there is no associated head injury, I will anaesthetise him once he has sobered and achieved the starvation status.

There are no other associated injuries, and the chance of head injury has been ruled out. He is presented for isolated mandible fracture.

STEPS	KEY POINTS
How would you anaesthetise him?	• Prepare for a potential difficult intubation (i.e. senior help, skilled assistant, difficult airway trolley). • The route of repair also needs consideration, as it can be intraoral, subconjunctival, or via a scalp flap. • Induction: If any forewarning sign of problems with mask ventilation or endotracheal intubation is observed, the airway should be secured prior to anaesthesia induction. This process may involve fibreoptic nasal or oral intubation or tracheostomy. • Different endotracheal tubes (ETT) may be used: In this patient, after discussing with the surgeon for options, my consideration would be to use a nasal tube as this gives room in the mouth for the surgeons to work in. Also this will be beneficial in patients with malocclusion or wedge fracture where insertion of an oral ETT would have been challenging. • The need for a throat pack, postoperative intermaxillary fixation, and facial nerve monitoring should also be discussed. Isolated mandible fractures usually do not make intubation more difficult. However, if it is associated with other facial injuries, the airway might be more difficult to manage. In these cases an inhalational induction might be considered. Remember the risk of an association with a fracture of the base of the skull in which case the nasal route has to be avoided.
What are the NICE guidelines regarding head injuries?	**Assessment** • In patients with GCS 15, assessment is done within 15 min. GCS 9–14 needs immediate assessment. GCS < 8: anaesthetist should be involved. **Investigation** • Exclude brain injury with CT scan before blaming the depressed level of consciousness on intoxication. **Transfer** • Transfer to a tertiary centre would benefit if the patient has a GCS < 8 regardless of the need for surgery. • If transfer is not possible, ongoing liaison with neuro unit is done for advice on management.

Further reading

1. Head injury: Triage, assessment, investigation and early management of head injury in children, young people and adults. *NICE Clinical Guideline* 176. guidance.nice.org.uk/cg176

05.3 SHORT CASE: RHEUMATOID ARTHRITIS

HISTORY *A 75-year-old female patient, suffering from severe Rheumatoid arthritis, is booked for a total knee replacement.*

STEPS	KEY POINTS
Can you tell me the positive findings on her chest X-ray.	See Figure 5.4

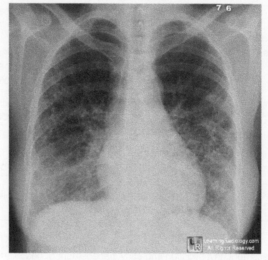

Fig. 5.4

Published with permission from LearningRadiology.com

Bilateral airspace disease with:
- Extensive reticular change throughout both lungs
- Reduced volume
- Honeycomb pattern
- Shaggy heart border

Diagnosis: Pulmonary fibrosis. This can be because of the disease progression or as a side effect of drugs for rheumatoid disease.

STEPS	KEY POINTS

What does her C spine X-ray show? See Figure 5.5

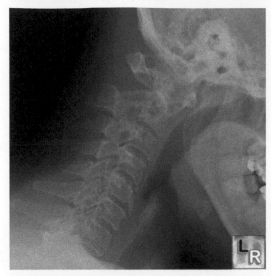

Fig. 5.5

Published with permission from LearningRadiology.com

Lateral radiograph of the neck with the head in flexion shows an increased distance between the anterior border of the dens and the posterior border of the anterior tubercle of C1. This "pre-dentate space," should be less than 3 mm in the adult. Also there is forward suluxation of C1 on C2.

Mainly two types of changes might be seen: *Atlanto-axial subluxation and sub-axial subluxation.*

Atlanto-axial subluxation
- *Anterior*: Most common (80%) finding in rheumatoid arthritis involving the neck, where C1 vertebra is moved forward on body of C2 vertebra due to damage to transverse ligament and can cause spinal cord compression by odontoid peg. Subluxation occurs when distance between atlas and odontoid is > 4 mm in adults and > 3 mm in children.

It is best seen in lateral neck X-ray with neck flexion (which makes subluxation worse).

- *Posterior*: Occurs in 5% of the patients and is due to destruction of odontoid peg, which causes backward movement of C1 vertebra over C2 vertebra. It is best seen in lateral X-ray with neck extension, which makes the condition much worse.

Sub-axial subluxation
It is not very common, occurs below C2 level, and can cause fixed flexion deformity due to ankylosis and osteoporosis.

What is rheumatoid arthritis?

It is an autoimmune, systemic chronic inflammatory disease associated with:
- Polyarthritis of joints with pannus formation
- Synovitis of joints and tendon sheaths
- Loss of articular cartilage and erosion of bone and joint destruction

Women are affected more than men.
Age group is 30–55 years.
Seventy percent are HLA DR4 +ve & seropositive for rheumatoid factor.

STEPS	KEY POINTS

What are the other system manifestations in rheumatoid arthritis?

RS
- Pulmonary fibrosis, vasculitis
- Pulmonary hypertension, nodules

CVS
- Arteriosclerosis, MI, stroke
- Mitral valve disease, pericardial effusion, conduction defects

Blood
- Anaemia

Nervous system
- Peripheral neuropathy
- Autonomic dysfunction
- Compression neuropathy, myelopathy

Renal
- Amyloid, nephropathy

Liver
- Felty's syndrome

Eye/skin
- Episcleritis, rheumatoid nodules, thin papery skin

Due to drugs
- NSAIDS—renal and GI impairment
- Methotrexate, gold, pencillamine—immunosuppression, pancytopenia, liver and renal dysfunction
- Steroids—hypertension, osteoporosis

Joints
- Pain and morning stiffness due to inflammation of synovium
- Reduced bone density, cartilage loss

Should you be worried about this patient's airway?

- Anterior or posterior subluxation and spinal cord compression
- Sub-axial subluxation—fixed flexion deformity
- TMJ involvement—reduced mouth opening
- Cricoarytenoid involvement—stridor
- Steroids—cause osteoporosis

How will you anaesthetise this patient?

Regional anaesthesia in form of spinal is the best for this patient, if there is no absolute contraindication. It is also ideal from the surgical (enhanced recovery pathway in major arthroplasty) point of view.

Preassessment
- Routine anaesthetic history and examination
- Airway assessment—Mallampati assessment, thyromental distance, mouth opening, jaw protrusion, neck extension
- Drug history and its effect on various organ systems

Investigations
- FBC, renal, and liver function tests to assess type of anaemia and for a baseline function
- Chest X-ray to look for pulmonary involvement
- Because of the nature and effect of the disease on cervical spine, lateral C spine X-ray is deemed necessary both in neck extension and flexion view
- Routine ECG and echocardiography if any significant cardiac symptoms

STEPS	KEY POINTS

Intraoperative
- Position during the procedure needs extra care and take precautions for pressure area to be protected to prevent any injury
- Full asepsis is maintained, as a general measure and also due to the state of immunocompromise in this group of patients
- Warming and fluid management to prevent any renal failure in the postoperative period
- Steroid replacement during surgery
- Good pain relief in postoperative period; exercise caution with the use of NSAIDs for fear of renal dysfunction and gastric ulcer
- Patient control analgesia may not be appropriate if hand deformities are present

Postoperative
- ITU/HDU care in patients with severe respiratory disease
- Early mobilisation and postoperative physiotherapy is useful in preventing postoperative respiratory and other complications

Further reading

1. Kwek TK, Lew TWK, Thoo FL. The role of preoperative cervical spine X-rays in rheumatoid arthritis. *Anaesth Int Care* 1998; **26**: 636–41.
2. Fombon FN and Thompson, JP. Anaesthesia for the adult patient with rheumatoid arthritis. *Contin Educ Anaesth Crit Care Pain* (2006) **(6)**6: 235–39.

05.4 SHORT CASE: INADVERTENT DURAL PUNCTURE

HISTORY *You are administering an epidural for labour analgesia in a 25-year-old primigravida, with a 16 G Tuohy needle when a wet tap occurs.*

STEPS	KEY POINTS
What is your immediate course of management?	• Resite: Take the needle out and reinsert in an adjacent space (OR) • Spinal catheter: Insert the epidural catheter into the subarachnoid space • General: document, explain to patient, explain to team

State the advantages and disadvantages of both techniques.

	Advantages	Disadvantages
Spinal catheter	• Prevents another dural puncture • Rapid and predictable analgesia	• Risk of infection • Cauda equina syndrome
Resite	• Less chance of intrathecal dosing • Operator expertise not very important	• Risk of another dural puncture • Procedure can be difficult and may need more expertise

STEPS	KEY POINTS
What special precautions would you take if you had inserted a spinal catheter?	• Labeling the catheter • Handover to the team • All top-ups given by the anaesthetist • Regular neurological observations • Aseptic precautions
What top-up would you give if you were inserting a spinal catheter?	2–3 mLs of the low dose mix (0.1% bupivacaine + 2mcg/mL fentanyl) or 1 mL of 0.25% Bupivacaine +/− fentanyl 15–25 mcg
What is the chance of this patient developing a post-dural puncture headache (PDPH)?	There is a 80% chance of her developing PDPH as the Tuohy needle is wide-bore needle • 16 G: 80% • 20 G: 40% • < 25 G: 1%–2%
What are the characteristics of PDPH?	• Fronto-occipital headache increasing in upright posture (due to higher CSF pressure in upright posture) • Nausea, vomiting, visual disturbances, general malaise • Presents in < 3 days and lasts for 14 days • Usually self-limiting

STEPS	KEY POINTS

What are the risk factors that predispose one to the development of PDPH?

Patient factors	Needle factors	Operator factors
Young age	> 25 G needle	Experience
Female	Cutting or non-atraumatic needle	Fatigue, stress
Obstetric population	Rotating the needle in the epidural space	Use of loss of resistance to air

What is the mechanism of pain in PDPH?

CSF leakage leading to
- Loss of buoyancy—sagging of brain causing traction on pain-sensitive meninges, nerves, and veins
- Compensatory dilation of cerebral veins causing direct pressure on meninges

You are called to see the same patient in the postnatal ward. She is Day 2 postpartum and is complaining of a headache.

How would you approach this patient?

- Obtain history
- General examination
- Neurological examination

What is the differential diagnosis of postpartum headache?

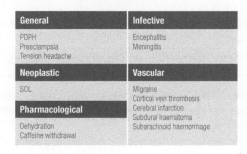

General	Infective
PDPH	Encephalitis
Preeclampsia	Meningitis
Tension headache	
Neoplastic	**Vascular**
SOL	Migraine
	Cortical vein thrombosis
Pharmacological	Cerebral infarction
	Subdural haematoma
Dehydration	Subarachnoid haemorrhage
Caffeine withdrawal	

You have diagnosed PDPH in this patient. What is your management plan?

- Adequate hydration
- Avoid abdominal binders as they are shown to be ineffective
- Conventional analgesics—paracetamol, NSAIDS, codeine, opioids
- Analgesic adjuvants—caffeine, sumatriptan, theophylline, ACTH
- Gold standard treatment—homologous Epidural Blood Patch (EBP)

What is the mode of action of caffeine?

- Methyl xanthine analogue
- Cerebral vasoconstrictor
- 150–300 mgs oral every 6 to 8 hours
- 500 mgs intravenous infusion over one hour. Repeat if needed.
- Adverse effects (which are rare): Cardiac arrhythmias, seizures if dose > 300 mgs
- Cerebral irritability in neonates

When is the suitable time to perform EBP?

24–48 hours. Not effective if performed in less than 24 hours.

STEPS	KEY POINTS
How would you perform EBP after establishing the diagnosis and having assessed the suitability?	• Explain to patient • Two personnel with experience • Strict aseptic precautions • Locate epidural space as per usual technique—a space higher • 10–20 mls of homologous blood • Blood for culture, as per department policy—no consensus • STOP if pain/discomfort on injection • Supine—2 hours and no straining for 1–2 weeks to prevent patch blow-off • Follow-up
Name any three complications of EBP.	• Back pain • Meningeal irritation • Radicular pain • Cranial nerve palsy • Infection
What is the success rate with EBP?	First attempt: 60% Subsequent attempts: up to 80% *The patient is very apprehensive that EBP would be a contraindication if she were to have epidurals in the future.*
What is your view regarding this?	EBP is not a contraindication for subsequent epidurals. She should inform the anaesthetist in the future pregnancies about PDPH so extreme care and expert advice (use of ultrasound guided epidural) would be sorted in case of dural puncture due to difficult procedure.

Further reading

1. Postpartum headache: diagnosis and management. *Contin Educ Anaesth Crit Care and Pain* first published online July 14, 2011 doi:10.1093/bjaceaccp/mkr025.
2. Effective management of the post dural puncture headache. *Anaesthesia Tutorial of the Week*. May 2010.

section 05

BASIC SCIENCE VIVA

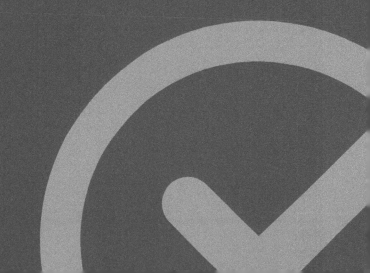

05.5 ANATOMY: CAUDAL BLOCK

Possible questions: *Consider analgesic options in a child having hypospadias repair, anatomy of the caudal space, indications and technique, complications of caudal block. What are the differences in the anatomy of caudal space in adults and children?*

STEPS	KEY POINTS
What are your analgesic options for a child who is booked for hypospadias surgery?	**Multimodal analgesia (WHO ladder)** • Simple analgesics • NSAIDS • Opioids—oral/IV • Wound infiltration • Nerve blocks—dorsal penile block/caudal block
What is the nerve supply of the scrotum and penis?	**Scrotum** • Anterior 1/3—ilioinguinal nerve (L1) • Posterior 2/3—perineal nerve (S2) • Lateral—posterior cutaneous nerve of thigh (S3) **Penis** • Dorsal nerve of penis (S2,3,4) • Ilioinguinal nerve (L1)
What are the indications of caudal block?	It is the commonest regional technique in children and the first means of administering local anaesthetic in the epidural space dating back as early as 1901.

Indications	***Acute pain***
	• Surgical: To cover area innervated by lower lumbar and sacral roots. In younger children, the caudal block effectively covers T10-S5, although only sacral roots are blocked in older children and adults. Caudal anaesthesia is also recommended for upper abdominal surgery, but higher doses are needed to attain a high block
	  ○ Elective: anorectal, genitourinary procedures—inguinal hernia, hypospadias, orchidopexy, circumcision
	  ○ Emergency: testicular torsion, strangulated hernia
	• Nonsurgical: To provide sympathetic block in vascular insufficiency of lower extremities secondary to vasospastic disease, unrelieved perineal pain in labour (historical)

STEPS	KEY POINTS

Chronic pain
- Complex regional pain syndromes (CRPS)
- Lumbar radiculopathy secondary to herniated discs and spinal stenosis
- Backache with sciatica after failed conservative or surgical treatment
- Coccydynia
- Diabetic polyneuropathy

Cancer pain
- Primary genital, pelvic, and rectal malignancy
- Bony metastasis to the pelvis

What are the advantages of caudal over lumbar epidural analgesia?

Onset: The onset of perineal anaesthesia and muscle relaxation after caudal anaesthesia is rapid compared to epidural.

Extent: It is good for ankle and foot surgery as it covers S1 reliably, whereas the lumbar epidural fails to block S1 in 10%–20% of patients.

Indications: Can be performed where lumbar epidural cannot be done, especially after spinal surgeries.

Complications: The incidence of postdural puncture headache (PDPH) is negligible.

Caudal epidural uses a larger volume of local anaesthetic compared to the lumbar epidural, and there is a similar failure rate due to anatomical variation.

Describe the anatomy relevant to caudal anaesthesia.

Sacrum (Latin for sacred) is believed to have played a key part in ancient pagan sacrificial rites and also it was thought as the last bone of the body to decay and the body resurrects around it. It is a triangular bone (▼) composed of five fused sacral vertebrae forming a median crest.

Sacral hiatus is a triangular defect in the lower part of the posterior wall of sacrum formed by the failure of the fifth sacral laminae to fuse in the midline. It is bounded above by the fused laminae of S_4, laterally by the margins of the deficient laminae of S_5, inferiorly by the posterior surface of the body of S_5, and covered posteriorly by the dense sacrococcygeal ligament (formed from supraspinous ligament, interspinous ligament, and ligamentum flavum). It is about 5 cms above the tip of the coccyx.

Sacral canal is the prismatic cavity running through the length of the sacrum following from the lumbar spinal canal and terminating at the sacral hiatus.

The left and right lateral walls of the canal contain the four intervertebral foramina.

What are the contents of sacral canal?

- Terminal part of dural sac ending at S_1–S_3
- Sacral and coccygeal nerves making up cauda equina
- Sacral epidural veins end at S_4 but may extend throughout the canal
- Filum terminale—final part of spinal cord, which does not contain nerves
- Epidural fat—loose in children and fibrosed close-meshed texture in adults

STEPS	KEY POINTS

Describe the technique of performing the block.	Preparation: Informed consent, intravenous access, monitoring, resuscitation equipment, and equipment needed for the block.
	Full asepsis: Similar to any central neuraxial block.
	Personnel: Trained anaesthetist and skilled assistant.
	Calculation: Calculate the local anaesthetic dose using the Armitage regimen.
	• Drug: 0.25% L—Bupivacaine
	• Dose: Infraumbilical operation – 0.5 mL/kg
	   - Lower thoracic operation – 1 mL/kg
	   - Higher thoracic operation – 1.25 mL/kg
	• In our patient: 0.5 mL/kg of 0.25% L—Bupivacaine
	
	Position: The lateral position is efficacious in paediatrics because it permits easy access to the airway when general anaesthesia has been administered.
	
	Prone position is preferable in adults, as the caudal space is made prominent by internal rotation of the ankles.
	
	Landmarks: Locate the sacral hiatus.
	
	• The sacral hiatus forms the apex of an equilateral triangle drawn joining posterior superior iliac spines.
	• When the curve of the sacrum is followed in the midline with the tip of the finger from the tip of the coccyx, the sacral hiatus is felt as a depression.
	
	Procedure: A 22 G short beveled cannula is inserted at 45 degrees until a 'click' is felt, indicating the sacrococcygeal ligament has been pierced. Then the needle is directed cephalad at the angle approaching the long axis of sacral canal. Careful aspiration for blood or CSF should be performed before injection of local anaesthetic although negative aspiration does not always exclude intravascular or intrathecal placement. For this reason, the cannula is left in place whilst the drugs are being drawn, thus giving adequate time for the passive flow of CSF/blood with any inadvertent puncture. After confirming position, drugs are injected slowly.
	
	Test to confirm: Introduction of small amounts of air would produce subcutaneous emphysema if the needle were superficial. A 'whoosh' sound is heard when a stethoscope is placed further up the lumbar spine in successful blocks.

What are the additive drugs that can be used along with the local anaesthetics whilst performing a caudal block?	Preservative-free additives are used to prolong the duration of analgesia, improve the quality of the block, and reduce the unwanted side effects. Opioids—fentanyl, morphine, and diamorphine: Injection of opioids enables provision of analgesia due to a local action of the opioid at the spinal cord level rather than due to systemic absorption. It increases the duration of the block by up to 24 hours, but at the expense of nausea, pruritus, urinary retention, and late respiratory depression. The use of opioids has been replaced by clonidine and ketamine as they significantly prolong the duration of 'single-shot' caudal injections with minimal risk of side effects. The addition of clonidine to plain bupivacaine 0.25% can extend the duration of postoperative analgesia by 4 h, whereas ketamine and bupivacaine are even more effective, providing analgesia for up to 12 h. The main side effects of epidurally administered clonidine are hypotension, bradycardia, and sedation.

STEPS	KEY POINTS
	Clonidine (1–2 mcg/kg): α_2 adrenoceptor agonist. It acts by stimulating the descending noradrenergic medullospinal pathway, thereby inhibiting the release of nociceptive neurotransmitters in the dorsal horn of spinal cord.
	S(+)Ketamine (0.5–1 mg/kg): NMDA receptor antagonist that binds to a subset of glutamate receptor and decreases the activity of dorsal horn neurons.

What are the complications of this block?

Serious or catastrophic complications are rare and can be related to the procedure or the drug injected.
- Absent/patchy block
- Subcutaneous injection
- Hypotension
- Urinary retention
- Intravenous or intraosseous injection—seizures and cardiac arrest
- Dural puncture—resulting in total spinal block if not recognised
- Rectal perforation
- Sepsis
- Haematoma

What are the differences in the anatomy of the caudal epidural space between adults and children?

Adults	Children
• Dura ends at S_2.	• Dura ends at S_4 at birth.
• Sacral fat pad, making it difficult to feel hiatus.	• No fat and thus easy anatomy.
• Epidural fat is dense, making it difficult to achieve a high block.	• Epidural fat is loose, so drug spreads well.
• Sympathetic blockade causes pronounced hypotension.	• Delay in autonomic maturation, so there is cardiovascular stability.

05.6 PHYSIOLOGY: PREECLAMPSIA

STEPS	KEY POINTS
How do you define preeclampsia?	Preeclampsia is described as hypertension (> 140/90 mmHg) and significant proteinuria* that develops after 20 weeks of gestation; although preeclampsia can develop without proteinuria and eclamptic fits can occur with a minimally elevated blood pressure. Oedema is no longer part of the definition although it is often present. *Significant proteinuria: • Urine Protein: Creatinine (PCR) > 30 mg/mmol (OR) • Total protein excretion ≥ 300 mg per 24-hr collection of urine (OR) • Two specimens of urine collected ≥ 4 hours apart with ≥ 2+ on the protein reagent strip. 24-hour proteinuria is difficult to measure and has been replaced by PCR (protein creatinine ratio). What is important is the fact that preeclampsia is linked to eclampsia, HELLP (haemolysis, elevated liver enzymes, and low platelet count) and most probably AFLP (acute fatty liver disease of pregnancy). **Some statistics** • Preeclampsia occurring before 30 weeks of pregnancy is associated with severe morbidity • Up to 30% can occur after delivery (up to 6 weeks post-delivery) • Occurs in 5%–6% of pregnancies overall and up to 25% of hypertensive mothers • 1%–2% women with PET will develop eclampsia
Could you explain the pathophysiology?	A two-stage process into the pathogenesis has been explained. An abnormal placentation along with endothelial dysfunction gives rise to the spectrum of the disease. Preeclampsia is linked to a failure of placentation, which occurs early in pregnancy and results in the placenta becoming hypoxic. This leads to an immune reaction with secretion of upregulated inflammatory mediators from the placenta causing vascular endothelial cell damage and dysfunction.

STEPS	KEY POINTS
Stage I	Abnormal placentation and vascular remodeling ⟶ decreased placental perfusion

Maternal factors

- Genetic
- Behavioral
- Environmental

| **Stage II** | Maternal syndrome of preeclampsia with endothelial dysfunction |

Resulting endothelial dysfunction produces an imbalance of pro- and anti-angiogenic factors, with an increase in anti-angiogenic factors. It should be noted that these biomarkers do not have sufficiently high positive predictive value when used alone.

Pro-angiogenic factors	Anti-angiogenic factors
Vascular Endothelial Growth Factor (VEGF) Placental Growth Factor (PlGF) Placental protein 13 (PP-13) Pregnancy-associated plasma protein A (PAPP-A)	Soluble fms-like tyrosine kinase-1 receptor (sFlt-1) Soluble Endoglin (sEng) Asymmetric Dimethylarginine (ADMA)

The maternal syndrome of preeclampsia is characterised by decreased perfusion due to vasospasm and activation of coagulation cascade with microthrombi formation and end organ damage.

- *Fluid shift*: Leaky capillaries together with a low oncotic pressure result in a low intravascular volume and fluid shift into the interstitial compartment
- *Vasoconstriction*: The generalised vasoconstriction will mean increased systemic vascular resistance and in severe preeclampsia increased pulmonary pressure; also renal, hepatic, and pancreatic dysfunction. Vasospasm in the cerebral vasculature causes seizures and intracerebral bleeds.
- *Decreased placental blood flow*: The compromised placental blood flow will result in IUGR (intrauterine growth retardation), fetal distress, and the high blood pressure increases the risk of placental abruption

What risk factors are associated with the development of preeclampsia?

Pregnancy associated factors
First pregnancy Multiple pregnancy Donor insemination Molar pregnancy Chromosomal abnormalities

Maternal factors
> 35 years < 25 years Family history of preeclampsia Prior history of preeclampsia (20% will develop PET in subsequent pregnancy, 2% eclampsia) Booking diastolic blood pressure of 80 mmHg or more Associated diabetes, obesity, chronic hypertension, and renal disease Antiphospholipid antibodies/factor V Leiden

Paternal factors
First-time father Previous history of preeclampsia

STEPS	KEY POINTS
How would you manage a preeclamptic woman?	Preeclampsia requires multidisciplinary team management, and effective communication with midwives and obstetrician is crucial. The mother should be reviewed regularly by the whole team and the treatment plan clearly written in the notes.

Aim
The aim is to stabilise the blood pressure until the decision to deliver is taken whilst monitoring for signs of severe preeclampsia. Before 34 weeks, two doses of steroids are given to the mother to improve fetal lung maturity.

Monitoring
- BP, RR, SpO_2, urine output recorded on a MEOWS chart
- Strict input/output chart (fluid balance)
- Fetal monitoring in the form of cardiotocography

Vigilance
Clinical examination looking for photophobia, headache, epigastric pain, hyperreflexia and other signs and symptoms of eclampsia

Treatment
- Control of hypertension
- Prevention and control of eclamptic seizures

The Royal College of Obstetricians and Gynaecologists (Green top guideline 10A) and National Institute for Health and Care Excellence (NICE CG 107) have produced guidelines setting specific criteria for the treatment of preeclampsia including the method for measuring blood pressure.

Discuss the medical management of hypertension in pregnancy.

The evidence base for treatment of mild to moderate chronic hypertension in pregnancy resides in maternal benefit rather than clear evidence of an enhanced perinatal outcome for the baby. NICE suggests treating only moderate and severe hypertension (BP > 150 mmHg systolic and 100 mmHg diastolic pressure) and recommends Labetalol as the first line.

- Labetalol
  Route and dose: Oral—200–1600 mg in divided doses; IV—50 mg bolus followed by titrated infusion
  Mode of action: Combined specific α_1 and nonspecific β adrenoceptor antagonist. The ratio of α:β blocking effects depend on the route of administration—1:3 for oral and 1:7 for intravenous
  Side effects: Bradycardia, fatigue, bronchospasm, gastrointestinal disturbances
  Contraindication and caution: Asthma, cardiac disease, phaeochromocytoma

- Methyldopa
  Route and dose: Oral only—250 mg–3 g/day in divided doses
  Mode of action: Acts as false neurotransmitter to norepinephrine
  Side effects: Postural hypotension, bradycardia, headache, haemolytic anaemia
  Contraindication and caution: Liver disease, risk of postnatal depression

- Nifedipine
  Route and dose: Oral only—20–90 mg od (Avoid sublingual route)
  Mode of action: Calcium channel antagonist. Blocks the entry of calcium ions through the L-type channels.
  Side effects: Headache, tachycardia, flushing, and visual disturbances
  Contraindication and caution: Aortic stenosis, liver disease

STEPS	KEY POINTS

- Hydralazine
  Route and dose: IV only 5 mg slow bolus followed by 5 mg/hr
  Mode of action: Activation of guanylate cyclase and increase in intracellular cyclic GMP leading to decrease in intracellular calcium, causing vasodilatation
  Side effects: Fluid retention, flushing, palpitations, headache, dizziness, tachycardia, systemic lupus-like syndrome, peripheral neuropathy
  Contraindication and caution: Severe tachycardia

- α Blockers (Prazosin/Doxazosin)
  Mode of action: Highly selective α_1 adrenoceptor blocker
  Side effects: Syncope, headache, postural hypotension
  Contraindication and caution: No true evidence of teratogenicity but use only if benefit outweighs risk.

- β Blockers
  Mode of action: β adrenoceptor antagonists
  Side effects: Bradycardia, neonatal hypoglycaemia
  Contraindication and caution: May cause IUGR; avoid in pregnancy

- Diuretics
  Mode of action: Various sites of nephron; only use in pulmonary oedema
  Side effects: Neonatal thrombocytopenia
  Contraindication and caution: Do not cause fetal malformations; generally avoided in pregnancy as its use might prevent the physiologic volume expansion in normal pregnancy.

- Magnesium Sulphate
  Route and dose: IV only—4 g bolus over 10 min followed by 1 g/hr infusion for 24 hours or 0.5 g/hr if oliguric. (Further bolus of 2–4g over 10 min if seizures recur.)

  Mode of action:
  o Antagonist at calcium channels reducing systemic and cerebral vasospasm
  o N-methyl D-aspartate receptor antagonist—anticonvulsant action
  o Increased production of endothelial prostacyclin may restore thromboxane—prostacyclin imbalance

Caution: Due to its vasodilatory effects, it increases blood loss and, if given prior to general anaesthetic, will also increase the duration of neuromuscular blocking agents. Care when using along with Nifedipine as they may interact synergistically. Magnesium crosses the placenta leading to neonatal hypotonia and respiratory depression.

When the decision is made to deliver the baby, what anaesthetic technique would you use?

The decision to deliver is made by the consultant obstetrician and usually depends largely on the maternal rather than the fetal well-being as delivery improves the maternal disease.

The mother's safety is paramount, and the blood pressure has to be under control to avoid complications.

The choice between general anaesthesia (GA) and regional technique will be guided by:
- Platelets level ($> 80 \times 10^9$/L on a recent blood result)
- Blood pressure control
- CTG

STEPS	KEY POINTS
	And also influenced by:
	• Mother's anaesthetic history
	• Airway assessment
	• BMI
	The choice is between spinal anaesthetic and GA. There is no evidence that an epidural technique confers more cardiovascular stability than a spinal. Providing there are no contraindications (i.e. low platelets or fetal bradycardia), a regional technique is the preferred option.
What are the indications for magnesium?	The MAGPIE trial in 2002 has shown that magnesium is effective in reducing the incidence of eclampsia. The Collaborative Eclampsia Trial in 1995 has proved it to be more efficient in treating eclamptic seizures than diazepam or phenytoin.
	The loading dose is 4 g over 10 to15 min followed by 1 g/hr infusion for 24 hours or 0.5 g/hr if oliguric. A further bolus of 2–4 g over 10 min is repeated if seizures recur.
How does magnesium work in preeclampsia?	• Antagonist at calcium channels reducing systemic and cerebral vasospasm
	• N-methyl D-aspartate receptor antagonist—anticonvulsant action
	• Increased production of endothelial prostacyclin may restore thromboxane—prostacyclin imbalance
How and why is the magnesium level monitored? What are the side effects of hypermagnesaemia?	Higher magnesium levels in the blood lead to undesirable and life-threatening complications, and hence the level should be monitored. The adequacy of treatment is assessed by regular checking of deep tendon reflexes and by blood levels.
	The therapeutic range is 2–4 mmol/L.
	• Loss of deep tendon reflexes, blurred vision > 5 mmol/L
	• Respiratory depression > 7 mmol/L
	• Cardiac conduction defects > 7.5 mmol/L
	• Cardiorespiratory arrest >10 mmol/L
	Loss of patellar reflexes should prompt a blood level and the stopping of the infusion.
	Toxicity is more likely to occur if renal impairment is present.
How is magnesium-induced cardiac arrest treated?	In the case of cardiac arrest:
	• Stop infusion
	• Start CPR
	• Give 10 ml of 10% calcium gluconate intravenously
	• Send blood for magnesium levels to lab immediately
	• Employ further symptomatic treatment

Further reading

1. Hypertensive disorders of pregnancy. *ATOTW*. March 2014.
2. Po W, Li J, et al. Pre-eclampsia and the anaesthetist. *Anaesthesia & Intensive Care Medicine, Volume 14*, Issue 7, 283–286.
3. Hypertension in pregnancy: The management of hypertensive disorders during pregnancy. *CG107*. August 2010.

05.7 PHARMACOLOGY: TRICYCLIC ANTIDEPRESSANTS

STEPS	KEY POINTS
What are the features of a tricyclic antidepressant (TCA) drug poisoning?	**Cardiovascular** • Palpitations, chest pain, tachycardia, hypotension • ECG changes include nonspecific ST or T wave changes, prolongation of QT, PR and QRS interval, right bundle branch block, right axis deviation, atrioventricular block, Brugada wave (ST elevation in V1–V3 and right bundle branch block) **Central Nervous System** • Agitation, hallucinations, blurred vision, convulsions, hyperreflexia, myoclonus, and coma in severe cases **Peripheral autonomic system** • Dry mouth, dry skin, urinary retention, and pyrexia
What is the mechanism of action of TCA drugs?	The pharmacological effects of tricyclic antidepressant drugs at therapeutic doses are complex and include: • Anticholinergic effects • Competitive antagonism of H_1 and H_2 receptors • Blockade of presynaptic uptake of amines (norepinephrine, dopamine, and serotonin) • Antagonism of α_1 adrenergic receptors • Blockade of the cardiac fast sodium channel • Blockade of the cardiac delayed rectifier potassium channel
Describe the pharmacokinetics of TCA drugs.	Absorption: TCA drugs are well absorbed from the gastrointestinal tract, and peak plasma levels occur 2 to 4 hours after ingestion. Distribution: The large volume of distribution reflects high concentrations in tissues. Less than 10% of TCA circulates as free drug; the rest is bound to circulating proteins (albumin and α_1 acid glycoprotein) or dissolved in circulating free fatty acids. Metabolism: TCA drugs are metabolised in the liver by hydroxylation and methylation. Many TCAs have active metabolites. Both the parent drug and the active metabolites may undergo enterohepatic circulation. Excretion: Renal excretion is low and is usually less than 10%.

STEPS	KEY POINTS
Why do TCA drugs cause arrhythmias and hypotension?	Tricyclic antidepressants slow phase 0 of cardiac depolarisation by inhibiting sodium channels. The resulting delay in propagation of depolarisation in the atrioventricular node, His-Purkinje fibres, and ventricular myocardium leads to prolongation of the PR and QRS interval. Abnormal atrial and ventricular repolarisation may give rise to ECG changes mimicking myocardial infarction (ST segment elevation and T wave inversion).
	The blood pressure may be elevated in the early stages after overdose, presumably due to the inhibition of norepinephrine uptake. Subsequently, the blood pressure is reduced, often to very low levels and may be due to a number of causes. TCAs themselves can cause direct myocardial depression or it relates to relative volume depletion and α receptor blockade induced vasodilatation. Thus, it usually responds rapidly to intravenous fluids.
What is the management of acute TCAD overdose?	ABC approach

Specific measures
- Preventing gastric absorption with activated charcoal
- Induced alkalemia with sodium bicarbonate as this reduces the amount of free drug in circulation
- Treatment of arrhythmias: Ventricular tachyarrhythmias are treated with blockade and severe bradyarrhythmias may need pacing
- Treatment of seizures with benzodiazepines

Supportive care in a HDU/ICU setting. Ventilation may be required for a low GCS.

ECG monitoring is recommended for the first 24 hours.

Further reading
1. http://www.emed.ie/Toxicology

05.8 PHYSICS: OSMOLARITY

STEPS	KEY POINTS
What is osmosis?	The process of net movement of water molecules due to diffusion between areas of different concentration separated by a semipermeable membrane.
What is osmotic pressure?	The pressure exerted within a sealed system of solution in response to the presence of osmotically active particles on one side of a semipermeable membrane (kPa).
Define osmolarity and osmolality.	• Osmolarity is the number of osmoles of solute per litre of solution • Expressed as osm/L and is influenced by temperature Volume of solution changes with the amount of solute added and the changes in temperature and pressure, making it difficult to determine. • Osmolality is the number of osmoles per kilogram of solution and is not dependent on temperature • Expressed in osm/kg Amount of the solvent would not change with temperature and pressure changes, and for this property, osmolality is easier to evaluate.
What is an osmole?	An osmole is a unit of measurement that describes the number of moles of a compound that contribute to the osmotic pressure of a chemical solution [number of particles equal to Avogadro's number (6×10^{23})] and that would depress the freezing point of the solvent by 1.86 Kelvin.
What is used clinically: osmolarity or osmolality and why?	The two terms refer to similar concepts; however, osmolality is the preferred term. When temperature changes, volumes will change but mass remains the same. Under most physiological conditions, temperature is fairly constant and the two are functionally very similar but technically different. Osmolality is used in clinical practice to remove a source of error.
What is the formula for calculation of estimated osmolarity?	Formula for calculated osmolarity = 2 Na + 2 K + Urea + Glucose *Sodium and potassium*: Sodium and potassium along with chloride are the most abundant ions in the body and are hence used in the equation. As chloride normally tags along sodium and potassium, they are multiplied by a factor of two to account for the chloride in the body fluids. *Urea*: Urea is added for a historical reason as it does decrease the freezing point, although it is not osmotically active. *Glucose*: This makes a big difference to osmolarity especially in diabetics. Proteins are NOT used in the calculation as they are not ionic although osmotically active.

STEPS	KEY POINTS
How is it measured in the lab?	Osmometers utilise the colligative properties of the osmotically active substances. The most commonly used osmometers work on the freezing point depression technique as they are quick, easy, and measure the volatile alcohol along with the other solutes.
What are colligative properties?	The properties of a solution that vary according to the osmolarity of the solution. • Depression of the freezing point: Depressed by 1.86 K per osmole of solute per kilogram of solvent • Reduction of vapour pressure (Raoult's Law) by 0.3 mmHg The depression of freezing point or reduction of the vapour pressure of a solvent is proportional to the molar concentration of the solute. • Elevation of the boiling point by 0.52°C • Increase in osmotic pressure by 17 000 mmHg
Why is there a difference between the estimated and the calculated osmolarity?	Osmolar gap is the difference between measured and calculated osmolarity, which is a measure of an osmotically active particle that is not normally found in the plasma (e.g. ethanol).
What are some conditions that affect osmolarity?	SIADH: defined by the nonosmotic release of ADH with consequent water retention and hypotonicity (ADH: Osmoreceptors in the supraoptic nuclei of the hypothalamus has a threshold of 289+/−2.3 mosmol/kg. Above this plasma level, ADH is released) Diabetes insipidus: neurogenic (deficiency of ADH synthesis or impaired release), nephrogenic (renal resistance of action of ADH); massive diuresis and hypovolaemia TUR syndrome: excessive absorption of irrigating fluid Water intoxication: Self-inflicted, or excess glucose solution Hyperosmolar states: Hyperglycaemic nonketotic hyperosmolar coma
What is oncotic pressure (colloid osmotic pressure)?	The osmotic pressure exerted by plasma proteins. Measured with an oncometer, comprising a semipermeable membrane, which separates the plasma sample from a saline reference solution. Thus, change of oncotic pressure can be transduced and measured.
What is meant by tonicity?	Osmolality measures the total number of solute particles within a solution, but tonicity is only influenced by those solute particles that are not able to cross the membrane separating two solutions. Urea and glucose freely permeate and therefore are not included in the calculation of tonicity. (A very dry question with lots of definitions; however, a recurring favourite in the viva)

section 06

CLINICAL
VIVA

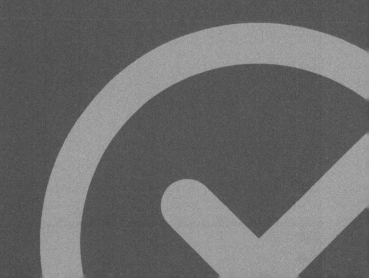

06.1 LONG CASE: PREGNANT WOMAN WITH AORTIC STENOSIS

HISTORY *You are on-call on labour ward and are alerted of a pregnant woman who had been admitted earlier that day with complaints of chest pain and breathlessness. She is 23-years-old in her first pregnancy at 32 weeks gestation. She had been seen by the senior Obstetric registrar and has had blood investigations, ECG, and an urgent ECHO. The consultant Obstetrician is on her way from home.*

STEPS	KEY POINTS
Past medical history	She has a background of bicuspid aortic valve disease but had no cardiology follow-up due to social reasons. She gets breathless on moderate exertion and does only minimal household work.
Obstetric history	She had seen the community midwife at 12 weeks and was then referred for a consultant-led obstetric clinic due to the 'heart condition'. The patient failed to attend further antenatal follow-ups for the fear of being told to terminate the pregnancy.
No significant past surgical history.	On examination: Looks unsettled and anxious Heart rate: 95/min Respiratory rate: 34/min Blood Pressure: 80/60 mmHg

Blood tests						
Hb	11.1 g/dL	(13–16)	Na	138 mmol/L	(137–145)
WCC	3.0×10^9/L	(4–11)	K	4.8 mmol/L	(3.6–5.0)
Platelets	242×10^9/L	(140–400)	Urea	2.5 mmol/L	(1.7–8.3)
PCV	0.28	(0.38–0.56)	Creat	42 umol/L	(62–124)

STEPS	KEY POINTS

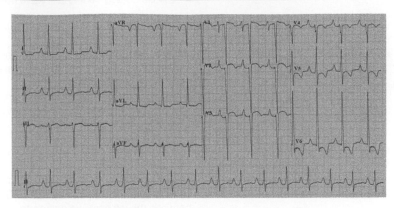

Fig. 6.1 ECG

ECHO report

LA: dilated
LV: hypertrophied
RA: Normal size and function
RV: Normal size and function
Aortic valve: Thickened, possibility of a bicuspid valve cannot be excluded; no calcification
Valve area: 0.8 cm^2
Peak gradient: 75 mmHg
Mitral valve: Minimal mitral regurgitation
Tricuspid Valve/Pulmonary Valve: Normal
Systolic pulmonary artery pressure: 35 mmHg

Summarise the case.

A high-risk primiparous pregnant woman in her third gestation, admitted with signs of decompensation with a background of underlying aortic valvular heart disease. The problems are:
- Congenital bicuspid aortic valve with severe aortic stenosis with a high gradient between the LV and aorta
- Signs of left ventricular hypertrophy with strain
- Pulmonary hypertension
- Poor social history and medical follow-up

Describe the ECG.

Rate: 90
Rhythm: Regular sinus rhythm
Axis: Left axis

Intervals:
- PR—Normal
- QRS—Normal

Segments:
- ST Elevation lead V1–3
- ST Depression leads I, V5–6

Additional:
- Voltage criteria left ventricular hypertrophy
  - R wave lead I + S wave lead III > 25 mm
  - R wave V5 + S wave V1 > 45 mm
  - T wave inversion V1–6

STEPS	KEY POINTS

Interpretation:
- Voltage criteria for LVH
- Diffuse ST segment and T wave changes, indicating strain

What findings can be diagnosed with a Doppler ECHO in a patient with valvular heart disease?

- Chambers—size and function, wall motion abnormalities, presence of thrombus
- Septum—thickening or thinning, motion abnormalities
- Valves—structural anatomy, thickening, number of cusps, calcification, stenosis, or regurgitation
- Measurements—pressures in chambers, aorta and pulmonary vasculature, peak velocity across valves and peak/mean gradients, ejection fraction

How does a Doppler ECHO determine the valve area and the gradient?

Gradient: Doppler echocardiography takes advantage of the acceleration of flow across a restrictive orifice based on Doppler shift. Blood flow velocities can be converted to pressure gradients to yield mean and peak gradients according to the Bernoulli equation. The gradient is the difference in pressure between the left ventricle and aorta in systole.

Valve area: There are various ways to determine aortic valve area. The most commonly used is the continuity equation.

By law of conservation of mass, flow in one area (i.e. left ventricular outflow tract, LVOT) should be equal to the flow in the second area (i.e. valve orifice) provided there are no shunts between the two areas. Flow is derived from the cross-sectional area and the velocity of flow.

Applying the law of conservation of mass

Area of LVOT $\times$ Velocity in LVOT = Aortic Valve Area $\times$ Velocity at Valve

$$\text{Aortic Valve Area (A2)} = \frac{A_{LVOT}\,(A1) \times V_{LVOT}\,(V1)}{V_{valve}\,(V2)}$$

See Figure 6.2.

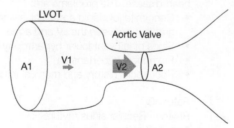

Fig. 6.2

Is there any difference in the gradient values when measured using Doppler echocardiography and cardiac catheterisation techniques?

Doppler measurements overestimate the gradient, due to 'pressure recovery' based on fluid mechanics theory.

Explanation: In fluid mechanics, flow equates to kinetic energy and pressure is potential energy. According to the law of conservation of energy, the sum of kinetic and potential energy remains constant.

Kinetic energy (KE) + Potential energy (PE) = Constant

Proximal to stenosis: The blood flow in the left ventricle is such that there is a higher pressure and lower flow.

Stenosis: As the blood passes through the valve, there is an increase in KE and a decrease in PE. This increased velocity of blood across the stenotic valve accounts for a reduced pressure.

STEPS	KEY POINTS

Post stenosis: Distal to the orifice, the flow decelerates again. KE is reconverted into PE with a corresponding increase in static pressure. This increased pressure immediately distal to the orifice due to the reduction of KE is called pressure recovery.

Doppler measures the highest velocity across the stenosis; hence, the Doppler gradients are markedly greater, whereas catheterisation measures a more or less recovered pressure at some distance from stenosis.

This pressure recovery depends on:
- Aortic valve area
- Ascending aortic area
- Transvalvular velocity

What is aortic stenosis?

Aortic stenosis is a fixed output state, where the narrowing of the aortic valve impedes delivery of blood from the heart to the aorta.

How can you classify aortic stenosis?

There are four grades of severity according to the valve area and the mean gradient.

Grade of severity	Valve area	Mean gradient
Normal	3.0–4.0 cm²	
Mild	1.2–1.8 cm²	12–25 mmHg
Moderate	0.8–1.2 cm²	25–40 mmHg
Severe	0.6–0.8 cm²	40–50 mmHg
Critical	0.6 cm²	> 50 mmHg

It should be remembered that classifying by gradient, rather than area, would underestimate disease severity once the left ventricle starts to fail.

What are the symptoms and signs of aortic stenosis?

The classic triad of symptoms are:
- Angina
- Heart failure: dyspnoea, orthopnoea, paroxysmal nocturnal dyspnoea
- Syncope

Also associated with palpitations, hypertension, and oedema
The signs are:
- Slow-rising pulse of decreased amplitude (pulsus parvus et tardus)
- Hypertension
- Absent S2 or paradoxical splitting of S2 due to late closure of aortic valve
- Prominent S4 due to forceful atrial contraction against a hypertrophied ventricle
- Classic systolic murmur radiating to the carotids

What does pregnancy do to maternal physiology that makes valvular diseases an important concern?

Pregnancy is associated with significant haemodynamic changes such as:
- 30%–50% increase in stroke volume and cardiac output
- Increase in heart rate

Normal pregnancy is a volume overloaded state where the valvular heart diseases mainly severe stenotic lesions are not tolerated. Also, the symptoms and signs that arise during the course of normal pregnancy are similar to those reported by patients with cardiac disease; hence the difficulty in diagnosing deterioration.

What are the causes of aortic stenosis?

- Congenital bicuspid aortic valve
- Rheumatic heart disease leading to mixed valve disease
- Degenerative calcific aortic stenosis

STEPS	KEY POINTS

Describe the pathophysiology of aortic stenosis. See Figure 6.3.

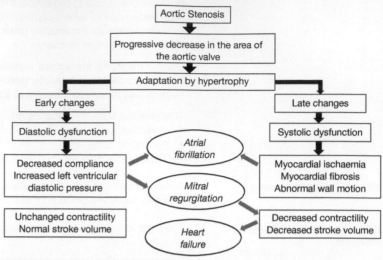

Fig. 6.3

Right ventricular function is normally maintained even in severe cases.

What other conditions are associated with congenital bicuspid valve?

It can occur with other congenital heart diseases but mainly coarctation of aorta (COA) and VSD.

What is the concern in COA?

Medial thickening and infolding of the intimal tissue of the descending aorta distal to the origin of the left subclavian artery (juxta-ductal position).

Also associated with VSD are berry aneurysms in brain and retina, Turner's syndrome, and other congenital abnormalities.

What are the symptoms and signs of COA?

- Symptoms include headache, chest pain, fatigue and weak legs.
- Signs:
  o Hypertension
  o Prominent brachial and absent/weak femoral pulses
  o Differential cyanosis
  o Systolic or continuous murmur in the left infraclavicular and infrascapular areas

What are the findings of COA on chest radiograph?

- Cardiomegaly due to LVH
- Signs of pulmonary oedema and failure
- '3' sign (or inverted '3' sign on barium studies)—coarctation with pre- and post-stenotic dilatation
- Rib notching of the fourth through eighth ribs due to presence of long-standing dilated intercostal collateral vessels

What are the cardiac conditions where pregnancy is contraindicated?

Absolute
- Primary pulmonary hypertension
- Secondary pulmonary hypertension—Eisenmenger's syndrome
- NYHA III/IV patients (New York Heart Association functional classification)

Relative
- Severe aortic and mitral stenosis
- Marfan's syndrome with significant aortic root dilatation
- Prosthetic valves requiring anticoagulation
- Cyanotic heart diseases

STEPS	KEY POINTS

How can you risk stratify pregnant patients with cardiac diseases?

The WHO risk stratification seems an excellent model to predict pregnancy outcome in patients with structural heart disease. With an increasing level of risk score, more cardiac, obstetric, and neonatal complications were encountered. A WHO score of 1 indicates low risk, while a WHO score of 3 indicates a high risk and a WHO score of 4 is a contraindication for pregnancy.

I: No detectable increased risk in maternal mortality ($<$ 1%) and no/mild increase in morbidity
- Uncomplicated PS, PDA, or mitral valve prolapse
- Successfully repaired simple lesions (ASD, VSD, TAPVD)

II: Small increased risk of maternal mortality (5%–15%) and moderate increase in morbidity
- Unoperated ASD or VSD
- Repaired TOF/COA
- Most arrhythmias
- Marfan's syndrome without aortic dilatation

III: Significantly increased risk of maternal mortality (25%–50%) or severe morbidity
- Expert counseling required. If pregnancy is decided upon, intensive specialist, cardiac, and obstetric monitoring needed throughout pregnancy, childbirth, and puerperium.
  - Mechanical valve
  - Fontan circulation
  - Unrepaired cyanotic heart disease
  - Other complex congenital heart diseases
  - Marfan's syndrome with aortic root dilatation 40–45 mm

IV: Extremely high risk of maternal mortality or severe morbidity

- Pregnancy contraindicated. If pregnancy occurs, termination should be discussed.
  - Pulmonary arterial hypertension of any cause
  - Severe systemic ventricular dysfunction (LVEF $<$ 30%, NYHA class III–IV)
  - Severe symptomatic MS and AS
  - Marfan's syndrome with aortic root dilation $>$ 45 mm
  - Native severe COA

How would you manage this patient?

Preconception
- European Society of Cardiology guidelines on 'Management of Cardiovascular Disease During Pregnancy' recommends that patients with severe aortic stenosis should undergo intervention preconception if they are symptomatic and have ventricular dysfunction (EF $<$ 50%).
- Careful cardiac exam and assessment of functional capacity to determine the likelihood of patients to tolerate the haemodynamic changes of pregnancy.
- Serial echocardiographic assessment to see disease progression.
- Patient education and lifestyle changes.
- Other investigations as needed.
- Medical treatment to optimise functional capacity.
- Aortic valve replacement (AVR) is the definitive treatment, and ideally this patient should have had an AVR preconception.

Antepartum
- Joint care with cardiology, obstetrics, and anaesthesia in a tertiary care setup.
- Optimisation of medical therapy (discussed below).

STEPS	KEY POINTS

Intrapartum

- The timing and mode of delivery are discussed and are dictated by medical and obstetric condition; vaginal delivery is indicated unless obstetric indication for caesarean delivery.
- Position: Avoid supine and lithotomy position as they are poorly tolerated. Nurse the patient in cardiac (legs lower than abdomen) or lateral position.
- Monitoring: Invasive arterial and central venous pressure monitoring in severe cases. Pulmonary floatation catheter is used in patients with severe and critical stenosis with symptoms of heart failure.
- Avoid pain and pushing: Sympathetic overactivity causes tachycardia, and the increased venous return with pushing causes decompensation. A short assisted second stage is recommended.
- Syntocinon is given as a diluted infusion.
- Auto transfusion is not tolerated; blood loss to some extent is beneficial as long as venous return is maintained.

Postpartum

- Monitoring is continued until 24–48 hours postpartum.
- Cardiology follow-up for a definitive management.

Anaesthetic management

The goal is to maintain blood pressure and prevent maternal and foetal distress, by maintaining preload, heart rate, and afterload.

$$BP = SV \times HR \times SVR$$

- Preload
  - Maintain preload by optimal positioning, avoiding aortocaval compression, and adequate fluid balance.
  - Vasodilatation with regional and general anaesthesia can decrease the venous return, jeopardising the situation.

- Contractility
  - Maintain contractility: General anaesthesia causes myocardial depression whereas regional techniques do not.

- Afterload
  - Both general and regional anaesthesia decreases the afterload.
  - As long as contractility is maintained, a decrease in SVR is beneficial as this would aid forward flow. For this reason regional anaesthesia is a good option as it does not have any effect on cardiac contractility.

- Heart rate
  - Slow/normal heart rate is maintained and tachyarrhythmias are avoided.
  - Tachycardia reduces the coronary perfusion as diastolic time is reduced, and also the preload is highly dependent on the 'atrial kick' and arrhythmias obviate this factor.

There is *no absolute contraindication for any anaesthetic technique*. Understanding the pathophysiology aids management.

Traditionally GA was advocated for these patients. It should be borne in mind that most anaesthetic agents cause vasodilatation and it is the conduct of anaesthesia that is important rather than the specific technique. The safe use of carefully titrated regional blocks using epidural and spinal catheters is currently increasing.

STEPS	KEY POINTS

Key goals
- Slow/normal heart rate
- Adequate preload
- Preserve contractility
- Maintain afterload
- Treat anaemia and careful fluid management
- Prevent triggers that increase pulmonary vascular resistance—hypercarbia, hypoxia, acidosis, and pain
- Adequate invasive monitoring
- Transfer to tertiary care with progressive symptoms

What medical management can you offer this patient?

The treatment options are limited. There is no solid evidence that pathological course of aortic stenosis is prevented with any medical therapy; rather, it is symptomatic treatment that is considered to 'buy time'. There is equivocal evidence regarding the use of statins in preventing disease progression.

Hypertension
- Vasodilators like ACE inhibitors and Angiotensin Receptor blockers (ARBs) are well tolerated in mild/moderate aortic stenosis. They are used in severe aortic stenosis with extreme caution to avoid critically reducing preload or systemic arterial blood pressure. Be aware of the teratogenic effects of these drugs.
- β blockers: Used with caution in pulmonary oedema, the prevention of atrial fibrillation, and prevention of aortic root dilation.

Angina
- Bed rest, oxygen
- β blockers to decrease myocardial oxygen consumption
- Nitrates to dilate coronary vessels
- Prevent reduction of preload and blood pressure

Syncope
- If syncope is due to brady/tachy arrhythmias, then pacemaker or anti-arrhythmic drugs are used.

Pulmonary congestion
- Digoxin
- Diuretics—used with utmost care because they can precipitate life-threatening haemodynamic compromise in patients who are preload dependent
- Careful titration of ACE inhibitors and ARBs

This patient is symptomatic with signs of heart failure.
- Cautious use of diuretics and nitrates to treat pulmonary congestion
- Ideally dealt with in tertiary hospital with expert help
- Invasive monitoring—ideally pulmonary artery pressure monitoring
- Careful fluid management

Further deterioration despite optimal medical treatment warrants surgical intervention.

In cases where patients remain severely symptomatic (in particular, if they have signs of heart failure), aortic stenosis should be relieved before delivery.

This patient would benefit from a percutaneous balloon aortic valvuloplasty.

STEPS	KEY POINTS
What are the surgical interventions in severe aortic stenosis?	The surgical options are • Percutaneous Balloon Aortic Valvuloplasty (PBAV) • Aortic Valve Replacement (AVR) • Transcatheter Aortic Valve Implantation (TAVI) PBAV is ideal in this patient because it precludes the need for an open bypass surgery in pregnancy and TAVI is done only in specialist centres. *This patient then comes in with a successful pregnancy 3 years later having had a mechanical prosthetic valve after her first pregnancy.*
What is the risk of prosthetic valve thrombosis in this patient?	Prosthetic valve thrombosis is a potentially devastating complication with an incidence of 0.7%–6% per patient per year. The risk is higher in this patient because of: • Presence of mechanical, rather than biological, prosthetic valve • Hypercoagulable state of pregnancy • Chance of interruption of anticoagulation in pregnancy
How could her anticoagulation be managed during pregnancy?	Risk of valve thrombosis due to inadequate anticoagulation is weighed against the risk of direct harm due to the teratogenic drugs on the fetus. **Warfarin** • Good for mother • Bad for fetus as it crosses placenta and causes fetal embryopathy—nasal cartilage hypoplasia, brachydactyly, IUGR—when administered between 6 and 12 weeks of gestation. **Heparin – unfractionated (UFH) or low molecular weight heparin (LMWH)** • Good for foetus • Bad for mother due to increase in the risk of valve thrombosis. Three treatment choices according to the current recommendations are suggested. 1. Treatment dose: subcutaneous UFH throughout pregnancy. 2. Treatment dose: subcutaneous LMWH throughout pregnancy. 3. UFH/LMWH until 13 weeks followed by warfarin. UFH/LMWH restarted at 36 weeks of gestation. Monitoring anticoagulation with appropriate tests is important in pregnancy, especially in high-risk patients with renal impairment.

Further reading

1. ESC Guidelines on the management of cardiovascular diseases during pregnancy. *European Heart Journal* (2011) **32,** 3147–3197; doi:10.1093/eurheartj/ehr218

06.2 SHORT CASE: HOARSENESS AND MICROLARYNGOSCOPY

HISTORY *You are asked to see a 70-year-old man with a hoarse voice who is booked for an elective micro laryngoscopy and excision of vocal cord lesion.*

STEPS	KEY POINTS
What are the causes of a hoarse voice?	• Vocal cord pathology—paralysis, nodules, etc. • Extrinsic airway compression • Nerve lesions • Functional dysphonia • Laryngeal papilloma • Reflux laryngitis • Laryngeal carcinoma
What is the nerve supply of the larynx?	Motor and sensory supply is by branches of the Vagus nerve. **Motor** • Recurrent laryngeal nerve supplies all muscles except cricothyroid. • External laryngeal nerve supplies cricothyroid muscle. **Sensory** • Recurrent laryngeal nerve: sensation below vocal cords • Internal laryngeal nerve: sensation above the vocal cords
What are the effects of laryngeal nerve damage?	*Partial recurrent laryngeal nerve damage* The vocal cords are held in midline position as abductors are more affected than adductors (Semon's law). • Unilateral lesion may lead to hoarseness. • Bilateral lesions can lead to complete airway obstruction. *Complete recurrent laryngeal nerve damage* The vocal cords are held midway between the midline and abducted position. • Unilateral lesion can lead to stridor. • Bilateral lesions result in loss of voice and aspiration. *Superior laryngeal nerve damage* • Leads to a weak voice because of slack vocal cords.
What are the issues anaesthetising this patient?	**Patient factors** • Likely to be a smoker • Cardiovascular and respiratory comorbidities

STEPS	KEY POINTS

Anaesthetic factors
- Difficult airway risk
- Need for airway that allows surgery with possible use of jet ventilation and lasers during surgery

Surgical factors
- Shared airway
- Head end distant from anaesthetic machine

What special investigations would you like this patient to have?

- Flexible nasendoscopy to know vocal cord movement
- CT scan of neck
- Pulmonary function tests if indicated

Your airway assessment on the patient does not show the presence of a difficult airway.

What are the airway options in this case?

Standard intravenous induction with insertion of a micro laryngoscopy tube (MLT) or jet ventilation.

What are the features of a micro laryngoscopy tube?

It is longer than standard endotracheal tubes of this diameter (usually a small diameter to aid surgery) with a high-volume, low-pressure cuff.

This is the micro laryngoscopy picture of the vocal cord lesion that the surgeon decides to excise with laser.

See Figure 6.4. *Published with permission from Department of Pathology, University of Washington*

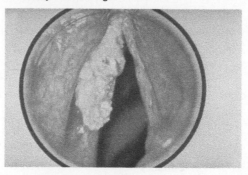

Fig. 6.4

What can this lesion be?

- Laryngeal carcinoma (more likely)
- Vocal cord nodules, polyps, or cysts
- Laryngeal papilloma
- Granuloma

What are the risks of laser surgery?

- Ocular damage
  The nondivergent beam of laser light, even when reflected, may be focused on the fovea and cause irreversible blindness. CO_2 lasers will not penetrate farther than cornea. Staff should wear goggles to protect them from specific wavelength that is being generated.

- Explosions and fires
  Instruments should have a matte finish to minimise reflection. Special hazard associated with laser surgery to upper airway. Surgical swabs and packs can also ignite and thus must be kept moistened with saline.

What precautions are suggested in laser surgery?

- Flexible metallic or metallic coated tubes
- Cuff inflation with saline instead of air
- Use of nonexplosive mixture of gases
- Limitation of LASER power and duration of bursts
- Avoidance of tracheal intubation (e.g. HFJV)

STEPS	KEY POINTS
What are the pros and cons of jet ventilation?	**Advantages** • Improved surgical access • Reduced peak airway pressure • Reduced cardiovascular compromise • Avoidance of endotracheal tube ignition if laser is used **Disadvantages** • Barotrauma—pneumothorax, pneumomediastinum, pneumopericardium, pneumoperitoneum, subcutaneous emphysema • Malposition—gastric distension, rupture • Dysrhythmias • Airway soiling during surgery • Inhalational anaesthesia impossible • Efficacy of gas exchange less predictable
What types of jet ventilation are available?	• Low-frequency jet ventilation delivered via Sanders or Manujet • High-frequency jet ventilation (HFJV)
What are the basic settings on a jet ventilator?	• Driving pressure (DP) The DP is the operating pressure for the jet ventilation that may range from 103–405 kPa. 'Start low, go slow' is the appropriate approach for initiating jet ventilation. In an adult, one can start with a DP of 150–200 kPa, apply a few manual breaths, watching chest movement, airway pressure, and expiratory CO_2. • Frequency of breaths (respiratory rate) Automatic jet ventilators are capable of delivering jets at 1–10 Hz. An initial rate of 100–150 breaths/min is commonly chosen. It is then adjusted depending on the limits of other interacting parameters and the adequacy of ventilation. • Inspiratory to Expiratory (I:E) Ratio A longer expiratory time is normally chosen with a typical 1:E ratio of 1:3 for better emptying of the lungs. • End Expiratory Pressure (EEP) Limit Rate dependent gas trapping is due to inadequate time for full expiration of gases and altered lung mechanics. The EEP is an indicator of alveolar distension or the state of FRC. The value for EEP limit on the ventilator is set at a similar level to the PEEP during IPPV (5–10 cm of H_2O).
What is the mechanism of gas exchange in HFJV?	• Pendelluft occurs as a result of regional variation in airway resistance and compliance causing some areas of the lung to fill or empty more rapidly than others. • Convective streaming/Taylor dispersion occurs as a result of the asymmetrical velocity profile of the inspired gas front as it moves through the bronchial tree. Molecules in the central zones where axial velocities are higher diffuse to lateral zones with lower axial velocities. • Cardiogenic mixing where beating heart enhances gas exchange through agitation of surrounding lung tissue and molecular diffusion. • Bulk flow—partial contribution.

Further reading

1. Evans E, Biro P, Bedforth N. Jet ventilation. *Contin Educ Anaesth Crit Care Pain* (2007) **(1)**7: 2–5.

06.3 SHORT CASE: HEAD INJURY

HISTORY *A 25-year-old patient has been involved in a RTA and brought to A&E with GCS of 11.*

STEPS	KEY POINTS
Discuss the prevalence of head injury and its main causes.	**Prevalence and causes** • 70%–80% male. • 10%–20% aged more than 65 yrs, 40%–50% children. • Death due to head injury is 6–10 per 100 000 per annum. **Minor injury** • Falls (22%–43%) and assaults (30%–50%) are commonest cause of minor head injury, followed by road traffic accident (25%). **Major injury** • Road traffic accident is the major cause of moderate to severe injury.
How will you manage this patient?	• Principal of management of head injury is to prevent secondary brain injury due to hypoxia, hyper/hypocarbia, hypovolaemia, hypotension, and increased ICP. • Initial assessment and management as per ATLS guidelines. • Primary survey and management of other life-threatening injury (tension pneumothorax, cardiac tamponade, airway obstruction, etc.). • Secondary survey.
Can you tell me the criteria for a CT scan in adult trauma patient?	• GCS < 13 on presentation • Suspected open or depressed skull fracture • Signs of basal skull fracture (haemotympanum, CSF leak from ear or nose, battle's sign, panda eyes) • Focal neurological signs **Others** • More than one episode of vomiting following head injury • History of loss of consciousness following injury or more than 30 minutes of retrograde amnesia of events immediately prior to injury • Mechanism of injury (e.g. cyclist or pedestrian struck by motor vehicle, occupant ejected from a motor vehicle)

STEPS	KEY POINTS
How will you rule out cervical spine injury in trauma patient?	The cervical spine may be cleared clinically if the following preconditions are met. **Alert and awake patient** • Fully orientated • No head injury • Not under influence of drugs or alcohol • No neck pain • No abnormal neurology • No significant injury that may 'distract' the patient from complaining about a possible spinal injury Provided these preconditions are met, the neck may then be examined. If there is no bruising or deformity, no tenderness and a pain-free range of active movements, the cervical spine can be cleared. Radiographic studies of the cervical spine are not indicated. **Unconscious, intubated patients** The standard radiological examinations of the cervical spine in the unconscious, intubated patient are: • Lateral cervical spine film. • Antero-posterior cervical spine film. • CT scan of occiput—C3. • The open-mouth odontoid radiograph is inadequate in intubated patients and will miss up to 17% of injuries to the upper cervical spine. Axial CT scanning with sagittal and coronal reconstruction should be used to evaluate abnormal, suspicious, or poorly visualised areas on plain radiology. With technically adequate studies and experienced interpretation, the combination of plain radiology and directed CT scanning provides a false negative rate of less than 0.1%.
What are the indications for intubation in a head injury patient?	• GCS < 8 in adult and < 9 in paediatric patients • Seizure after trauma • Airway obstruction, airway injury • Severe facial injury (Le Fort fracture, mandible fracture) • Inability to maintain oxygenation/ventilation (PaO_2 < 9 kPa on air or < 13 kPa with oxygen, $PaCO_2$ < 4 kPa or > 6 kPa) • To facilitate transfer of patient to tertiary centre • Alcohol or other drug intoxication plus signs of head injury
This patient has sustained an extradural haematoma and needs urgent transfer to a neurosurgical centre. How will you manage this transfer?	**Ensure** **Patient** • Airway is secured and the patient is ventilated as indicated. • Any life-threatening injury is dealt with and patient is optimally resuscitated. **Personnel** • Fully trained doctor and assistant who are experienced in transferring critically ill patient. • Receiving team is aware and awaiting.

STEPS	KEY POINTS

Equipment

- Monitoring equipment are all fully charged or replacement batteries taken. Minimal monitor for transfer of patient with head injury are ECG, SpO_2, invasive arterial blood pressure, $EtCO_2$, GCS, and pupillary reflex.
- Infusion pumps and ventilators are adequately charged and spare batteries are taken for transfer.
- Oxygen cylinders are full and spares available.
- Cannulation and intubation kits.

Drugs

- For intubation
- Emergency drugs in case of decompensation
- Anti-seizure drugs
- Drugs that decrease ICP
- Fluids, blood, and blood products (if deemed necessary)

Notes

- Patient notes and CT scan report plus hard copy in place
- All available blood results

Maintain

General

- 30–45 degree head up
- Neck is midline and free from any tight ties
- Cervical spine immobilisation

Ventilation

- $PaO_2 > 13$ kPa and $PaCO_2$ around 4.5 kPa

Circulation

- MAP > 90 mmHg (to maintain CPP 60–70 mmHg, assuming that ICP is 20 mmHg)
- Use vasopressor to maintain MAP

Others

- Treat hyperpyrexia
- Maintain blood glucose level

How will you manage a sudden rise of ICP if it occurs during transfer?	Steps to treat sudden increase in ICP (dilated pupil and direct absent light reflex)

General

- Ensure that patient is 30 degree head up.
- Make sure that patient is adequately sedated and ventilated (bucking and coughing increases ICP).
- ETT is in place and taped properly but not obstructing any venous drainage.

Numbers

- $PaO_2 > 13$ kPa and $PaCO_2$ around 4.5 kPa
- MAP > 90 mmHg
- Temperature and blood glucose are within normal limits

STEPS	KEY POINTS

Drugs
- Phenytoin if convulsion is present.
- Mannitol: 0.25–0.5 gm/kg bolus over 5–10 minutes and repeated once again if indicated, but always communicate with neurosurgeon before second dose. Maximum 1 gm/kg, as above that it is not beneficial. Hypertonic saline may also be used.

Expert help
- Communicate with neurosurgeon in charge.

Can you tell me the role of hypothermia in a head injury patient?

Any hyperpyrexia increases cerebral metabolic rate of oxygen ($CMRO_2$) and should be aggressively treated.

Equally hypothermia reduces $CMRO_2$, which can be beneficial for neurological outcome but hypothermia below 35°C affects enzyme systems and can cause clotting abnormality. This can result in further bleeding in injured patient, which ultimately increases ICP; so, routinely there is no role of active cooling of head injury patient.

Future reading

1. Head injury: Triage, assessment, investigation and early management of head injury in children, young people and adults. *NICE Clinical Guideline* **176**. guidance.nice.org.uk/cg176
2. Hoffman JR, Mower JR, et al. Validity of a set of clinical criteria to rule out injury to cervical spine in patients with blunt trauma. National Emergency X-Radiology Utilization Study Group (NEXUS). *N Eng J Med* 2000 July 13; **343(2):** 94–9.

06.4 SHORT CASE: CHRONIC OBSTRUCTIVE PULMONARY DISEASE

HISTORY *You take a telephone call from a concerned nurse regarding a 70-year-old female patient with COPD being admitted on the surgical ward. The patient has a productive cough, respiratory rate of 32/min, and sats 88% (on oxygen). The patient is awaiting an incisonal hernia repair.*

STEPS	KEY POINTS
Can you define COPD?	COPD is a chronic lung disease characterised by airflow limitation due to progressive inflammatory disease, which is not fully reversible, and often complicated by significant systemic manifestations and comorbidities.
	Classic symptoms include productive cough, dyspnoea, wheeze, frequent winter bronchitis, and exercise intolerance. The pathogenesis of COPD is thought to arise from the combined effects of inflammation, increased oxidative stress, and an imbalance between proteinases and antiproteinases. Historically there are two types: emphysema and chronic bronchitis.
	Pathologic changes of COPD are present throughout the lung. • Large central airways: enlarged mucous glands, loss of cilia, and decreased ciliary function, increased smooth muscle and connective tissue deposition in the airway walls • Small airways: collagen deposition and airway remodeling

How do you diagnose COPD?	Spirometry is used to confirm the diagnosis and classify the severity of COPD but will be more robust when complemented with clinical status and radiology investigations. Both the NICE and the GOLD offer guidelines for the diagnosis and assessment of COPD.
	 • Airflow obstruction [defined by a ratio of forced expired volume in one second to forced vital capacity (FEV_1/FVC) < 0.7] is used to diagnose COPD.
	    ○ If FEV_1 is > 80% of the predicted value, then COPD is diagnosed only in presence of respiratory symptoms.
	    ○ Reversibility testing with corticosteroids or bronchodilators is unnecessary for the diagnosis but they are used to differentiate COPD from asthma.

STEPS	KEY POINTS

FEV$_1$% predicted	GOLD criteria (2008)	NICE (2010)
< 80%	Mild	Stage 1—mild
50%–79%	Moderate	Stage 2—moderate
30%–49%	Severe	Stage 3—severe
< 30%	Very severe	Stage 4—very severe

National Institute for Clinical Excellence
Global Initiative for Chronic Obstructive Lung Disease

What are the complications in untreated COPD patients?

- Expiratory airflow limitation arises due to airway inflammation and hyperplasia, mucus accumulation, fibrosis, and bronchospasm. Expiratory flow is decreased and expiratory time prolonged with resultant hyperinflation, which increases total lung capacity, functional residual capacity, and residual volume, giving rise to exertional dyspnoea.
- V/Q mismatch due to increase in physiologic dead space and shunt.
- Chronic hypoxia leads to secondary polycythemia, pulmonary hypertension, and eventually right ventricular dysfunction and cor pulmonale.

How do you manage COPD?

Preventive
- Smoking cessation is the only intervention that slows the progression.
- Yearly influenza vaccination has been shown to significantly reduce morbidity and mortality and is recommended for all patients with COPD.

Pharmacologic management
- Early-stage COPD: Short-acting inhaled bronchodilators
- Severe COPD:
  - Long-acting inhaled bronchodilators (tiotropium) improve lung function and relieve dyspnoea.
  - Inhaled corticosteroids decrease frequency of exacerbations and slow the rate of decline in FEV$_1$.
  - Combination therapy seems to show additive benefits.

Treatment of acute exacerbations:
Oxygen
- Domiciliary oxygen therapy for patients with hypoxia

Drugs
- Appropriate antibiotics if suspected infection
- Escalate bronchodilator therapy
- Systemic corticosteroids to shorten the recovery time

Ventilation
- Progressive hypercarbia and respiratory acidosis warrant noninvasive mechanical ventilation to avoid the need for intubation.
- Patients with severe acidosis, refractory hypoxemia, or respiratory arrest require intubation and mechanical ventilation.

Treatment of end-stage disease
Treatment options for advanced COPD are limited.
- Domiciliary oxygen therapy. Aim for sats > 90%
- Lung volume reduction surgery—high-risk palliative treatment, which is performed especially for upper-lobe emphysema
- Lung transplantation

STEPS	KEY POINTS
How will you manage this patient?	Patients with COPD have a two- to five-fold increase in risk of perioperative pulmonary complications such as atelectasis, pneumonia, and respiratory failure.

Preoperative management
- ABCD approach; optimise oxygen and drug therapy.
- Risk assessment—patient and surgical factors.
- Investigations—besides routine investigations, a bedside spirometry and a chest radiograph is obtained to influence clinical management. Consider echocardiography if ECG reveals right heart disease (right ventricular hypertrophy or strain). A baseline ABG on room air with $PaCO_2$ > 5.9 kPa and PaO_2 < 7.9 kPa predict a worse outcome.
- Advice smoking cessation.
- Appropriate antibiotics for suspected bacterial infection, systemic corticosteroid, and escalate bronchodilator therapy. If permissible, delay surgery until after full recovery from an acute COPD exacerbation.

Intraoperative management
- Where possible, neuraxial analgesia and peripheral nerve blockade for postoperative pain relief are offered.
- Airway manipulation can worsen the condition and may be treated with short-acting bronchodilators such as β2 agonists or anticholinergics. Bronchodilating volatile anaesthetics (isoflurane, sevoflurane, halothane, enflurane) also may reverse acute bronchospasm.
- Titrated dose of neuromuscular blockers is crucial as is adequate reversal at the end of operation.
- Ventilation strategy: Avoidance of dynamic hyperinflation by the use of a slow respiratory rate, long expiratory time, and minimal tidal volume to avoid excessive hypercapnia. Use extrinsic PEEP judiciously to replace intrinsic PEEP.
- Fluid balance is crucial in patients with cor pulmonale where appropriate right ventricular preload is essential to produce adequate cardiac output when the right ventricular afterload is high.

Postoperative care
- HDU/ITU care
- Adequate pain control
- Lung expansion maneuvers such as deep breathing, chest physiotherapy, and incentive spirometry
- Thromboprophylaxis and early ambulation to help restore baseline lung volumes and to aid in clearing secretions
- Careful administration of oxygen to avoid suppressing ventilatory drives in patients who are dependent on hypoxia

Further reading

1. Lumb A, Biercamp C. Chronic obstructive pulmonary disease and anaesthesia. *Contin Educ Anaesth Crit Care Pain 2014;* **14** (1): 1–5.
2. Henzler D, Rossaint R, Kuhlen R. Anaesthetic considerations in patients with chronic pulmonary disease. *Curr Opin Anaesthesiol* 2003; **16**: 323–30.

BASIC SCIENCE
VIVA

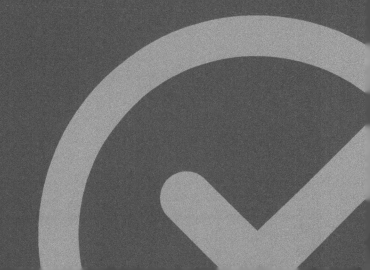

06.5 ANATOMY: CORONARY CIRCULATION

Possible questions to ask are:

- *What symptoms would a patient have with a blocked left coronary artery, coronary circulation including venous drainage, and chronological ECG changes post MI? How does MI present and progress?*

- *What structures are supplied by the LAD?*

- *What factors affect coronary blood flow?*

- *What changes occur during cardiac cycle, and how do they differ between left and right sides?*

- *What differences exist between systemic circulation and coronary circulation?*

STEPS	KEY POINTS
What symptoms would a patient have with a blocked left coronary artery?	Acute coronary syndrome is the term used to describe the spectrum of clinical presentation attributed to occlusion of coronary arteries. The symptoms and signs depend on extent and duration of the obstruction, volume of the affected myocardium and its complications. They can be very varied and generally include • Chest pain—squeezing or burning, often radiating to the left arm or jaw • Nausea, vomiting, and sweating due to vagal stimulation • Dyspnoea, mainly because of cardiac failure • Sense of impending doom • Arrhythmias • Hypo or hypertension • Signs and symptoms of complications: ventricular aneurysm and rupture of interventricular septum, papillary muscle or ventricular wall leading to pulmonary oedema, and valvular incompetence

STEPS

KEY POINTS

Describe the coronary arterial supply in detail. See Figure 6.5.

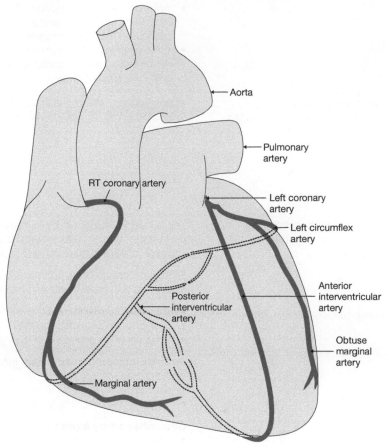

Fig. 6.5 Coronary circulation

The heart receives its blood supply from the right and left coronary arteries.
- The total coronary blood flow is about 250 mls/min, which equates to 5% of the cardiac output. The blood flow increases by 5 times in strenuous exercise.

Right coronary artery: arises from the right aortic sinus, runs between the right atrium and the pulmonary trunk to descend in the right atrioventricular groove. It winds around the inferior border to reach the diaphragmatic surface of heart and runs backwards and left to reach posterior interventricular groove. It terminates by anastomosing with left coronary artery.
- Marginal branch
- Posterior interventricular artery (PIVA): This anastomoses with the AIVA in the posterior interventricular groove. It is the PIVA that determines the dominance of the arterial system. In this case the right coronary is dominant.

STEPS	KEY POINTS

Left coronary artery: After originating from the left aortic sinus, it passes forwards and to the left and emerges between pulmonary trunk and the left atrium and gives off two main branches.

- Anterior interventricular artery (AIVA), which runs downwards in anterior interventricular groove and anastomose with the PIVA. This is the major branch, as it supplies most of the muscle bulk.
- Circumflex branch, which runs to the left in the left atrioventricular sulcus, winds around the left border of heart and terminates by anastomosing with right coronary artery.

What are the structures supplied by the left and right coronary arteries?

Structure	Right Coronary	Left Coronary
Musculature	Rt atrium Rt ventricle Part of the IV septum	Lt atrium Lt and Rt ventricle Part of the IV septum
SA node	65%	35%
AV node	80%	20%
Rest of the conducting system	80%	20%

What is the importance of knowing the coronary blood supply?

The ischaemic vessel can be identified from the clinical and ECG presentation which would prevent delay in treatment. Also, ischaemia/infarction of the ventricle can lead to abnormal conduction.

Example: Right coronary artery involvement leads to inferior MI and is also associated with bradycardia and heart block.

Rt Coronary artery infarct
- Inferior MI (ECG leads II, III, aVF)
- Posterior MI (prominent R in V_1, V_2)

Anterior Interventricular artery infarct
- Anteroseptal MI (V_1, V_2)
- Anterior MI (V_2–V_4)
- Anterolateral MI (I, aVL, V_4–V_6)

Circumflex artery infarct
- Lateral MI (I, aVL, V_5, V_6)

What can you tell me about the venous drainage?

Two thirds of the venous drainage is by veins that accompany the coronary arteries and open into the coronary sinus in the right atrium. The remaining one third drains the endocardium and inner myocardium directly into the cardiac cavity.

The coronary sinus lies in the right atrium between the superior and inferior vena caval openings. The main veins draining into the coronary sinus are:
- Great cardiac vein, which accompanies the AIVA
- Middle cardiac vein, which lies in the inferior interventricular groove near the anastomosis of circumflex and right coronary arteries
- Small cardiac vein, which accompanies the marginal branch of the right coronary artery
- Oblique vein, which drains the posterior half of left atrium.

The anterior cardiac vein drains most of the anterior surface of the heart and opens into the right atrium directly.

The venae cordis minimae (Thebesian veins) drains the endocardium and inner myocardium directly into the cardiac cavity and is an example of physiological shunt as venous blood enters the left heart.

STEPS	KEY POINTS

How does the coronary blood supply relate to cardiac cycle in right and left ventricles?

Left ventricle
- During systole, intramuscular blood vessels are compressed and twisted by the contracting heart muscle and blood flow is at its lowest of only 10% to 30% of that during diastole. The force is greatest in the subendocardial layers where it approximates to intramyocardial pressure. It is important to note that the layers of the heart, excluding the subendocardium, receive blood supply even in systole.
- In diastole, the heart musculature is relaxed and cardiac muscle effects do not impede blood flow to the heart.

Right ventricle:
The compression effect of systole on blood flow is minimal as a result of the lower pressures developed by that chamber.

The heart is perfused from the epicardial (outside) to the endocardial (inside) surface. The mechanical compression of systole has a more negative effect on the blood flow through the endocardial layers, where compressive forces are higher and microvascular pressures are lower. Therefore, subendocardial layers of the heart suffer more impairment and ischemia than do the epicardial layers.

What are the ECG changes associated with myocardial infarction in increasing chronology?

- Hyperacute changes (within minutes)
  - Tall T waves and progressive ST elevation
- Acute changes (minutes to hours)
  - ST elevation and gradual loss of R wave
- Early changes (hours to days)
  - < 24 hours: inversion of T wave and the resolution of ST elevation
  - Within days: pathological Q wave begins to form
- Indeterminate changes (days to weeks)
  - Q waves and persistent T wave inversion
- Old changes (weeks to months)
  - Persisting Q waves and normalised T waves

What are the determinants of coronary circulation?

- Factors inherent to the circulation
- Pressure or myogenic autoregulation
- Chemical/metabolic factors
- Neural factors
- Humoral factors

Factors inherent to the circulation
- Coronary perfusion pressure (CoPP) is the difference between aortic diastolic pressure (ADP) and left ventricular end diastolic pressure (LVEDP). Any factor that increases the ADP and decreases the LVEDP would increase the CoPP.
- Heart rate—lower heart rate increases the diastole and thus the coronary filling time.
- Cardiac output—directly proportional to the coronary blood flow.
- State of the cardiac cycle—coronary blood flow is the highest during the isovolumetric relaxation phase.

Pressure or myogenic autoregulation
Coronary blood flow is autoregulated between a mean arterial pressure of 60–140 mmHg. This is by the myogenic constriction and dilatation of the coronary vessels in response to changes in the blood flow and pressure.

Chemical and metabolic
- O_2, CO_2, K^+, H^+, prostaglandins, endothelium-derived relaxing factor (EDRF), nitric oxide, and adenosine
- Drugs that influence coronary blood flow include nitrates, aminophylline, etc.

STEPS	KEY POINTS

Neural

Autonomic innervation has minimal influence on the vessel wall diameter but can increase the blood flow by improving contractility and metabolism.

Hormonal

Angiotensin receptors present in the vessel wall can cause vasoconstriction, thereby decreasing the coronary blood flow. T_3/T_4 increases cardiac muscle metabolism, and thus coronary blood flow improves due to vasodilation.

What are the differences between systemic and coronary circulation?

Coronary circulation is a part of the systemic circulation that supplies the heart.
- Coronary blood flow changes with cardiac cycle and is minimum during systole, whereas the converse is true for systemic circulation.
- The second major difference is the myocardial oxygen extraction ratio of 80% when compared to around 25% in the rest of the body.

What is the myocardial oxygen consumption and oxygen extraction ratio?

Myocardial oxygen consumption is defined as the actual amount of oxygen consumed by the heart muscle per minute. It is normally expressed as MVO_2 and is about 30 mLs/min for a resting heart. Owing to the obligatory aerobic nature of myocardial metabolism, MVO_2 serves as a measure of the total energy utilisation of the heart.

The myocardial oxygen extraction ratio is about 70%–80%, which means increased oxygen demand therefore has to be met by an increase in coronary perfusion.

What is meant by the terms DPTI and TTI?

Diastolic pressure time (DPTI) and tension time (TTI) indices are measures of myocardial supply and demand, respectively, collectively depicted as endocardial viability.

$$\text{Endocardial viability ratio (EVR)} = \frac{\text{DPTI}}{\text{TTI}} \times \text{HR}$$

EVR < 0.7 denotes a high likelihood of ischaemia. See Figure 6.6.

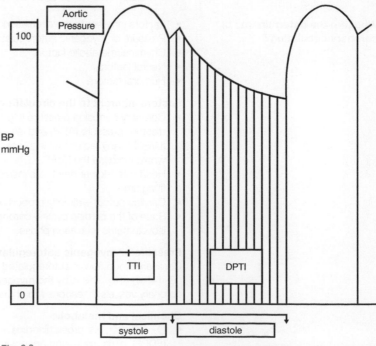

Fig. 6.6

06.6 PHYSIOLOGY: LIVER DISEASE

STEPS	KEY POINTS
How would end stage hepatic disease present to anaesthetists?	**Acute decompensation secondary to** • Infection • Hypovolemia • Hypotension • Diuretics • Gastrointestinal haemorrhage • Excess dietary protein • Electrolyte imbalance **Infection** • Flare-up of hepatitis (A, B, or C) • Prone to acquiring fungal infections, TB **Portal hypertension** • Ascites—diaphragmatic splinting and respiratory distress • Spontaneous bacterial peritonitis • Varices—variceal bleeding • Splenomegaly—thrombocytopenia **Bleeding** • Due to decreased production of clotting factors (II, VII, IX, X) and splenomegaly-related thrombocytopenia • Haematemesis **Hepatic encephalopathy**

What is the pathophysiology of liver injury in alcoholic liver disease?	Conventionally divided into three histological types, although may co-exist:
	• Steatosis
	  ○ Metabolism of ethanol causes the accumulation of lipid in liver cells.
	
	• Alcoholic hepatitis
	  ○ Ethanol metabolism generates reactive oxygen species and neoantigens, which promote inflammation.
	
	• Cirrhosis
	  ○ Prolonged hepatocellular damage generates myofibroblast-like cells that produce collagen, resulting in fibrosis.
	  ○ As hepatocytes are destroyed and liver architecture changes, hepatic function falls and increased resistance to portal blood flow produces portal hypertension.

STEPS	KEY POINTS

List the common clinical findings in patients with alcoholic liver disease.	• Signs of acute hepatitis
	    ○ Jaundice
	    ○ Tender hepatomegaly
	    ○ Fever (< 38.5°C, often sawtooth)
	
	 • Signs of chronic liver disease
	    ○ Leuconychia/palmar erythema/dupuytren's contracture/spider naevi
	    ○ Telangactasia/bruising
	    ○ Oedema (hypoalbuminaemia)
	    ○ Parotid swelling/hepatomegaly
	    ○ Gynaecomastia/testicular atrophy
	    ○ Encephalopathy
	
	 • Portal hypertension
	    ○ Ascites/splenomegaly/caput medusa
	
	 • Poor nutrition
	    ○ Muscle wasting/weight loss/cachexia/glossitis

What is hepatorenal syndrome?	• Hepatorenal syndrome (HRS) is the reduced glomerular filtration rate (GFR) and consequent decline in renal function caused by advanced liver disease. • Serum creatinine of > 133 µmol/litre in a patient with cirrhosis and ascites that persists after all possible pathologies have been excluded or treated. • Due to generalised vasodilatation and altered hormone release (renin–angiotensin, ADH, and sympathetic systems) subjecting the kidney to hypotension, hypovolaemia, and local vasoconstriction. **HRS type 1**: A rapid and severe progressive renal failure occurring in under 2 weeks. • As a result of some precipitating factors, (e.g. Alcoholic hepatitis, gastrointestinal bleeding, NSAIDs, aminoglycosides, or infection). **HRS type 2**: A slowly progressive moderate deterioration in function. Refractory ascites is the dominant clinical feature.
What is hepatic encephalopathy?	Occurrence of confusion, altered level of consciousness, and coma due to liver failure Grading: I: Confused, altered mood II: Inappropriate, drowsy III: Stuporose, but rousable, very confused, agitated IV: Coma, unresponsive to painful stimulus
How would you assess the prognosis of liver disease and how is this assessment tool useful?	• The Model for End-Stage Liver Disease (MELD) score uses bilirubin, INR, and creatinine. • The Child-Pugh score [Pugh's modification (1972) of Child's criteria (1964)] is used to determine the prognosis, as well as the required strength of treatment and the necessity of liver transplantation.

STEPS	KEY POINTS

Pugh's modification of Child's criteria

Variable	Points scored for increasing abnormality		
	1	2	3
Encephalopathy grade	None	Minimal (1&2)	Advanced (3&4)
Ascites	None	Easily controlled	Poor control
Serum bilirubin mg/dL	< 2	2–3	> 3
Serum albumin g/dL	> 3.5	2.8–3.5	< 2.8
Prothrombin time (seconds > control)	1–4	4–6	> 6

What are the anaesthetic implications for anaesthetising patients with end-stage liver failure (for nonhepatic surgery)?

Preoperative
- Comprehensive assessment of suitability and work-up for procedure—multidisciplinary approach
- Preoperative optimisation of fluid and nutritional status, as well as any electrolyte disturbance or coagulopathy
- Consider preoperative abdominal paracentesis
- Delayed gastric emptying—antacid prophylaxis +/− rapid sequence induction

Intraoperative
- Drugs
  - Altered drug handling
  - Increased sensitivity to sedative agents
  - Reduced metabolism of many drugs including opioids
  - Increased volume of distribution and altered protein binding
  - Short-acting drugs preferred (desflurane, remifentanil)

- Technique
  - Extreme caution with epidural anaesthesia and other regional procedures due to associated coagulopathy

- Monitoring
  - Invasive monitoring for major surgery (oesophageal doppler contraindicated in the presence of varices)
- Others
  - Glycaemic control
  - Thermoregulation
  - Antibiotic prophylaxis and strict adherence to aseptic technique

Postoperative
Care on high-dependency unit or ITU

06.7 PHARMACOLOGY: DRUGS USED FOR SECONDARY PREVENTION

STEPS	KEY POINTS
What is secondary prevention post myocardial infarction (MI)?	Patients who have had a ST elevation myocardial infarction (STEMI) or non-ST elevation myocardial infarction (NSTEMI) benefit from treatment to reduce the risk of further MI or other manifestations of vascular disease. This is known as secondary prevention.
	NICE provides comprehensive guidelines to prevent further MI and progression of vascular disease in patients who have had an MI either recently or in the past (> 12 months ago).

What drugs are used as secondary prevention after an MI?

Angiotensin-converting enzyme inhibitor (ACE-i)
- Offered to patients who present acutely with an MI as soon as they are haemodynamically stable and continued indefinitely.
- Titrate dose upwards at short intervals (e.g. 12–24 hours before discharge from hospital until maximum dose tolerated).
- If unable to titrate dose upwards during admission, this should be completed within 4 to 6 weeks of hospital discharge.
- ACE-i is not to be combined with angiotensin II receptor blocker (ARB).
- Monitor renal function, serum electrolytes, and blood pressure.

Dual platelet therapy (aspirin plus second antiplatelet agent)
- Aspirin is offered to all patients after an MI and to continue indefinitely unless aspirin intolerant or have indication for anticoagulation.
- Patients who have had an MI > 12 months ago should also be offered aspirin.
- Ticagrelor in combination with low-dose aspirin is recommended for up to 12 months.
- Alternative is Clopidogrel for up to 12 months in patients who have had NSTEMI or STEMI with bare metal or drug-eluting stents.

Beta blocker
- Offered as soon as possible after an MI, when patient is haemodynamically stable.
- Continue for at least 12 months in patients with and without left ventricular systolic dysfunction or heart failure.
- Continue indefinitely in patients with left ventricular systolic dysfunction.

Statin
- Offered to all patients with clinical evidence of cardiovascular disease.

STEPS	KEY POINTS
Is calcium channel blocker routinely offered?	No, It is offered only if beta blockers are contraindicated or need to be discontinued. Commonly used drugs are diltiazem or verapamil.
What is ACE-i?	ACE-i inhibits the angiotensin-converting enzyme in the renin—angiotensin—aldosterone system.

Angiotensinogen (from liver)
Renin (from juxtaglomerular apparatus in kidney)

Angiotensin I
ACE (from surface of pulmonary and renal endothelium)

Angiotensin II
- Increase sympathetic activity.
- Increase tubular sodium and chloride reabsorption and water retention.
- Increase tubular potassium excretion.
- Increase aldosterone secretion in adrenal cortex.
- Arteriolar vasoconstriction—increase blood pressure.
- Increase antidiuretic hormone (ADH) in posterior pituitary to increase water absorption in the collecting duct.

STEPS	KEY POINTS
Can you give some examples of ACE-i?	Ramipril Lisinopril Captopril Enalapril
What clinical situations require use of ACE-i?	• After an MI • Hypertension– first-line treatment for patients < 55 years old or non-Afro-Caribbean origin • Heart failure • Diabetic nephropathy—renal protective • Chronic kidney disease—slows the progress of kidney disease

What are the common side effects of ACE-i?

Renal impairment
- Under normal circumstances, angiotensin II maintains renal perfusion by altering the caliber of the efferent glomerular arterioles. ACE-i inhibits this causing drop in renal perfusion pressure, which can lead to renal failure in patients with pre-existing impaired renal circulation. ACE-i is therefore contraindicated in patients with renal artery stenosis.

Dry cough
- Due to increased bradykinin, which is normally degraded by ACE

Hypotension
- First-dose hypotension—test dose should be given at night.
- Can cause refractory hypotension with anaesthesia. ACE-i is usually omitted for 24 hours prior to surgery.

Angioedema
- Swelling of lips, eyes, and tongue
- More common in Afro-Caribbean patients

Further reading
1. *NICE Clinical Guideline 172* (Nov 2013).

06.8
PHYSICS: SCAVENGING

STEPS	KEY POINTS
What are the sources of pollution in the operating theatre complex?	• Gas induction • Spillage • Leaks from breathing circuit • Facemasks • Laryngeal masks • T-piece or other open circuits • Post-anaesthetic exhalation of vapour • Failure to turn off vapour or gas flow after anaesthesia
What are the concerns?	• Reports of increased spontaneous abortion rates in female staff • Increased rates of malignancy • Decreased fertility • Mortality • Staff particularly at risk: paediatric anaesthetists, bronchoscopists, recovery staff • Pollution and global warming
What are the effects of nitrous oxide?	*Bone marrow toxicity and neurotoxicity* • Methionine synthetase inhibition can prevent production of methionine and tetrahydrofolate. • Methionine is a precursor of S-adenosyl methionine (SAM), which is incorporated into myelin. Its absence can lead to subacute combined degeneration of the spinal cord in chronic B12 deficiency and acutely to dorsal column dysfunction and peripheral neuropathy. • Tetrahydrofolate is required for nucleotide and DNA synthesis. • Megaloblastic anaemia can occur in folate and B12 deficiency. *Teratogenicity* • Association is not strong. *Spontaneous miscarriage* • Reports suggesting an increased incidence of miscarriages in dental practice nurses working with nitrous oxide. *Substance abuse*

STEPS	KEY POINTS
How may anaesthetic gas pollution be reduced or prevented?	• Ensuring operating theatres are efficiently ventilated (minimum 15 exchanges/hour) • Use of closed circuits with soda lime • Use of TIVA with oxygen/air • Use of regional anaesthesia • Consideration when using nitrous oxide and inhalational agents—consider low flow • Careful filling of vaporizers avoiding spillage and using keyed fillers • Monitoring of theatre pollution levels • Use of scavenging • Use of low flow and ultra low flow breathing systems

What are the current recommendations for theatre pollution levels?

Control of Substances Hazardous to Health (COSHH) sets maximum exposure limits to chemicals and other hazardous substances. Currently the maximum anaesthetic pollutant levels (based on 8-hour time weighted average, parts per million) are as follows:

Halothane	10 ppm
Enflurane	50 ppm
Isoflurane	50 ppm
Nitrous oxide	100 ppm

In the USA, the maximum exposure limit for all halogenated volatiles is 2 ppm.

What are the features of a scavenging system?

Scavenging systems can be classified into passive and active.

Passive:
• Patient dependent.
• No active positive or negative pressure.
• 30 mm connector used between patient and system.
• Gases are vented to atmosphere either by patient's spontaneous respiratory efforts or by mechanical ventilator.
• These are rarely used in modern theatres.
• Cardiff Aldasorber: canister containing charcoal particles that absorb halogenated volatile agents. Absorption does not render agents inert. Inhalational agents are released into atmosphere when canister is disposed of by incineration. Device does not absorb nitrous oxide.

Active:
Collecting system: Collection of expired gases from breathing system or ventilator via 30 mm connector so that misconnection is prevented.

Transfer system: Wide-bore 30 mm tubing.

Receiving system: Reservoir with visual flow indicator. Consists of two springloaded valves guarding against excessive positive pressure (1000 Pa) and negative pressure (–50 Pa) developing in the scavenging system.

Disposal system: Air pump or fan generates a vacuum. Connected to the wall and vented outside. Able to cope with flows up to 120 L/min.

Exterior

What are the disadvantages of an active system?

• Excessive positive pressure may lead to barotrauma.
• Excessive negative pressure can deflate reservoir bag of breathing system, leading to rebreathing.

STEPS	KEY POINTS
What other systems are available to ensure efficient ventilation?	**Laminar flow** • Can be used to create an ultra clean environment • Recommended for prosthetic implant surgery • Provides over 400 air changes per hour by recirculating air after passing it through high-efficiency filters (0.5 µm) All ventilation systems should provide a positive pressure across any openings so that when doors are opened, there is less chance of bacterial escape. Opening of doors can make system less efficient.
What other factors need to be taken into consideration when designing a theatre?	• Temperature control • Humidity

section 07

CLINICAL VIVA

07.1 LONG CASE: CHILD FOR FUNDOPLICATION

HISTORY *A 4-year-old boy with a past medical history of birth asphyxia, developmental delay, and poorly controlled epilepsy is scheduled for a Nissen's fundoplication due to chronic reflux.*

He suffers from gastro-oesophageal reflux disease and gets recurrent chest infections; roughly three admissions per year. The child had to be admitted to the paediatric intensive care unit 4 months ago with chest infection.

STEPS	KEY POINTS		
Medication	Lamotrigine and Sodium valproate		
On Examination	Weight: 12 kg		
	Afebrile Heart rate: 140/min; regular Heart sounds: normal Respiratory rate: 32/min Crackles right base		
Blood Investigations	Hb	10 g/dL	(13–16)
	Haematocrit	0.45	(0.38–0.56)
	WCC	21.1 × 10⁹/L	(4–11)
	Platelets	221 × 10⁹/L	(140–400)
	MCV	70 femtolitres	(80–100)
	Na	128 mmol/L	(137–145)
	K	4.8 mmol/L	(3.6–5.0)
	Urea	6.1 mmol/L	(1.7–8.3)
	Creat	72 µmol/L	(62–124)

CXR. See Figure 7.1.

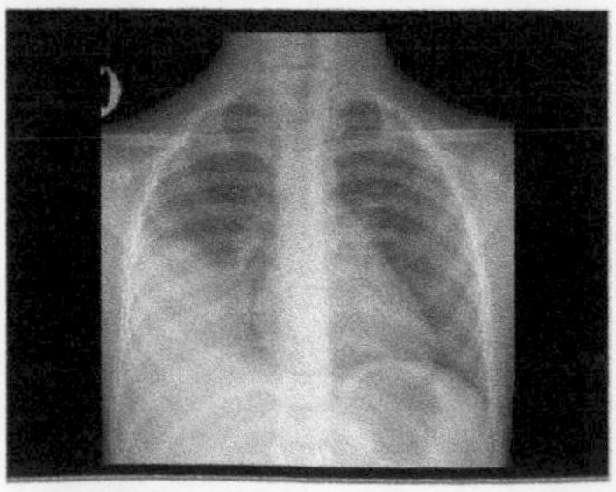

Fig. 7.1

STEPS	KEY POINTS
Summarise the case.	A 4-year-old child for elective major surgery, probably laparoscopic with multiple comorbidities, exhibits: • Poorly controlled epilepsy • Significant chest infection • Anaemia and hyponatremia • Small stature for his age These need to be optimised before going ahead with surgery.
Why do you think he is small for his age? What would be his ideal weight?	The commonly used formula to calculate weight from age is Weight = 2(age + 4) This means the ideal weight of this child should be 16 kg. The Luscombe and Owens formula [Weight = (3 × age) + 7] probably reflects the actual weight in this country. It can be used over a larger age range (from one year to puberty) and allows a safe and more accurate estimate of the weight of children today and prevents underestimation and hence under-resuscitation. The main reason for poor weight gain in this child might be the gastrooesophageal reflux disease (GORD) and chronic chest infection.
Describe the blood and CXR results.	Blood: Microcytic anaemia, raised WCC, and low sodium CXR: Frontal chest radiograph shows right lower lobe consolidation and the silhouette sign—the adjacent diaphragm is obscured, the right cardiac silhouette, anterior to the consolidation, is preserved. Diagnosis: Right lower lobe pneumonia.
What are the causes of anaemia?	The causes of anaemia can be broadly grouped as: 1. Etiological classification 　a) Impaired RBC production 　b) Excessive destruction 　c) Blood loss 2. Morphological classification 　a) Macrocytic anaemia 　b) Microcytic hypochromic anaemia 　c) Normochromic normocytic anaemia
Etiological classification	**Impaired RBC production** 1. Abnormal bone marrow 　a) Aplastic anaemia 　b) Myelofibrosis 2. Essential factors deficiency 　a) Iron deficiency anaemia 　b) B12 deficiency 　c) Folate deficiency 　d) Erythropoietin deficiency, as in renal disease

STEPS	KEY POINTS

3. Stimulation factor deficiency
   a) Anaemia in chronic disease
   b) Anaemia in hypothyroidism
   c) Anaemia in hypopituitarism

Excessive destruction
1. Intracorpuscular defect
   a) Membrane: hereditary spherocytosis
   b) Enzyme: G-6 PD deficiency
   c) Haemoglobin: thalassemia, haemoglobinopathies

2. Extracorpuscular defect
   a) Mechanical: microangiopathic haemolytic anaemia
   b) Infective: Clostridium tetani
   c) Antibodies: SLE
   d) Hypersplenism

Blood loss
1. Acute: trauma, acute GI bleed
2. Chronic: parasitic infestation, chronic NSAIDS

Morphological classification

MCV – mean corpuscular volume; MCHC – mean corpuscular Hb concentration

Macrocytic/megaloblastic anaemia
MCV > 94; MCHC > 31
- Vitamin B12 deficiency: Pernicious anaemia
- Folate deficiency: Nutritional megaloblastic anaemia
- Drug-induced abnormal DNA synthesis: anticonvulsant, chemotherapy agents, etc.

Microcytic hypochromic anaemia
MCV < 80; MCHC < 31
- Iron deficiency anaemia: chronic blood loss, dietary inadequacy, malabsorption, increased demand, etc.
- Abnormal globin synthesis: thalassemia

Normocytic normochromic anaemia
MCV 82–92; MCHC > 30
- Blood loss
- Increased plasma volume
- Hypoplastic marrow
- Endocrine: hypothyroidism, adrenal insufficiency
- Renal and liver disease

Why do you think the patient's sodium is low?

Sodium valproate can cause this.

Hyponatremia is the most common electrolyte disturbance in hospitalised children. This is usually due to hypotonic intravenous fluids. It can be due to renal causes or rarely because of poor dietary intake.

Would you anaesthetise him now?

No. He needs optimisation with paediatric and neurology reviews for
- Treatment of chest infection with antibiotics and physiotherapy
- Further investigation and correction of low sodium
- Further investigation and treatment of anaemia
- Optimisation of the epilepsy medications

Also one should bear in mind that these cannot be corrected to normal, as his nutrition is not going to improve without surgery due to his underlying problem resulting in recurrent chest infections.

STEPS	KEY POINTS
What do you know about this surgery?	Nissen's fundoplication is the most common operation to stop reflux. More than half the patients presenting for this procedure are neurologically impaired, have cerebral palsy, epilepsy, or chronic pulmonary aspiration.

The operation is usually done by laparoscopic route and involves the tightening of the lower oesophageal sphincter by wrapping the fundus of stomach around it. Complications include chest infection, port site hernia, and adhesions.

Failure rate for surgery is 5%–10%.

The child now comes back after a month having been seen by the paediatric team in view of treatment of chest infection and optimisation of epileptic medication. |
| **Discuss your anaesthetic management.** | **Preoperative assessment**
• Careful airway evaluation as patient needs rapid sequence induction and there might be difficulties due to congenital deformities.
• History of previous anaesthetics, allergies, and fasting status should be established.
• Parental anxieties should be addressed carefully, and detailed discussion about the perioperative care should be discussed.
• Premedication in the form of antacids and topical local anaesthetic cream to aid cannulation should be prescribed.
• Preoperative pulmonary assessment to identify risk factors for postoperative respiratory compromise.

Conduct of anaesthesia
• Mode of induction: Intravenous mode is preferred due to need for rapid sequence induction, but small child with recurrent hospital admissions might be a challenge!
• Drugs: Thiopentone 5 mg/kg (60 mg) and Suxamethonium 2 mg/kg (25 mg). A nondepolarising muscle relaxant (Atracurium 0.5 mg/kg) is added once the effect of suxamethonium wears off.
• Tube: 5 mm cuffed tube due to risk of reflux and laparoscopic surgery.
• Maintenance: Oxygen in air with inhalational agent is the routine. Nitrous oxide is generally not used, as it can cause bowel distension and increase nausea and vomiting. Total intravenous anaesthesia using propofol and remifentanil infusion can also be safely employed.
• Analgesia: See below.
• Antiemetics: Ondansetron 0.1 mg/kg (max 4 mg) is given routinely to prevent retching.
• Monitoring: Routine monitoring of ECG, pulse oximetry, noninvasive blood pressure and temperature along with capnography and gas measurement. An arterial line might be useful in this case due to poor premorbid condition. |
| **How will you manage intravenous cannulation?** | **At preassessment**
• Building rapport with the child and the parents.
• Premedication and topical anaesthesia

a) Premedication: Oral midazolam (0.5 mg/kg) is widely used. Ketamine and temazepam are alternatives.
b) Topical: <u>EMLA cream 5% emulsion</u>—eutectic mixture of 2.5% lidocaine and 2.5% prilocaine in 1:1 ratio. Applied 45 min before and lasts for 60 min. <u>Ametop</u>—4% gel formulation of amethocaine. Onset in 30 min and lasts for 4 hours. Usually causes vasodilation and higher chance of allergy. |

STEPS	KEY POINTS

In anaesthetic room
- Distraction technique—distraction of child's attention by the parent and nurse/play specialist, hiding the needle, and asking to cough while cannulating are some of the various techniques used.

During the operation, patient develops bradycardia.

What are the causes and how will you manage this?

Heart rate < 60 per min is bradycardia in age group 2 to 10 years.
- Anaesthetic factors: hypoxia, deep plane of anaesthesia
- Surgical factors: surgical stimulation leading to parasympathetic activation
- Drugs: suxamethonium, remifentanil, clonidine, neostigmine, and β blockers
- Patient factors: congenital cardiac problems

Common causes during this operation are hypoxia and reflux bradycardia due to handling and traction of abdominal contents.
Management includes:
- Correction of hypoxia if present
- Lightening/deepening the level of anaesthesia as required
- Asking the surgeons to stop traction
- Treating with atropine (20 mcg/kg) if bradycardia is sustained and compromising the blood pressure.

If patient is hypoxic, what is your management?

- Administer 100% oxygen.
- Call for help.
- Ask the surgeons to stop.
- Release pneumoperitoneum if possible.
- Check tube position—exclude accidental extubation or endobronchial intubation
- Check the circuit for disconnection, kink, or obstruction.
- Hand ventilation with 100% oxygen might be needed if ventilation is inadequate.
- Endotracheal suctioning of secretions obstructing the bronchi, trachea, and ET tube which may cause hypoxia.

What is your plan for pain control?

Multimodal analgesia tailored to the needs of the patient and procedure.

Intraoperative
- IV paracetamol (15 mg/kg), diclofenac (1 mg/kg), and morphine (0.1–0.3 mg/kg). Remifentanil infusion is useful.
- Local infiltration with bupivacaine (maximum 2 mg/kg) will reduce the morphine requirement. If it is an open procedure, thoracic epidural might be useful in this patient, especially because of his respiratory comorbidity.

Postoperative
- Paracetamol 20 mg/kg 6 hourly and ibuprofen 5–10 mg/kg 8 hourly
- Morphine oral 0.3–0.5 mg/kg 4 hourly. Morphine NCA (nurse-controlled analgesia) in open procedures.

There is marked difference in analgesic requirements between open and laparoscopic Nissen's fundoplication. With the open procedure, the need for an intensive care unit bed on account of respiratory complications is significant, but is less so with epidural infusion compared to morphine infusion.

STEPS	KEY POINTS
The procedure is now complete and was successful laparoscopically. Would you extubate this patient?	This decision depends on the condition of the patient. If the child had pre-existing chronic lung disease and had poor gas exchange during the operation, he would benefit from postoperative ventilation in ITU. If there were no significant issues and if the surgery was uneventful, he can be extubated and warded.

Reasons for mechanical ventilation postoperatively:
- Need for airway control
- Abnormal lung function
- Assurance of stability during the immediate postoperative period
- Due to neurological concerns or residual anaesthesia

Mechanical ventilation is continued until there is adequate haemostasis, the heart rate and rhythm are stable, cardiac output is adequate with minimal inotropic support, oxygen saturation is adequate, lung function is close to normal, and the patient is awake enough to have adequate respiratory drive and airway protective reflexes.

In order to facilitate successful extubation, the patient must have the following: a patent airway, return of muscle strength, ability to cough and protect the airway, spontaneous respiratory drive, adequate blood oxygenation, and cardiovascular stability with minimal support.

Paediatric formulae

General
- Estimated weight (kg) = 2 × (Age + 4)

Respiratory
- Endotracheal tube inner diameter (mm) = (> 1 year) = Age/4 + 4
- Oral Endotracheal tube length (cm): age/2 + 12
- Nasal Endotracheal tube length (cm): age/2 + 15
- LMA size
  Size 1 for < 5 kg; size 1.5 for 5–10 kg; size 2 for 10–20 kg; size 2.5 for 20–30 kg; size 3 for 30–50 kg

Circulation
- Systolic BP = (Age × 2) + 80
- Adrenaline: 10 mcg/kg (0.1 ml/kg of 1:10,000 solution)
- Atropine: 20 mcg/kg
- Blood volume: 75 mL/kg
- Defibrillation: 4 J/kg

Fluids
- Crystalloid: 20 ml/kg for resuscitation (4:2:1 for maintenance)
- RBC units: 10 ml/kg
- Platelets: 10 ml/kg
- FFP: 15 ml/kg
- Cryoprecipitate: 5 ml/kg
- Glucose: 2 mls/kg of 10% dextrose

Drugs
- Propofol: 4 mg/kg
- Thiopentone: 3–6 mg/kg
- Suxamethonium: 2 mg/kg
- Rocuronium: 0.5–1 mg/kg
- Atracurium: 0.5–1 mg/kg

07.2 SHORT CASE: EPIDURAL ABSCESS

HISTORY *You are asked to see a 67-year-old patient 8 hours after having a cystectomy under general anaesthetic and an epidural block. The nurses in the ward are concerned that she is unable to move her legs since admission postoperatively.*

STEPS	KEY POINTS
What are the causes of nonreceding motor block after epidural anaesthesia?	***Factors related to neuraxial block*** • Use of large volume of high concentration local anaesthetic • Inadvertent subarachnoid placement • Migration of the catheter into the subdural/subarachnoid space • Direct nerve trauma • Epidural haematoma • Epidural abscess ***Factors unrelated to neuraxial block*** • Pregnancy, surgical, etc. • Disc herniation • Tumours • Transverse myelitis • Vascular and neurological disease • Meningitis
How can you prevent epidural abscess?	• Basic precautions—surgical scrubbing and donning of gloves and mask. Operating department practitioner also wears a mask. • Skin disinfectant—chlorhexidine (0.5%) in ethanol (70%) being fully bactericidal in 15 seconds. • Catheter dressing—opsite spray, semipermeable clear dressing. • Infusion systems—large volume reservoirs better than repeated changing of syringes; avoiding disconnection. • Epidural filters. • Identifying high-risk patients.
What is the incidence of epidural abscess?	• Rare complication; different incidence in different studies • 0.2–1.2/10 000 hospital admissions/year (not necessarily intervention related) • 1:100 000–1:500 000 in one study • 1:45 000 of all neuraxial blocks according to NAP 3

STEPS	KEY POINTS
What are the risk factors for the development of epidural abscess?	• Compromised immunity—diabetes, HIV, intake of alcohol, steroids, and immunosuppressants • Disruption of spinal column—trauma, intervention, and surgery • Source of infection—respiratory, urinary, etc., prolonged duration of catheterisation
What are the signs and symptoms?	• Back pain 90% • Feeling unwell and fever • Neurological deficits • Signs of meningism • Localised pain and temperature
What are the most common causative organisms?	• Gram +ve cocci—Staphylococcus aureus and epidermidis, Streptococcus pneumonia • Gram −ve rods—pyogenes • Aspergillus and mycobacterium
How would you manage it?	**Diagnosis by clinical suspicion** • Blood tests and cultures—inflammatory markers and antibiotic sensitivity • MRI—90% sensitivity **Management** • ABC approach • Early surgical decompression • Prolonged antibiotics (6–12 weeks) • Conservative management only in cases without neurological complications
Describe the epidural filter.	• It is disc-shaped with hydrophilic supported membrane. • Filter pore size is usually 0.22 microns. • It filters viruses, bacteria, and foreign bodies.
What others filters do you know that you use every day at work?	**Heat and Moisture Exchanger/Filter (HMEF)** • Hygroscopic membrane pleated to decrease the dead space • Mode of action—mechanical filters or electrostatic filters • 0.2 microns pore size [relative size of organisms—HIV ($0.14\ \mu m$), HCV ($0.06\ \mu m$), and *M. tuberculosis* ($0.4\ \mu m$)] • 60%–70% relative humidity and adds up to 100 mls dead space • Can increase positive end expiratory pressure **Filter needles** • Prevents particulate and organism contamination • Size: 0.2 microns **Fluid filter** • 15 microns to prevent particulate contamination **Blood filter** • I generation: 170–250 microns; for whole blood • II generation: 20–50 microns; 70%–80% of leucocytes depleted • III generation: electrostatic filters (100% leucodepletion) **Filters used in renal haemofiltration**

07.3 SHORT CASE: CARDIOMYOPATHY

HISTORY *A 36-year-old man is scheduled for elective nasal polypectomy. The nurse in the preoperative assessment unit tells you that he has got a murmur loudest at the sternal edge. He had been informed of the murmur many years ago, when he fainted as a teenager on a hot summer day. But he had remained asymptomatic and never been investigated.*

STEPS	KEY POINTS
How would you proceed?	It is wise to attend preassessment to see the patient. • History—about the fainting incident, family history, and current medical history focusing on cardiac symptoms of exertional dyspnoea, fatigue, angina, syncope • Examination—thorough systemic examination with particular emphasis to the cardiovascular system • Investigations—to assess the cause and pathology of the murmur
What investigations would you do?	The various investigations that might be necessary are 12 lead ECG, ECHO, cardiac catheterisation, and radionuclide imaging to study associated coronary artery disease. MRI is increasingly used nowadays.
Comment on the ECG shown in Figure 7.2.	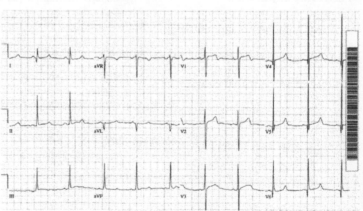

Fig. 7.2

STEPS	KEY POINTS
	• Voltage criteria for left ventricular hypertrophy (LVH).
	• Deep narrow Q waves < 40 ms wide in the lateral leads I, aVL, and V4–6
	These two features are suggestive of LVH with an old lateral infarct.
	• In an asymptomatic young patient, this ECG raises suspicion of an alternate pathology and not 'prior lateral infarction'. An ECG that meets LVH criteria in a young person with suspected syncope, think "Hypertrophic Cardiomyopathy"!
What is the differential diagnosis?	• Aortic valve stenosis • Mitral valve insufficiency • Hypertrophic Cardiomyopathy (HCM) • Glycogen storage diseases—Pompe's disease • Lysosomal storage disease—Fabry's diseas
What are the ECHO findings of HCM?	Asymmetric septal hypertrophy and nondilated left ventricular cavity. Echo confirms the size of the heart, the pattern of ventricular hypertrophy, contractile function of heart, and severity of outflow tract obstruction.
	Two-dimensional (2-D) echocardiography is diagnostic for hypertrophic cardiomyopathy. The common findings are abnormal systolic anterior leaflet motion (SAM) of the mitral valve, LV hypertrophy, left atrial enlargement, small ventricular chamber size, septal hypertrophy, mitral valve prolapse, and mitral regurgitation. A narrowing of the LV outflow tract occurs in many patients with HCM, contributing to the creation of a pressure gradient.
	Cardiac magnetic resonance imaging (MRI) is very useful in the diagnosis and assessment of hypertrophic cardiomyopathy, particularly apical hypertrophy.
What is HCM?	HCM is an intrinsic myocardial disorder characterised by unexplained LVH that is inappropriate and often asymmetrical and occurs in the absence of an obvious hypertrophic stimulus such as pressure overload or storage/infiltrative disease. It is classified as the most common purely genetic cardiovascular disease causing sudden death in young people with a prevalence of 1:500 and affecting twice as many men as women.
What is primary and secondary cardiomyopathy?	Primary cardiomyopathy (intrinsic) is due to weakness in the myocardium due to intrinsic cause. • Genetic: HCM, arrythmogenic right ventricular cardiomyopathy (ARVC) • Mixed: dilated and restrictive cardiomyopathy • Acquired: peripartum cardiomyopathy
	Secondary cardiomyopathy (extrinsic) is where the primary pathology is outside the myocardium. • Ischemia: coronary artery disease • Metabolic: amyloidosis, haemochromatosis • Endocrine: diabetic, acromegaly • Toxicity: alcohol, chemotherapy • Inflammatory: viral myocarditis • Neuromuscular: muscular dystrophy
What is the inheritance of HCM?	It is a genetic disorder that is typically inherited in an autosomal dominant fashion with variable penetrance and variable expressivity. It is attributed to mutations of genes that encode for sarcomere proteins such as myosin heavy chain, actin, and tropomyosin.

STEPS	KEY POINTS
What is the clinical presentation?	• Can be asymptomatic in many patients and diagnosed during a routine examination or investigation. • Dizziness, fainting, chest pain, and shortness of breath after exercise, blackouts, fatigue, and palpitations are present when symptomatic. • Signs include hypotension, low-volume pulse, left ventricular heave, ejection systolic murmur, and a mitral regurgitation murmur. • Dysrhythmias and heart failure can present in some patients. • Sudden collapse and death. The major risk factors for sudden cardiac death are: • Family history of sudden death • Extreme hypertrophy of the left ventricular wall (> 30 mm) • Unexplained syncope • Nonsustained ventricular tachycardia
Explain the pathophysiology.	The pathophysiology involves these interrelated processes. • Ventricular hypertrophy with poor ventricular compliance and diastolic dysfunction characterised by impaired left ventricular filling with subsequent raised LV filling pressures. • Hypertrophy of septum with left ventricular outflow tract (LVOT) obstruction in 20% of cases. • Mitral regurgitation due to anterior motion of the mitral valve in systole. • Familial hypertrophy occurs due to defects in sarcomeric proteins. This leads to myofibril disarray and fibrosis. This can be pro-arrythmogenic and leads to ventricular arrhythmias. • Myocardial ischaemia (see below).
What is the mechanism leading to ischaemia?	**Decreased supply** • Abnormally small partially obliterated intramural coronary arteries as a result of hypertrophy. • Inadequate number of capillaries for the degree of LV mass. • Diastolic dysfunction leads to an increase in end-diastolic pressure and decrease in the coronary perfusion pressure. • Any decrease in systemic vascular resistance can lead to a further reduction in coronary blood flow. **Increased demand** • In addition, the hypertrophied muscle, with a higher oxygen demand, makes the ventricle prone to ischaemia. In summary, myocardial ischaemia is due to septal/ventricular wall hypertrophy, elevated diastolic pressures, and increased O_2 demand.
Why do they get outflow obstruction?	HCM can be obstructive or nonobstructive. Obstructive HCM is due to midsystolic obstruction of flow through the LVOT. The two main reasons for this are: • Prominent hypertrophy of the interventricular septum causing a dynamic LVOT in the subaortic region. • The velocity of blood in the outflow tract draws the anterior mitral valve leaflet towards the interventricular septum (Venturi effect), thereby resulting in complete obstruction of the outflow tract.
What are the treatment options?	The main goals of treatment include: • Decreasing ventricular contractility • Increasing ventricular volume • Increasing ventricular compliance and LVOT dimensions • Vasoconstriction • Prevention of arrhythmias

STEPS	KEY POINTS

General

Screening echocardiography/genetic counseling of first-degree relatives

Medical therapy

- β blockers
- Calcium channel blockers
- β disopyramide
- Diuretics
- Amiodarone

Nonresponders to medical therapy

- Surgery to relieve obstruction—myotomy/myectomy with mitral valve replacement
- Internal cardio-defibrillator (ICD)—in patients with high risk of sudden death
- Dual chamber pacemaker—may favorably alter diastolic function and can also cause LVH regression
- Septal ablation—controlled myocardial infarction of the basal ventricular septum
- Heart transplant

What are the main anaesthetic considerations?

Preoperative period

- Good preoperative workup and adequate preoptimisation with drug therapy
- Premedication to reduce sympathetic activity
- Adequate hydration to maintain preload

Intraoperative period

- Induction
  - Invasive arterial monitoring prior to induction.
  - Choice of anaesthetic agents—minimise the decrease in SVR, prevent tachycardia or sympathetic surges.
  - Regional anaesthesia is relatively contraindicated as it can cause a decrease in systemic vascular resistance and potentially lead to outflow obstruction. But it has been successfully used in selective patients.
- Maintenance
  - Ventilation through frequent and small tidal volumes—minimise reduction in venous return.
  - Appropriate monitoring—transoesophageal echocardiography to monitor the adequacy of left ventricular filling and development of LVOT obstruction.
  - The application of external defibrillator pads is recommended before induction of anaesthesia to effectively treat intraoperative arrhythmias.
  - Adequate analgesia and anaesthesia to prevent sympathetic activity.
  - Hypotension should be treated with judicious volume resuscitation and α agonists such as phenylephrine. The use of agents with inotropic or chronotropic actions can increase myocardial oxygen demand and should be avoided.
  - Hypertension should be treated with β blockade rather than vasodilator agents such as GTN.

Postoperative period

- Avoid sympathetic stimulation by providing good pain control and avoidance of hypothermia.
- In the case of cardiac arrest, the use of inotropic agents is contraindicated if the arrest is thought to be due to LVOT obstruction, as this will only increase the obstruction. α agonists, IV fluids, and rapid correction of arrhythmias are more appropriate measures.

Key points

Preload: Normal/high normal
Contractility: slight negative inotropy is beneficial
Heart rate: around 60–80/min; avoid tachycardia
Afterload: normal/high normal

Avoid

Increased sympathetic activity and contractility, tachycardia, and reduced afterload.
Drugs – digoxin and nitrates as they decrease preload; β1 agonists as they increase inotropy and chronotropy.
Arrhythmias, hypovolemia, hypothermia.

Additional content: Other ECGs in HOCM. See Figure 7.3.

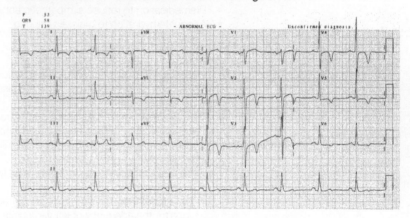

Fig. 7.3

- High precordial voltages.
- Deep T wave inversions in the precordial and lateral leads.
- There is also evidence of left atrial enlargement (P mitrale).

STEPS	KEY POINTS

ECG in HOCM does not have any distinct pattern. However, the most common abnormality includes deep S waves in V2 and V3, ST depression, T wave inversion and pathological Q waves, left bundle branch block and left axis deviation.

- Left ventricular hypertrophy results in increased precordial voltages and nonspecific ST segment and T-wave abnormalities.
- Asymmetrical septal hypertrophy produces deep, narrow ('dagger-like') Q waves in the lateral (V5–6, I, aVL) and inferior (II, III, aVF) leads. These may mimic prior myocardial infarction, although the Q-wave morphology is different: Infarction Q waves are typically > 40 ms duration, while septal Q waves in HOCM are < 40 ms. Lateral Q waves are more common than inferior Q waves in HCM.
- Apical hypertrophy leads to giant T wave inversion in the precordial leads.
- Left ventricular diastolic dysfunction may lead to compensatory left atrial hypertrophy, with signs of left atrial enlargement (P mitrale) on the ECG.
- Atrial fibrillation and supraventricular tachycardias are common. Ventricular dysrhythmias (e.g. VT) also occur and may be a cause of sudden death.

Other questions: How is HCM different from dilated and restrictive cardiomyopathy, and what are the anaesthetic implications?

Further reading

1. Ho CY. Hypertrophic cardiomyopathy in 2012. Clinician update. *Circulation*. 2012; **125**: 1432–1438.
2. Davies MR, Cousins J. Cardiomyopathy and anaesthesia. Continuing Education in Anaesthesia, *Critical Care & Pain*. 2009; **9**(6).
3. Life in the fast lane (lifeinthefastlane.com) for excellent ECG review.

07.4 SHORT CASE: AUTONOMIC DYSREFLEXIA

HISTORY *A 26-year-old male is brought in by ambulance to A&E with a history of a fall from the eighth floor. The neck is immobilised with collar and sandbags.*

STEPS	KEY POINTS
At what levels are the cervical spines more vulnerable?	Most cervical spine fractures happen at C2 (one third of the cases) and C6/C7 (half the cases). Most fatal injuries occur at C1 or C2.

How would the patients with nonfatal injury present?	**Symptoms**
	• Limited range of movement associated with pain
	• Weakness, numbness, and paraesthesia along affected nerve roots
	
	Signs
	• Loss of diaphragm function in C1/2 injuries
	• Spinal shock
	  ○ Flaccidity
	  ○ Areflexia
	  ○ Loss of sphincter tone
	  ○ Priapism
	• Neurogenic shock
	  ○ Hypotension
	  ○ Paradoxical bradycardia
	  ○ Warm and flushed skin
	• Autonomic dysfunction
	  ○ Ileus
	  ○ Urinary retention

STEPS	KEY POINTS
How would you manage an acute C3/4 spinal cord injury?	• ATLS approach and ABCDE protocol. • Stabilise and immobilise the spine. • Airway and breathing: Indications for intubation are acute respiratory failure, decreased GCS, increased pCO_2, and decreased tidal volumes. In this patient with C3/4 injury, intubation and ventilation are often required. • Circulation: Treat any associated haemorrhagic shock or spinal shock with careful fluid replacement. • Steroids: High dose of methylprednisolone (30 mg/kg bolus over 15 min followed by an infusion at 5.4 mg/kg/hr for 23 hours) when given within 8 hours of injury decreases inflammation by suppressing the migration of polymorphonuclear leucocytes and reversing increased capillary permeability. The benefit of steroids remains an institutional preference. • Immediate referral to a neurosurgical centre for further management. *This patient suffered a complete C3/4 cord transection and is listed for debridement of ankle pressure sore 8 months later. He suffers from significant reflux.*
What are your main anaesthetic concerns?	• Risk of aspiration • Risk of hyperkalaemia with suxamethonium • Autonomic hyperreflexia • Choice of anaesthetic: GA or spinal? Any sensation on wound site? • Difficult airway secondary to tracheostomy and spine fixation • Latex sensitivity secondary to prolonged use of gloves during urinary catheterisation in a neurogenic bladder
What is autonomic hyperreflexia?	Autonomic hyperreflexia develops in individuals with a spinal cord injury above the T6 vertebral level. It is a medical emergency with complications resulting from sustained severe peripheral hypertension. A strong stimulus caused by bladder distension, urinary tract infection, bowel impaction, and various surgical procedures triggers this condition. A stimulus below the level of injury causes a peripheral sympathetic response through the spinal nerves resulting in vasoconstriction below the level of injury. The central nervous system, being not able to detect the stimuli below the cord due to lack of continuity, detects only sympathetic response and then sends inhibitory response down the spinal cord. This reaches only until the level of injury and does not cause a desired response in the sympathetic fibres below the injury, leaving the hypertension unchecked. Above the level of injury: Predominant unopposed parasympathetic response leading to flushing and sweating, pupillary constriction and nasal congestion, and bradycardia. Below the level of injury: Sympathetic overactivity giving a pale, cool skin.
Why T6?	The level depicts the autonomic supply to the biggest reservoir of blood, the splanchnic circulation. The greater splanchnic nerve arises at T5–9, and any lesions above T6 allow the strong uninhibited sympathetic tone to constrict the splanchnic bed, causing systemic hypertension. Lesions below T6 results in a good parasympathetic inhibitory control and prevents hypertension.

STEPS	KEY POINTS
What is the physiological explanation for this response?	Not fully known. One theory is that the peripheral alpha adrenergic receptors associated with the blood vessels become hyper-responsive below the level of spinal cord injury due to the low resting catecholamine levels. These 'orphaned' receptors have a decreased threshold to react to adrenergic stimuli with an increased responsiveness.

It has also been postulated that the loss of descending inhibition is responsible for this mechanism. |
| **How would you tailor your anaesthetic for this patient and minimise risk of hyperreflexia?** | • Seek senior help
• Use of general or regional anaesthesia +/– sedation

Regional anaesthesia
• Difficult positioning
• Prepare vasopressors

General anaesthesia
• Prepare vasopressors and atropine (excessive hypotension on induction)
• May need RSI because of reflux—avoid suxamethonium (increase in K^+!)
• Possible difficult intubation due to positioning
• Adequate anaesthesia and remifentanil to reduce stimulus

Others
• Careful temperature control due to altered temperature regulation
• Arterial line in severe cases
• Ensure bladder is not distended |
| **What drugs can be given if dysreflexia happens with severe hypertension?** | • Short-acting antihypertensives, such as nifedipine or nitrates
• Remifentanil or other short-acting opioids
• Deepening of anaesthesia |

BASIC SCIENCE
VIVA

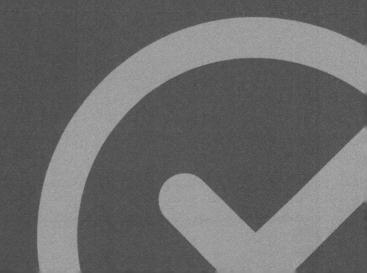

07.5 ANATOMY: PLEURA

Possible questions: *Pleural membranes, pleural space, its importance to anaesthetists, pneumothorax and pleural effusion, chest drain insertion, guidelines on using ultrasound for inserting the drains.*

STEPS	KEY POINTS
Describe the anatomy of the pleura.	Pleurae refer to the serous membranes covering the lung, mediastinum, diaphragm, and the inside of the chest wall.
	Two layers, visceral and parietal membranes, meet at the lung hilum.
	• *Visceral*: attached closely and adheres to the whole surface of the lung, enveloping the interlobar fissures.
	• *Parietal*: the outer layer, which is attached to the chest wall and the diaphragm and named as mediastinal, diaphragmatic, costal and cervical pleura, as per the association with the adjacent structures.
	The potential space between the two layers is called pleural space and is filled with a small amount of fluid amounting to around 0.2 mL/kg (5–10 mL). This is determined by the net result of opposing Starling's hydrostatic and oncotic forces and lymphatic drainage. Pleural fluid as little as 1 mL serves as a lubricant and decreases friction between the pleurae during respiration.
What are the constituents of pleural fluid?	• Clear ultrafiltrate of plasma
	• Quantity: 0.2 mL/kg (8.4+/− 4.3 mL)
	• Cellular contents: 75% macrophages, 25% lymphocytes
	• Biochemistry: Compared to plasma, the pleural fluid is alkaline (pH @ 7.6) and has higher albumin content but lower sodium, chloride, and LDH contents.
What is the blood supply of pleura?	• Visceral pleura is supplied by the bronchial arteries and drains into the pulmonary veins.
	• Parietal pleura gets its supply from systemic capillaries including intercostal, pericardiophrenic, musculophrenic, and internal mammary vessels. Venous drainage is via the intercostal veins and azygos veins, finally draining into the SVC and IVC.
How is pleura innervated?	The visceral pleura do not have pain fibres and is supplied by the pulmonary branch of vagus nerve and the sympathetic trunk.
	The parietal pleura receives an extensive innervation from the somatic intercostal and phrenic nerves.

STEPS	KEY POINTS
Explain the Starling's forces and describe the pathogenesis of pleural effusion.	The movement of pleural fluid between the pleural capillaries and the pleural space is governed by Starling's law of transcapillary exchange. Net filtration $= K_f [(P_c - P_i) - \sigma(\pi_c - \pi_i)]$ K_f: filtration coefficient and is dependent on the area of the capillary walls and the permeability to water. σ: reflection coefficient and is the ability of the membrane to restrict passage of proteins. P_c and P_i: Hydrostatic pressure in capillary and interstitium respectively. π_c and π_i: osmotic pressure in capillary and interstitium respectively.
Pathogenesis of pleural effusion	**Increased formation** • Increased interstitial fluid in the lung: LVF, PE, ARDS • Increased pressure in capillaries: LVF/RVF, SVC syndrome, pericardial effusion • Increased interstitial pressure: para pneumonic effusion • Decreased pleural pressure: lung atelectasis • Increased fluid in peritoneal cavity: ascites, peritoneal dialysis **Decreased reabsorption** • Obstruction of lymphatics: pleural malignancy • Increased systemic vascular pressures: SVC syndrome and RVF **Light's criteria** differentiates an exudate from transudate. The pleural fluid is an exudate if one or more of the following criteria are met: • Pleural fluid: serum protein > 0.5 • Pleural fluid: serum LDH > 0.6 • Pleural fluid LDH more than two-thirds the upper limits of normal serum LDH

Exudates	Transudates
Due to local pleural and pulmonary disease	Due to systemic factors that influence the formation and reabsorption of pleural fluid
Causes • Malignancy • Parapneumonic effusions • Pulmonary infarction • Rheumatoid arthritis • Autoimmune diseases • Pancreatitis • Postmyocardial infarction syndrome	Causes • Left ventricular failure • Liver cirrhosis • Hypoalbuminaemia • Peritoneal dialysis • Nephrotic syndrome • Mitral stenosis • Pulmonary embolism

STEPS	KEY POINTS
What drugs are known to cause pleural effusions?	• Amiodarone • Phenytoin • Methotrexate • Carbamazepine • Propylthiouracil • Penicillamine • Cyclophosphamide • Bromocriptine

STEPS	KEY POINTS

What are the effects of pneumothorax on pleural pressure?

Basic concepts

1. At FRC, due to the tendency of the lung to collapse and the chest wall to expand, the pleural pressure is maintained negative. This negative pressure holds the alveoli open.
2. Also due to gravity, the pleural pressure at the base of the lung is higher than that at the apex (more negative at the apex).

If chest wall is pierced (open pneumothorax) or the visceral pleura is breached (closed pneumothorax), air leaks into the pleural cavity causing a pneumothorax until the pressure gradient no longer exists. Because the thoracic cavity is below its resting volume and lung above its resting volume, with a pneumothorax, the thoracic cavity enlarges and the lung becomes smaller and hence collapses.

The pleural pressure is same throughout the entire pleural space, as per point (2), with the upper lobe being more affected than the lower lobe.

In tension pneumothorax, air enters into the pleural cavity with inspiration but cannot leave due to a flap of tissue acting as a one-way valve. The developed pressure collapses the affected lung and if high enough can cause a mediastinal shift.

What are the indications of intercostal drain in pneumothorax and pleural effusions?

Pneumothorax
- In any ventilated patient
- Tension pneumothorax after initial decompression
- Persistent or recurrent pneumothorax

Pleural effusion
- Large and symptomatic effusion
- Malignant pleural effusion, chylothorax
- Traumatic haemo pneumothorax
- Empyema
- Postoperative, for example, thoracotomy, oesophagectomy, cardiac surgery

What is the role of ultrasound in chest drain insertion?

Pleural procedures and thoracic ultrasound: British Thoracic Society Pleural disease guideline 2010.

Ultrasound-guided pleural aspiration is strongly recommended to increase success rates and reduce the risk of complications, particularly pneumothoraces and inadvertent organ puncture, and may not decrease the incidence of laceration of the intercostal vessels.

The evidence concludes that site selection for all pleural aspiration should be ultrasound-guided, with more emphasis when aspirating small or loculated pleural effusions or when a clinically guided attempt has been unsuccessful.

Describe the anatomy relevant to the insertion of chest drain.

Site

Safe triangle is bounded by the pectoralis major anteriorly, latissimus dorsi laterally, and fifth intercostal space inferiorly. The base of the axilla forms the apex of the triangle. This area is considered safe as it minimises risk to the underlying viscera, muscles, and internal mammary artery. Also the diaphragm rises to the fifth rib on expiration, and thus chest drains should be placed above this level.

STEPS

KEY POINTS

Occasionally the second intercostal space in the mid-clavicular line is chosen especially for apical pneumothorax, but its routine use is not recommended because of damage to internal mammary vessels.

If the drain is to be inserted into a loculated pleural collection, the site of puncture will be determined by imaging.

Intercostal space

The neurovascular bundle is situated between the internal and innermost intercostal muscles at the lower border of the rib. So to avoid the vessels, the needle is inserted in the space just above the rib.

Direction of the drain

Ideally the tip of the tube should be aimed apically to drain air and basally for fluid, but successful drainage can still be achieved when the drain is not placed in an ideal position.

Chest drainage system

Chest drain is connected to a drainage system containing a valve mechanism to prevent fluid or air from entering the pleural cavity. This is usually achieved by a Heimlich valve or underwater seal system.

In patients breathing spontaneously, the air/fluid is expelled during expiration whilst in IPPV the air/fluid exits in inspiration.

One-bottle system

Used in drainage of simple pneumothoraces.

When patient inspires, water in the bottle is drawn up the tube to a height equal to the negative intrathoracic pressure. So the collection bottle is placed at least 100 cm below the patient's chest to prevent water from being sucked back up.

The length of the tube under water should be limited to 2–3 cm to reduce any resistance to air drainage. See Figure 7.4.

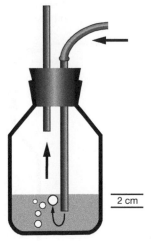

2 cm

Fig. 7.4

STEPS	KEY POINTS

Two-bottle system

In chest drains inserted for pleural effusion, the draining fluid might increase the depth in the bottle and increase the resistance to air flow. The first stage acts as a fluid drainage bottle, and the second stage then functions as an underwater seal that is not affected by the amount of fluid collecting in the first chamber. See Figure 7.5.

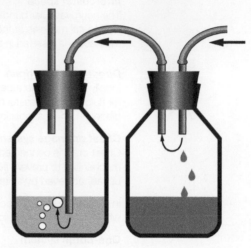

Fig. 7.5

Three-bottle system

If suction is required in case of persistent pneumothorax, this is provided by the use of underwater seal at the level of 10–20 cm H_2O or the application of a low-pressure suction adapter. The depth of the fluid in the third bottle determines the amount of negative pressure that can be transmitted to the chest. To obtain a suction of 20 cm H_2O, the tip of the tube should be 20 cm below the surface of fluid.

There is very little evidence to suggest the use or nonuse of suction in improving the resolution and altering the outcome. See Figure 7.6.

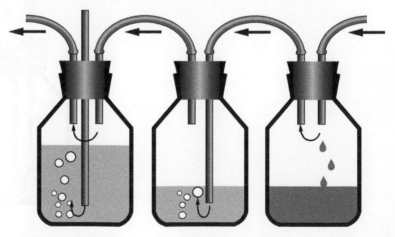

Fig. 7.6

Further reading

1. BTS Pleural Disease Guideline 2010. A Quick Reference Guide. *Thorax.* August 2010, **65,** Suppl 2

07.6 PHYSIOLOGY: DENERVATED HEART

HISTORY *A 65-year-old man is listed on the emergency list for incision and drainage of perianal abscess. He gives history of a heart transplant 3 years ago.*

STEPS	KEY POINTS
Where does the heart get its nerve supply?	**Autonomic innervation** • Sympathetic—T1–4 segment of the spinal cord—postganglionic cardio accelerator fibres form a cardiac plexus • Parasympathetic—branches of the Vagus
What is the effect of sympathetic stimulation on the heart?	• Positive chronotropy – increased heart rate • Positive inotropy – increased contractility • Positive dromotropy – increased electrical conductivity across atrioventricular node

What are the indications a heart transplant is in order?	The indication is end stage heart disease not remediable by conservative measures. The primary disease could be any of the following:
	• End stage cardiac failure
	• Cardiomyopathy
	• Congenital defects
	• Valvular heart disease
	
	According to the *UK guidelines for referral and assessment of adults for heart transplantation*, the conventional criteria for heart transplantation are as follows
	• Impaired LV systolic function
	• NYHA III/IV symptoms
	• Receiving optimal medical treatment (beta blockers, ACE inhibitors/ angiotensin receptor blocker and aldosterone antagonists)
	• Resynchronisation and/or defibrillator implanted (if indicated)
	• Evidence of a poor prognosis, defined as:
	  ○ VO_2 max <12 ml/kg/min if on β-blockade, <14 ml/kg/min if not on β-blockade, ensuring respiratory quotient ≥1.05
	  ○ Elevated B-type natriuretic peptide levels despite full medical treatment
	  ○ A poor prognosis indicated by the Heart Failure Survival Score (HFSS) or Seattle Heart Failure Model (SHFM)

STEPS	KEY POINTS

The contraindications are listed below
- Significant pulmonary hypertension (pulmonary arterial pressure > 60 mmHg).
- Severe, irreversible end organ damage—lung (FEV1< 50%), liver (bilirubin > 43 µmol/L), kidney (eGFR < 40 mL/min/1.73m^2).
- Diabetes mellitus with end organ damage.
- Active smoking, alcohol and other substance misuse.

Explain the physiology of a denervated (transplanted) heart.

- Absent sympathetic and parasympathetic innervation
  - Loss of vagal tone—resting heart rate at 90–100/min.
  - No response to direct autonomic influence or drugs that act via autononomic nervous system (atropine).
  - Absent rate response to baroreceptors, valsalva, carotid sinus stimulation, hypovolaemia, light anaesthesia.
  - Stimulated only through directly acting agents such as catecholamines.
  - Lack of catecholamine stores in myocardial neurons and loss of response to laryngoscopy/intubation.
- Absent sensory innervation
  - Increased incidence of silent myocardial ischaemia; hence the need for routine regular angiogram.
- Dependent on intrinsic regulation of cardiac output
  - Stroke volume is preload dependent; hence the need to maintain ventricular filling pressures.

Sympathetic neuronal reinnervation commences within 12 months after the transplant but the parasympathetic innervation is less extensive.

How does a denervated heart respond to direct and indirect sympathomimetics?

Direct sympathomimetics (adrenaline, noradrenaline, isoprenaline, dobutamine)
- Inotropic effects of adrenaline and noradrenaline are augmented; dobutamine and isoprenaline have normal response.

Indirect sympathomimetics (ephedrine)
- There is no catecholamine store in the myocardial neurones, so there is a decreased response.

What effect does atropine have?

Atropine and glycopyrollate (and digoxin) have no effect on the transplanted heart due to absence of vagal connection. Its use is still warranted as a neuromuscular reversal agent along with neostigmine to counteract the peripheral muscarinic effects such as miosis, nausea, bronchospasm, increased bronchial secretions, sweating and salivation.

What are the concerns when you are anaesthetising a patient with a heart transplant for a noncardiac surgery?

- Problems with physiology of denervation – as above.
- Related to progressive primary disease.
- Presence of defibrillator or pacemaker.
- Complications of transplant procedure such as leaky valves and conduction defects.
- Problems with rejection.
- Problems due to immune suppressants— nephrotoxicity, hepatotoxicity, hypertension, electrolyte imbalance, enhanced cytochrome P450.
- Infection - Cytomegalvirus, *Pneumocystis carinii, fungal and protozoal opportunistic infections.*
  - Need for meticulous aseptic technique.
  - Routine prophylactic antibiotics.
  - Use of irradiated, leucocyte depleted, CMV negative blood products if indicated.

STEPS	KEY POINTS

- Difficult venous and arterial access— avoid right internal jugular venous cannulation as this is the recommended route for endomyocardial biopsy.
- Need for extensive preoperative investigations and intraoperative monitoring.
  - Preoperative— ECG: beware of a double 'P' wave. Coronary angiogram might be indicated to rule out ischaemic heart disease.
  - Intraoperative— 5 lead ECG to monitor ischaemia and arrhythmias, cardiac output monitoring to evaluate cardiac function, volume status and aid fluid resuscitation, and peripheral nerve stimulator to assess the neuromuscular function.

Both general and regional anaesthesia have been used successfully in these patients and in the absence of significant cardiorespiratory, hepatic or renal dysfunction, there is no absolute contraindication to any anaesthetic technique. Titration of anaesthetic agents to avoid drastic reduction in preload and afterload is necessary due to the changes to normal physiological responses.

What are the problems with rejection?

Acute rejection: This is a cellular or antibody mediated response characterised by arrhythmias, fluid retention, dyspnoea, and pyrexia and happens in the first 3 months after transplant. Surveillance is by endomyocardial biopsy and the treatment is by augmenting the maintenance dose of immunosuppressants, high dose steroids and occasionally plasmapheresis and total lymphoid tissue irradiation.

Chronic rejection: Otherwise termed as allograft vasculopathy, it is immune-mediated and leads to an accelerated concentric intimal proliferation of the donor coronary vessels. It is a leading cause of late death in transplant recipient. Surveillance is by routine invasive angiogram and there is no specific treatment but the incidence is reduced by regular statin use.

What are the implications of the patient's immunosuppressant therapy for perioperative care?

Immunosuppression is usually achieved with the following drugs.

Drugs and mode of action	Side effects
Calcineurin inhibitor Eg. *Cyclosporin and Tacrolimus* Prevents T-cell activation and cell-mediated immune reactions such as delayed hypersensitivity and allograft rejection	• Metabolised by hepatic cytochrome P450—care with anaesthetic drugs • Nephro- and neuro-toxicity, dyslipidaemia, diabetes, pancreatitis, and hypertension • Hyperkalaemia, hypomagnesaemia, and hyperuricaemia • Enhances effects of neuromuscular blockers
Steroids Eg. *Methylprednisolone* Inhibition of T- cell lymphokines production	• Hypertension, cushingoid features, psychosis, hyperglycaemia, hyperkalaemia, osteoporosis • Adrenal suppression—need for intraoperative supplementation
Target of Rapamycin (TOR) inhibitors Eg. *Sirolimus* Prevention of T- and B- cell activation	• Minimal nephrotoxicity—so used in patients with renal dysfunction • Peripheral oedema, hypertension, dyslipidaemia, and diarrhoea
Antiproliferative drugs Eg. *Azathioprine and mycophenolate mofetil* Nonspecific inhibition of T- and B- lymphocytes	• Myelosuppression leading to pancytopaenia • Reduces effects of nondepolarising neuromuscular blocking agents • Hepatotoxicity and gastrointestinal side effects • Pulmonary infiltrates

In addition, all the drugs increase the incidence of skin and lympho-proliferative malignancy and propensity to infections.

The implications of immunosuppressant therapy are:
- Need for continuation intraoperatively to maintain the plasma levels.
- Steroid requires supplementation to account for stress response.
- Preoperative blood tests to rule out haematological, renal, and electrolyte impairment.

STEPS	KEY POINTS
	• Strict asepsis and appropriate antibiotic prophylaxis as these patients are at risk of infections—bacterial, viral, fungal, and protozoal.
	• Careful positioning due to presence of steroid induced osteoporosis and skin fragility.
	• Drug interactions:
	○ Cyclosporin enhances and azathioprine reduces aminosteroid neuromuscular blocking action.
	○ Cytochrome P450 interactions of anaesthetic drugs
	○ Avoid nephrotoxic drugs such as non-steroidal anti-inflammatory drugs and aminoglycoside
What long-term health issues may occur in these patients?	Between 85% and 90% of recipients live for at least a year after the transplant. The proportion decreases with around 50% survival rate at 10 years.
	There is also increased risk of infection, skin and lymphoproliferative malignancies, hepatic and renal impairment, allograft vasculopathy, diabetes mellitus, osteoporosis, etc.
	Health related quality of life is usually good, and improves rapidly after transplantation.
What are the issues associated with anaesthetising a lung transplant patient for subsequent surgery?	The control of breathing is usually preserved and hence there is little or no change in the pattern of breathing. Also the response to ventilation to CO_2 is normal. The goal is to maintain oxygenation with minimal airway pressures, optimal PEEP and FiO_2.
	• Complete transection of nerve supply with absent or very little reinnervation— loss of cough reflex and neurally mediated changes in bronchomotor tone.
	• Decreased mucociliary clearance— in the presence of impaired cough and immunosuppression, there is increased risk of perioperative chest infection. Strict asepsis, prophylactic antibiotics, incentive spirometry and physiotherapy in the immediate postoperative period is necessary.
	• Interruption of lymphatic drainage increases the susceptibility of pulmonary oedema stressing the importance of judicious fluid administration.
	• Drug-induced muscle weakness (steroid myopathy) can affect the muscles of respiration; hence the need for careful titration and monitoring of neuromuscular blocking drugs.
	• In single lung transplants, knowledge of underlying lung disease is important. In restrictive diseases of the native lung, increased airway pressures might be required to ventilate them, which can cause barotrauma and volutrauma in the transplant lung.
	• Hypoxic pulmonary vasoconstriction (HPV) response is intact in native and grafted lung. Positive pressure ventilation improves oxygenation to the native lung and obliterates HPV. This sudden increase in blood flow to the native lung can result in haemodynamic instability and problems with gas exchange. Also in case of allograft rejection blood flow to the transplant lung is reduced.

Further reading

1. Banner NR, Bonser RS, Clark AL, Clark S, et al. UK guidelines for referral and assessment of adults for heart transplantation. *Heart*. 2011; **97**(18):1520–1527.
2. Taylor DO, Stehlik J, Edwards LB, et al. Registry of the International Society for Heart and Lung Transplantation: Twenty-sixth official adult heart transplant report 2009. *J Heart Lung Transplant* 2009; **28**:1007–1022.

07.7 PHARMACOLOGY: HYPOTENSIVE DRUGS

STEPS	KEY POINTS
When would you decrease the blood pressure to induce hypotension intraoperatively?	Induced hypotension is the deliberate lowering of blood pressure by more than 30% of its resting value. Its use is highly controversial and is associated with dramatic consequences due to organ ischaemia and dysfunction of all vital organs.

Anaesthetic indications
- Nil
- Might be used in the preservation of blood in patients who are Jehovah's Witnesses

Surgical indications
- Types of surgery where the procedure might be hindered by bleeding, e.g. middle ear and neurosurgery

How would you decrease blood pressure during anaesthesia?

BP = Stroke volume (SV) × Heart rate (HR) × Systemic vascular resistance (SVR)

Mechanisms that decrease any of the above contributing factors can decrease blood pressure.

Non pharmacological
- Head-up positioning
- Use of intermittent positive pressure ventilation and preventing hypercarbia

Pharmacological
- Drugs with effect on heart rate
  - Beta blockers
- Drugs with effect on venous return
  - Neuraxial blockade
  - Venodilators
- Drugs with effect on myocardial contractility
  - Inhalational agents
- Drugs with effect on SVR
  - Vasodilators
  - Inhalational and intravenous anaesthetic agents
  - Neuraxial blockade

What drugs are commonly used for hypotensive anaesthesia?

β adrenoceptor blockers
Decreases heart rate and also inhibits the renin angiotensin system
- Esmolol—selective $β_1$ antagonist
- Labetolol—most commonly used α and β antagonist (1:7) resulting in decreased SVR without reflex tachycardia

STEPS	KEY POINTS

Vasodilators
- Glyceryl trinitrate (GTN)
  - Venodilator via cyclic GMP pathway resulting in decreased intracellular Ca^{2+}
  - Decreases venous return and stroke volume
- Sodium nitroprusside
  - Similar action to GTN but causes both arterial and venous dilatation, giving rise to hypotension and reflex tachycardia
- Hydralazine
  - Similar action to GTN and also a weak α inhibitory effect
  - Causes more arteriolar dilatation than venous and causes reflex tachycardia

α *adrenoceptor blockers*
- Phentolamine
  - Nonselective α antagonist with weak β agonist action

Ganglion-blocking drugs
- Trimetaphan
  - Antagonists at acetyl choline nicotinic receptors at the autonomic ganglia
  - Direct vasodilator effects on peripheral vessels

What are the problems with hypotensive anaesthesia?

- Need for invasive arterial monitoring
- CNS
  - Impaired cerebral perfusion, depending on associated comorbidities
  - Need for cerebral function monitors in 'at-risk' patients
- CVS
  - Hypotension can be useful by decreasing oxygen consumption, but in patients with ischaemic heart disease, it is detrimental because the coronary perfusion is pressure-dependent.
  - ECG monitoring is not helpful.
- Renal
  - Induced hypotension can impair renal perfusion especially in 'at-risk' patients.

Alternative answer: Drugs to treat hypertension can also be classified as

Centrally acting drugs
- Methyl dopa
- Clonidine
- Dexmedetomidine

Ganglion-blocking agents
- Trimetaphan

Adrenergic neuron blockade
- Guanethidine

Drugs affecting renin-angiotensin-aldosterone system
- ACE inhibitors
- Angiotensin II receptor blockers

β blockers
- Atenolol and others

Diuretics
- Loop diuretics
- Thiazides

STEPS	KEY POINTS

Vasodilators
- GTN
- Sodium nitroprusside
- Potassium channel activators—nicorandil
- Calcium channel blockers—verapamil, nifedipine, diltiazem

What level of mean arterial pressure (MAP) are you satisfied with intraoperatively in a patient who is normotensive?

Safe level of hypotension is no lower than about two-thirds of the resting blood pressure before inducing hypotension.

This number is obtained by various cerebral perfusion and EEG studies. The cerebral blood flow decreases to 60% normal with two-thirds MAP, with clinical manifestations of yawning, and inability to concentrate and carry out simple commands. With further decrease in MAP and cerebral blood flow, the slowing and flattening of EEG occurs with ischaemic irreversible brain damage ensuing.

Do not forget that the blood pressure decreases 2 mmHg for every 2.5 cm height above the point of measurement. So, mean arterial pressure in brain in a reclining or sitting patient under anaesthesia is about 12–16 mmHg lower than that measured at the upper arm.

Discuss sodium nitroprusside.

It is a vasodilator available as a reddish-brown powder that is reconstituted in 5% dextrose. The reconstituted solution is covered in an aluminium foil as it turns dark brown or blue on exposure to sunlight due to the production of cyanide ions.

Dose: 0.5–6 µg/kg/min and titrated to effect

Onset: 3 minutes and the effects are short-lived

Mechanism of action: Vasodilatation happens due to the production of NO, which activates the enzyme guanylate cyclase, leading to increased levels of intracellular cyclic GMP. This increases the uptake of Ca^{2+} into the endoplasmic reticulum, and hence the cytoplasmic calcium concentration falls, resulting in vasodilatation.

Pharmacodynamics:
CVS: Arteriolar and venous dilatation, decreased preload and reflex tachycardia

RS: Inhibition of hypoxic pulmonary vasoconstriction and increase of shunt

Cerebral: Cerebral vasodilatation and increased ICP

Others:
- Tachyphylaxis
- Toxicity due to thiocyanate (less toxic) and mainly cyanide ions, which bind to cytochrome oxidase and impair aerobic metabolism, causing a metabolic acidosis and histotoxic hypoxia.

Treat cyanide toxicity with oxygen, chelating agents, sodium thiosulphate (provide additional sulphydryl groups to aid conversion of cyanide to thiocyanate) and nitrites (converts oxyhaemoglobin to methaemoglobin and cyanide ions bind more avidly to methaemoglobin than cytochrome oxidase).

STEPS	KEY POINTS
Other questions: How will you anaesthetise for mastoidectomy?	*Anaesthesia for mastoidectomy – refer to Set 10.3*
What are the advantages of remifentanil in mastoidectomy?	*Advantages of remifentanil in mastoidectomy*

Intraoperative
- Controlled ventilation without neuromuscular blocking agents, thus permitting unimpeded facial nerve monitoring.
- Remifentanil provides a titratable degree of hypotension while maintaining a stable heart rate and provides superior operating conditions.
- Provides excellent analgesia and reduces the need for intraoperative morphine.

Postoperative
- Prevents airway irritation and coughing and provides smooth emergence.
- Rapid clearance of remifentanil due to metabolism by nonspecific plasma esterases results in a uniform and predictable onset and duration of action despite changes in the duration of infusion.
- Better recovery profiles – lesser pain, shivering, and PONV

Further reading

1. Jones A. Hypotensive anaesthesia. *Oxford Textbook of Anaesthesia for Oral and Maxillofacial Surgery.* Oxford University Press; DOI:10.1093/med/9780199564217.003.0020.

07.8 PHYSICS: RENAL REPLACEMENT THERAPY

STEPS	KEY POINTS
What are the ECG features of high potassium?	***Rate and rhythm*** • Bradycardia • Asystole • Ventricular tachycardia and fibrillation • Sine wave appearance ***Waves*** • Absent P waves • Wide QRS • Peaked T waves ***Intervals and segments*** • Slurring of ST segments
How would you treat this condition?	**Immediate measures to prevent cardiac arrest (especially if potassium > 6.5 mmol/L)** • Calcium: 5–10 mmol intravenously; repeated if necessary. ECG changes are reversed within 1 to 3 min. • Insulin to push the potassium into intracellular compartment. • Nebulised salbutamol increases cellular uptake of potassium. • Sodium bicarbonate: 50 mls of 8.4% intravenously in the presence of acidosis (exchanges potassium for hydrogen ions across cell membranes). • Diuretics if renal function is adequate. • Calcium resonium: polystyrene sulphonate resins orally or rectally. It might take 6 hours to achieve full effect. **Delayed measures depending on the cause of hyperkalaemia** • Aimed at correcting the disease and preventing further increase in plasma potassium

When would you institute renal replacement therapy (RRT)?	The indications of RRT can be
	• Acute kidney injury with
	  ○ K > 6.5 mmol/L
	  ○ Metabolic acidosis (pH < 7.1)
	  ○ Deteriorating renal parameters (urea > 30 mmol/L)
	  ○ Signs of fluid overload with oliguria/anuria
	• Drug poisoning
	  ○ Water-soluble and non-protein-bound drugs (e.g. salicylates)
	• Severe sepsis
	  ○ To remove inflammatory mediators

STEPS	KEY POINTS

What types of RRT are being used?

Depending on the mechanism of solute removal and the duration of treatment, RRT can be classified as:
- Intermittent haemodialysis (IHD)
- Continuous renal replacement therapy (CRRT)
  - Continuous venovenous haemofiltration (CVVH)
  - Continuous venovenous haemodialysis (CVVHD)
  - Continuous venovenous haemodiafiltration (CVVHDF)
  - Continuous arteriovenous haemofiltration (CAVHF)
- Peritoneal dialysis
- Sustained low-efficiency dialysis

Haemofiltration (filtration)
This method involves the use of a semipermeable membrane for ultrafiltration in an extracorporeal system. Blood is pumped through, and the hydrostatic pressure that is created on the blood-side of the filter drives plasma water across the membrane. Molecules that are small enough to pass through the membrane (< 50,000 Daltons) are dragged across the membrane with the water by the process of convection. The filtered fluid (ultrafiltrate) is discarded, and a replacement fluid is added in an adjustable fashion according to the desired fluid balance.

Haemodialysis (diffusion)
Blood is pumped through an extracorporeal system that has a dialyser, where blood is separated from a crystalloid solution (dialysate) by a semipermeable membrane. Solutes move across the membrane along their concentration gradient from one compartment to the other, obeying Fick's laws of diffusion. In order to maintain concentration gradients and therefore enhance the efficiency of the system, the dialysate flows counter-current to the flow of blood.

Haemodiafiltration
It is a combination of filtration and dialysis. It has the benefits of both techniques but to a lesser extent than when the individual techniques are used on their own.

Peritoneal dialysis
Same principle as haemodialysis, but peritoneum acts as the membrane. 2 L of sterile dialysate is placed in the peritoneal cavity via a catheter. The electrolyte movement is by osmosis, and the fluid is drained out at frequent intervals.

Sustained low-efficiency dialysis (SLED)
It is a hybrid therapy that aims to combine the logistic and cost advantages of IHD with the cardiovascular stability of CRRT. Treatments are intermittent but usually daily and with longer-session durations than conventional IHD. Solute and fluid removal are slower than IHD but faster than CRRT.

How would you determine the type of RRT to use?

This depends on:
- The size of particles to be removed from plasma

Urea, creatinine, K+	< 500 Daltons	Dialysis and Filtration
Large drugs	500–5000 D	Filtration
Cytokines, complement	5000–50000 D	Filtration
Water	18 D	Filtration

- Patient's cardiovascular status
  - Continuous RRT is better than IHD.
- Clinician experience
- Availability of resources
  - CRRT is labour intensive and expensive.

STEPS	KEY POINTS
What are the complications of RRT?	**Anticoagulation related** • Bleeding • Heparin-induced thrombocytopenia **Catheter related** • Sepsis • Thrombosis • Arterio-venous fistulae • Arrhythmia • Pneumothorax **Procedure related** • Hypothermia • Anaemia • Hypovolaemia • Hypotension • Electrolyte abnormalities (hypophosphataemia, hypokalaemia) **Drug related** • Altered pharmacokinetics
Do you know of any trials comparing different methods?	• The Randomised Evaluation of Normal versus Augmented Level (RENAL) of renal replacement therapy in ICU study randomised 1400 critically ill patients with acute kidney injury to intensive (35 ml/kg/hr) or nonintensive (20 ml/kg/hr) CRRT and no difference in mortality was seen in the two groups at 90 days. • The Acute Renal Failure Trial Network (ATN) study compared intensive or less-intensive dosing strategies for patients undergoing CRRT, IHD, and SLED. The recovery of renal function and the mortality at 60 days were the same in both arms of the trial. • HEMODIAFE study—multicentre RCT, randomised 184 patients to intermittent haemodialysis (IHD) and 175 patients to continuous veno-venous haemodiafiltration (CVVHDF) and concluded that CVVHDF and IHD may be used interchangeably for the critically ill patient in acute renal failure.
What is the role of RRT in sepsis?	The mediators involved in the inflammatory response such as tumour necrosis factor, interleukins (IL-1, IL-6, IL-8), platelet activating factor and complement are water-soluble middle-sized compounds. These compounds can be eliminated through the highly porous synthetic membranes used for convective filtration in CVVH with a high flow rate.

Further reading

1. Hall NA and Fox AJ. Renal replacement therapies in critical care. *Contin Educ Anaesth Crit Care Pain* (2006) **6** (5): 197–202.

CLINICAL VIVA

08.1 LONG CASE: PATIENT WITH VALVE REPLACEMENTS FOR URGENT SURGERY

HISTORY *You are asked to see a 63-year-old woman requiring hemiarthroplasty. She was found on the floor by her husband earlier that day and had sustained a fracture of neck of femur.*

STEPS	KEY POINTS
Past Medical History	Rheumatic heart disease diagnosed when she was about 30 years of age, and 2 years ago she had aortic and mitral valve replacements. She also had two strokes many years ago with no residual neurological deficit. Before the fracture, she was walking with a Zimmer frame but would get breathless after 100 yards when she would have to stop and 'take a breath'.
Social History	She gave up smoking 10 years ago after having smoked most of her life. She drinks socially and does not indulge in illicit drugs.
Drugs	Spironolactone 25 mg OD Bumetanide 1 mg OD Lisinopril 5 mg OD Digoxin 125 mcg OD Warfarin (variable dose over the week) Paracetamol and Tramadol prn
On Examination	Awake and alert Respiratory rate: 30/min Saturation: 94% on high flow oxygen Heart rate: 85/min Blood pressure: 110/70 mmHg BMI: 38.8 Raised JVP Reduced air entry bilaterally with bibasal crepitations

Investigations						
	Hb	10.1 g/dL	(13–16)	Na	128 mmol/L	(137–145)
	WCC	3.0×10^9/L	(4–11)	K	4.8 mmol/L	(3.6–5.0)
	Platelets	242×10^9/L	(140–400)	Urea	12 mmol/L	(1.7–8.3)
	PCV	0.35	(0.38–0.56)	Creat	150 umol/L	(62–124)
	MCV	88 femto Litres	(80–100)			
	MCH	30 pico grams	(26–34)	INR	3.6	(0.8–1.2)

STEPS	KEY POINTS
ECG	See Figure 8.1.

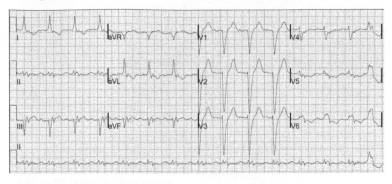

Fig. 8.1 CCF

| CXR | See Figure 8.2. |

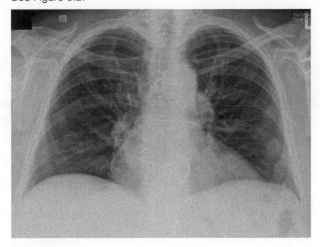

Fig. 8.2 CCF Valves

Some statistics

70 000 to 75 000 hip fractures per year in the UK

Mortality: 10% at one month, 20% at three months, 30% at one year. This is linked to the fact that neck of femur (NOF) fractures occur very often following a fall due to an 'event' (i.e. atrial fibrillation (AF), cerebrovascular accident (CVA), sick sinus syndrome).

(NICE guideline published in June 2011)

Summarise the case.

This is a relatively young obese patient who sustained a fracture of her neck of femur, the circumstances of which are unknown but could be linked to an acute event as this woman has multiple comorbidities.

Her medical history is mainly centred on her aortic and mitral valve replacements, which occurred 2 years ago and she is now presenting with clinical signs of cardiac failure and renal impairment for which she is treated. She is on two types of diuretics, digoxin, ACE inhibitors, and warfarin. She also suffered from two CVAs in the past.

STEPS	KEY POINTS
What are the pertinent features?	• Two metallic valves • Cardiac failure • Renal impairment • Obesity • Correction of high INR • Bridging therapy during surgery • High-risk case
What are the consequences of obesity?	**Anatomically** • Difficult IV access • Difficult airway • Increased risk of aspiration • Difficult procedures such as spinal, epidural, and any regional technique **Physiologically** • Increased oxygen demand and CO_2 production • Reduced FRC, chronic hypoxaemia, and hypoxic pulmonary vasoconstriction with increased pulmonary pressures leading to right-sided cardiac failure. In her case this is compounded by left-sided cardiac failure linked to her valve replacements. • Obstructive sleep apnoea • Hypertension (her BP is normal but she is on antihypertensives. In addition, her cardiac failure would not generate high blood pressures) Associated diseases: Diabetes and ischaemic heart disease. Increased risk of DVT, CVA, fatty liver disease Increased blood loss
Talk through the blood results.	Her preliminary investigations show that she is anaemic (normocytic and normochromic), has low sodium, raised urea, and an elevated creatinine. The most striking is her INR which is 3.6.
Looking at the results, what are the potential causes, in this particular case, for a low sodium, raised urea, and low haemoglobin?	• Hyponatraemia due to cardiac failure with subsequent fluid retention and diuretics. • Raised urea due partly to dehydration but is also indicative in this case of impaired renal function (creatinine 150). • The reason for her low haemoglobin is multi-factorial including blood loss from the fracture site but also chronic loss due to red cell damage by the valves and chronic insensitive loss as she is on warfarin.
What do the CXR and ECG show?	**CXR** Cardiomegaly Sternotomy wires Two metallic valves—mitral and aortic valves Bilateral increased lung markings Alveolar oedema Kerley B lines **ECG** Sinus rhythm rate 85/min Wide QRS complexes keeping with LBBB Left axis deviation QRS fragmentation in V4–5

STEPS	KEY POINTS
How would you identify these prosthetic valves as mitral and aortic?	Localising cardiac prosthetic valves can be difficult. The best strategy that can be employed to aid in characterising the type of prosthetic valve involves assessing the location of the valve and then determining the orientation and direction of flow (most accurate).

Location
On the frontal chest radiograph (either the AP or PA view), draw a longitudinal line through the mid sternal body and intersect it by a sagittal line. The aortic valve should overlie the intersection of these two lines, and the mitral valve will lie in the lower left quadrant (the patient's left).

Direction of flow
If the direction of flow is from inferior to superior (towards the aorta), then an aortic valve is likely. If the direction of flow is from superior to inferior (towards the apex) in the left chest, then the valve is likely a mitral valve.

What further investigations would you request prior to going to theatre?	• Group and save, cross match blood and blood products • Liver function tests as high BMI and potential right-sided cardiac failure • Echocardiogram prior to cardiology opinion
What will an ECHO show?	An echocardiogram will provide:

Qualitative assessment:
Establish the integrity of the valves and the gradients as well as any regurgitation.
The quality of the ventricular function, establishing any diastolic (ventricular compliance) and systolic dysfunction (ejection fraction).

Quantitative assessment:
Atrial and ventricular measurements
Filling pressures
Ejection fraction
Valve dimensions

Discuss the specific benefits of the various drugs the patient takes.	• Lisinopril—inhibits angiotensin-converting enzyme and decreases the formation of Angiotensin II → decreased sympathetic activity, reverses myocardial and vascular remodeling • Spironolactone—mineralocorticoid receptor blockade → natriuresis, diuresis, K retention, and also decreases the myocardial collagen formation and endothelial dysfunction • Bumetanide—loop diuretic for symptom control • Digoxin—rate control if patient is in atrial fibrillation • Warfarin—for thromboprophylaxis
What should the patient's normal INR be?	The presence of mechanical mitral valve calls for a maintenance of INR 2.5–3.5; but the history of CVAs while on warfarin warrants an INR of 3–4.

Target INR
• 2–3 for DVT prophylaxis, treatment of pulmonary embolus (PE), transient ischaemic attack (TIA), and AF with high risk of embolisation.
• 2.5–3.5 for mechanical mitral valve or aortic valve with additional risk factors.
• 3.0–4.0 for mechanical valve and systemic embolism despite therapeutic INR of 2.5–3.5.

STEPS	KEY POINTS

What INR is considered safe for a hemiarthroplasty? How would you correct this patient's high INR?

An INR of 1.5 is considered safe for surgery in these patients. Correction is required for surgery, but this has to be achieved for as short a period of time as possible due to the high risk of thromboembolism.

Base your answer on the way warfarin works (i.e. how it competes with vitamin K in the synthesis of factors II, VII, IX, and X and is highly protein bound).

- Vitamin K up to 5–10 mg IV, takes 4 to 8 hours to work and will interfere with anticoagulation for a long time.
- Prothrombin complex concentrate (Beriplex) is now preferred over FFP. Beriplex is made from blood and is a combination of factors II, VII, IX, and X with proteins C and S. It comes as a powder with a solvent to make a 100 ml solution containing 250 IU. The dose is calculated based on the patient's weight and current INR. The INR is normalised within 30 min, and the effect lasts 6 to 8 hours. Thus, if vitamin K has been administered at the same time, it should take effect when Beriplex stops working. Repeated monitoring of INR is compulsory.
- Fresh frozen plasma is no longer recommended. Also a large volume is needed (15 ml/kg), and this is detrimental in this patient with cardiac failure.

How would you prevent thromboembolic risks while you normalise the INR?

Perioperative management of patients on warfarin or antiplatelet therapy involves balancing individual risks for thromboembolism and bleeding.

Discontinuing anticoagulant therapy is necessary for major surgery, and to prevent thromboembolic events during this period, bridging therapy is advised.

Before surgery
- Discontinue warfarin 5 to 6 days before surgery.
- Start therapeutic low molecular weight heparin (LMWH) 36 hours after last dose of warfarin.
- Stop LMWH 24 hours prior to surgery.

After surgery
- Start therapeutic LMWH 24 hours after surgery.
- Restart anticoagulant after discussion with the surgeon and bleeding risks assessed
- Check INR daily.
- Discontinue LMWH once target INR is reached.

What is cardiac failure?

Cardiac failure is a complex clinical syndrome that results from any structural or functional impairment of ventricular filling or ejection of blood, secondary to hypertension, valvular heart disease, and ischaemic heart disease. It is a major clinical predictor of perioperative risk

Describe the pathophysiology of heart failure.

- Long-standing pressure or volume overload leads to cardiac myocyte remodeling and chamber enlargement and stiffness that impair filling.
- Decreased cardiac output leads to sympathetic activation of the renin-angiotensin-aldosterone system (RAAS) resulting in salt and water retention and an increase in circulating volume.

Initially this restores the cardiac output in accordance with the Frank Starling's law, but later it results in a myocardium vulnerable to ischaemia and a circulation that is dependent on sympathetic tone.

STEPS	KEY POINTS
Can you quantify heart failure?	**According to Ejection Fraction (EF)** Normal: EF of 60%–70% Mild: EF of 40%–50% Moderate: EF of 30%–40% Severe: EF < 30% **NYHA classification** I: Ordinary physical activity does not cause symptoms. II: Ordinary physical activity causes fatigue, dyspnoea, and angina. III: Comfortable at rest. IV: Symptomatic at rest.
How would you treat this patient's symptomatic cardiac failure?	This patient is already on cardiac failure treatment (i.e. diuretics, digoxin, ACE inhibitors); thus, any further improvement would require the involvement of a cardiologist who might consider adding vasodilators, β blockers, and angiotensin II receptor antagonists.
How would you anaesthetise her?	This is the difficult part of the question and relies on setting out a clear plan. This is a challenging patient who needs consultant input from a range of specialties—anaesthetic, surgical, cardiology, haematology, as well as postoperative ITU care. Consideration should be given to the resources available locally, and transfer to a tertiary centre might have to be considered in view of her complex cardiac history. The patient and her family should be made aware of the high risk of severe postoperative complications including death. The pertinent points as set above means that in order to decide between a regional technique or a general anaesthesia +/− nerve block, the following have to be taken into account: • There is no clear evidence to suggest one technique over the other. Weigh the benefits and risks and choose your anaesthetic method. • Although an INR of 1.5 does not preclude a spinal, a regional technique would not only be difficult (obese and positioning problem) but could lead to a potential catastrophic cardiovascular instability due to associated vasodilatation. • A general anaesthetic would allow for more control of blood pressure and cardiac output. But as discussed previously, choose one technique and explain the reasons behind your choice. **Preoperative** • Assessment—history and examination to look for decompensation • Optimisation of medical therapy—to decrease symptoms and prevent disease progression • Investigations—to assess cardiac function **Intraoperative** • Anaesthetic—GA or RA with application of general principles (see below). • Invasive monitoring—arterial line, CVP, oesophageal Doppler, or other method of cardiac output monitoring is useful. • Analgesia—regional block like fascia iliaca block with catheter can be considered for postoperative analgesia. Avoid NSAIDS due to susceptibility to renal failure and fluid retention. • Fluid balance—strict fluid balance guided by invasive monitoring is important. • Temperature control—maintains cardiac stability. • Antibiotics—for endocarditis and surgical prophylaxis.

STEPS	KEY POINTS

According to NICE guidelines, antibiotics should not be given routinely to patients with heart valve replacement but discussed on a case-by-case basis. This is a change from the past recommendations based on the increase in antibiotic resistance.

From the surgery point of view, the NICE guidelines have to be adhered to and antibiotics given at least 30 min prior to the start of the operation. Cefuroxime 1.5 g is commonly used and Teicoplanin 400 mg can also be given, as this patient group has a high MRSA contamination level.

Postoperative
ITU care is advisable due to chance of increased risk of:
- Cardiac failure
- Myocardial infarction
- Renal failure
- Endocarditis
- Valve failure
- TIA/CVA
- Death

General principles

Avoid
- Tachycardia and arrhythmias
- Hypotension/hypertension
- Hypovolemia
- Hypoxia and hypercarbia
- Anaemia
- Pain

Maintain
- Preload
- Contractility
- Afterload
- Fluid balance
- Tissue perfusion and cardiac output

Patient has advanced directive with DNAR status. Does this affect your management?

This does not affect the initial management as do not resuscitate doesn't mean do not treat, but it will help putting in place treatment ceilings if the patient deteriorates and is not responding to the therapy implemented.

What do you know about bone cement implantation (BCIS) syndrome?

BCIS is an important cause of intraoperative morbidity and mortality. It happens as a result of right ventricular failure due to increase in pulmonary vascular resistance and increased pulmonary artery pressure.

What is the composition of bone cement?

The important constituents of bone cement are:
Polymer—polymethyl methacrylate (PMMA) as a white powder
Liquid monomer—methyl methacrylate (MMA)
Activator—N, N-dimethyl-p-toluidine
Antibiotics—optional

Once mixed together, the powder particles become entrapped and glued within the net of the polymerised monomer.

What do you know about the pathophysiology?

Emboli theory
Reaming of the femur increases intramedullary pressure and releases debris such as marrow, bone, fat, and along with the cement particles, they embolise to the right heart and cause increased pulmonary artery pressure.

STEPS	KEY POINTS

Mediators theory

Systemic embolisation of the bone cement causes release of proinflammatory mediators such as histamine, complement factors, thrombin and tissue thromboplastin, which further increases the pulmonary vascular resistance and bronchoconstriction and V/Q mismatch.

How can you grade the BCIS according to severity?

I: Moderate hypoxia ($SpO_2 > 94\%$) or a decrease in systolic arterial pressure > 20%.

II: Severe hypoxia (SpO_2 44%) or unexpected loss of consciousness.

III: Cardiovascular collapse requiring cardiopulmonary resuscitation.

What are the risk factors for the development of BCIS?

Patient factors
ASA III/IV
Preexisting pulmonary hypertension
Significant cardiorespiratory disease
Osteoporosis

Surgical factors
Pathological fracture
Intertrochanteric fracture
Long-stem arthroplast

How would you prevent and treat BCIS?

Prevention

General
Identify high-risk patients
Avoid cemented arthroplasty in these patients

Anaesthetic management
Optimise the cardiovascular reserve
Maintain normovolaemia and high inspired oxygen
Avoid haemodynamic compromise

Surgical management
Thorough lavage of the medullary canal
Good haemostasis
Specific cement mixing method

Treatment
High flow oxygen
IV fluids
Pulmonary vasodilators
Inotropes (Dobutamine, Milrinone)
Invasive monitoring

BCIS is reversible, and the pulmonary artery pressures normalise within 24 hours. This means effective resuscitation is essential to decreasing the morbidity and mortality of this potentially life-threatening condition.

Further reading

1. Olsen F, Kotyra M, Houltz E, Ricksten SE. Bone cement implantation syndrome in cemented hemiarthroplasty for femoral neck fracture: incidence, risk factors, and effect of outcome. *Br. J. Anaesth.* first published online July 16, 2014 doi:10.1093/bja/aeu226.
2. The management of hip fracture in adults. *NICE Guideline CG124*. June 2011.
3. Antimicrobial prophylaxis against infective endocarditis. *NICE Clinical Guidelines, CG64*. March 2008.
4. Surgical site infection. *Quality Standards QS49*. October 2013.
5. 2013 ACCF/AHA *Guidelines for the Management of Heart Failure.*

08.2 SHORT CASE: SUPRAVENTRICULAR TACHYCARDIA

HISTORY *You are asked to review a 2-year-old child in recovery who is agitated and distressed after an elective myringotomy/grommets.*

STEPS	KEY POINTS
What is your differential diagnosis and management plan?	• Full history and examination • Full set of observations • Ensure parents/carers are present **Differential diagnosis** • Patient factors: separation anxiety, requiring feeding/water or nappy change, unfamiliar environment/people • Anaesthetic factors: Inadequate analgesia, hypoxia, hypothermia, inadequate ventilation, sore throat • Surgical factors: displacement of myringotomy tube • Unrelated medical problem **Management** • Ensure parent/carer present to reassure and comfort. • Assess ABC. • Give analgesia/antiemetic as indicated. • Ensure well oxygenated, not hypercarbic or hypothermic. • Allow to feed if appropriate. Check and change nappy. • Ask surgeons to review. • Reassess as required. *The recovery staff did an ECG as the child was 'very tachycardic'.*
What does the ECG in Figure 8.3 show?	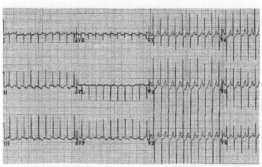 Fig. 8.3

The ECG shows a narrow complex tachycardia, rate ~ 300 bpm

STEPS	KEY POINTS
You are told the child is not decompensating (no evidence of shock) as yet. How do you manage?	See Figure 8.4.

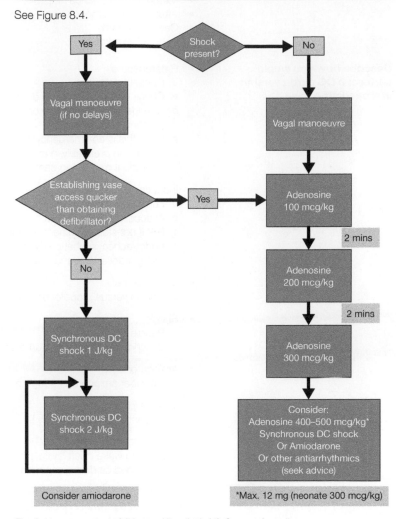

Fig. 8.4 Image courtesy of Advanced Paediatric Life Support Australia

How many joules would you shock with in this case?	Energy is calculated according to weight.
	Formula for weight in children of 1–5 years: Weight (in kgs) = (2 × age in years) + 8 In this case: Weight = (2 × 2) + 8 = 12 kg
	Therefore, energy for shocks is as follows: 1 J/kg = 12 J; 2 J/kg = 24 J (rounded to nearest J on defibrillator)
What is the dose of adenosine in this child?	Weight 12 kg based on formula above • Start dose 100 mcg/kg = 1200 mcg • Then 200 mcg/kg after 2 mins if no effect = 2400 mcg • Then 300 mcg/kg after 2 mins if no effect = 3600 mcg • Up to a max of 500 mcg/kg = 6000 mcg

STEPS	KEY POINTS
What are the potential causes of SVT in a 2-year-old?	• Re-entrant congenital conduction pathway abnormality (common) • Poisoning • Metabolic disturbance • After cardiac surgery • Cardiomyopathy • Long QT syndrome

Describe how you would perform a DC cardioversion in a paediatric case.	• Preprocedure
	  o Consent parents.
	  o Check electrolytes (could do a quick venous blood gas).
	  o Arrange for a second senior anaesthetist and paediatrician to be present.
	  o State this is an emergency if signs of decompensation are present.
	  o Performed preferably in an anaesthetic room, if not in an area where equivalent monitoring can occur.
	
	• Induction
	  o Full AAGBI monitoring
	  o IV access (if not going to distress the child)
	  o RSI if not starved, otherwise gas induction and maintenance
	  o Endotracheal intubation if aspiration risk; otherwise, may be able to use guedel airway and mask
	
	• Maintenance
	  o Volatile versus propofol boluses
	
	• Shock
	  o Paddles front to back
	  o Synchronised shock at 1 J/kg up to 2 J/kg
	
	• Amiodarone
	  o Consider amiodarone 5 mg/kg
	
	• 12-lead ECG
	  o To confirm no longer in SVT
	
	• Emergence/recovery
	  o Allow to wake in left lateral position
	  o Prolonged cardiac monitoring in recovery or on paediatric ward
	
	• Follow-up
	  o Will need review and follow-up by paediatricians and/or paediatric cardiologist

Future Reading

1. *Advanced Paediatric Life Support. The Practical Approach.* Fifth Edition 2011.
2. Doniger S, et al. Pediatric dysrhythmias. *Pediatr Clin N Am.* 2006; **53**: 85–105.

08.3 SHORT CASE: CYSTIC FIBROSIS

HISTORY *A 30-year-old female patient is listed for repair of median nerve and brachial artery on trauma list, and the orthopaedic surgeon informs you that this patient suffers from cystic fibrosis.*

STEPS	KEY POINTS
What do you know about cystic fibrosis?	Cystic fibrosis is an autosomal recessive genetic disorder that is characterised by abnormal transport of Na^+ and Cl^- ions across the epithelium of various organs causing thick viscous secretion. It can affect various organs, mainly lungs, pancreas, intestine, and liver.
What is the pathophysiology? How does chloride channel affect mucus?	The basic pathology is mutation in the cystic fibrosis transmembrane regulator (CFTR) gene located on chromosome 7, which creates a protein that does not normally fold on the membrane and is easily degraded by cells.
	The protein created by this gene is anchored to the outer membrane of cells in the sweat glands, lungs, pancreas, and all other remaining exocrine glands in the body and spans this membrane, acting as a channel that connects the inner part of the cell (cytoplasm) to the surrounding fluid. This channel is primarily responsible for controlling the movement of halogens from inside to outside the cell; however, in the sweat ducts, it facilitates the movement of chloride from the sweat into the cytoplasm. When the CFTR protein is faulty, chloride and thiocyanate are trapped inside the cells in the airway and outside in the skin. Because chloride is negatively charged, this creates a difference in the electrical potential inside and outside the cell, causing cations to cross into the cell. Sodium is the most common cation in the extracellular space, and the combination of sodium and chloride creates the salt, which is lost in high amounts in the sweat of individuals with CF. This lost salt forms the basis for the sweat test.
What are the effects of cystic fibrosis on different organs?	Cystic fibrosis causes blockage of narrow passage of the affected organ with thick secretions. **Respiratory system** • Presence of abnormal CFTR protein causes imbalance in Na absorption and inability to secret Cl^- ion, resulting in inadequate fluid secretion and dehydration of airways. • Dehydration of mucus and periciliary liquid layers produces adhesion of mucous to the airway surface, which leads to the failure to clear mucus. These retained secretions of mucus lead to chronic infections, which later result in bronchiectasis. • Eventually it leads to cor pulmonale, heart failure, and death.

STEPS	KEY POINTS

GIT
- Pancreas: Failure of secretion of sodium bicarbonate and water leads to retention of enzymes in the pancreas and destruction of pancreatic tissue and fibrosis of pancreatic tissue.
- Intestine: Because of the lack of secretion of Cl^- and water, the CF intestinal epithelium fails to flush secreted mucus from intestinal crypts, leading to dehydrated intraluminal contents and obstruction. Intestinal fluid contains less water and bicarbonate, which manifests as increased faecal fat excretion and steatorrhoea.
- Liver and gall bladder: Thickened biliary secretions, focal biliary cirrhosis, cholecystitis, and cholelithiasis.

Sweat glands
- Cystic fibrosis patients secrete nearly normal volumes of sweat in the sweat acinus but are not able to absorb NaCl from sweat ducts, resulting in higher concentration of salt in sweat.

Reproductive system
- Men: Infertility due to azoospermia and obliteration of vas deferens
- Women: Thick, tenacious cervical mucus blocks sperm migration

How is cystic fibrosis diagnosed?

Diagnosis is mainly based on a combination of clinical criteria and abnormal CFTR function as documented by sweat tests. Chloride concentration > 70 mEq/L differentiates between CF and other conditions.

Genetic testing for abnormal gene and protein is also definite diagnostic method.

How will you optimise this patient?

This is a trauma patient suffering from a neuro-vascular injury that requires urgent treatment, failture of which can lead to permanent damage. Although there is limited time for optimisation, the following measures may be undertaken:
- IV fluids, history, and long-term treatment review plus routine anaesthetic history, examination, and basic investigations including chest X-ray to rule out any active chest infection.
- Full blood count, urea and electrolytes, liver function test, clotting screening, and blood glucose level.
- Baseline arterial blood gas measurement and spirometry will guide the perioperative care.
- Make sure that the patient is adequately hydrated, bronchodilator treatment may be administered, mucolytic inhalation and preoperative chest physiotherapy help to minimise postoperative chest infections.
- Preoperative sputum culture will also be helpful for choosing appropriate antibiotics in postoperative period.
- Start insulin infusion if indicated to maintain blood glucose within normal limits

STEPS	KEY POINTS
What are the anaesthetic options for this patient?	As the respiratory system is involved in all cystic fibrosis patients, regional anaesthesia is more preferable whenever possible.
	This patient will benefit from regional anaesthesia in the form of interscalene block, but all disability or motor and sensory loss due to median nerve damage must be documented prior to theatres.
	Follow usual guidelines for any regional anaesthesia such as gaining consent, ruling out any contraindications, using resuscitation facilities, trained assistants, monitoring, and full asepsis technique.
	The interscalene block should be performed under ultrasound guidance as this will prevent complications such as pneumothorax, which can be detrimental in this patient.
	If there is any contraindication for regional anaesthesia over general anaesthesia, consider the following points: • Endotracheal intubation will give a better control of airway and will provide access for tracheal suctioning intraoperatively, which will improve gas exchange. • Use short-acting drugs. • Inhalation agents with bronchodilator properties such as sevoflurane are preferable. • Humidified gases and warm IV fluids. • Postoperative pain relief and HDU monitoring if necessary. • Bronchodilators, mucolytic agents, and regular physiotherapy in postoperative period is absolutely essential to prevent any chest infection.

Further Reading

1. Huffmyer JL, Littlewood KE, Nemergut EC. Perioperative management of the adult with cystic fibrosis. *Anesth Analg.* 2009; **109**: 1949–61.
2. Wiehe M, Arndt K. Cystic fibrosis: a systems review. *AANA J.* 2010; **78**: 246–51.
3. Fitzgerald M and Ryan D. Cystic fibrosis and anaesthesia. *Contin Educ Anaesth Crit Care Pain.* First published online September 29, 2011. doi:10.1093/bjaceaccp/mkr038

08.4 SHORT CASE: PNEUMOTHORAX

HISTORY *A 20-year-old male brought to the Accident and Emergency department following a traffic accident is complaining of pain in the pelvis.*

Vital Observations

Pulse: 100/min
Blood Pressure: 140/80 mmHg
Respiratory rate: 26/min
SpO$_2$ 96% on 8 litres of oxygen
GCS: E4V5M6
Chest X-ray provided in Figure 8.5.

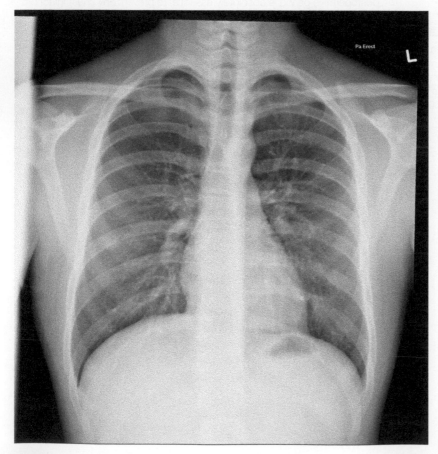

Fig. 8.5

STEPS	KEY POINTS
How will you manage this patient in A&E resus?	• ATLS approach • Primary survey, including monitoring and X-rays
Describe the chest X-ray.	• Simple right apical pneumothorax; the lung border is visible.
What is your management?	• ABC approach • Assess whether the airway is patent and if the patient has adequate effort of ventilation • Simple aspiration of the pneumothorax and intercostal tube drainage with an underwater seal
How would you perform this procedure?	• Determine site of insertion. (This is usually the 5th intercostal space anterior to the mid axillary line on the affected site. The second intercostal space in the midclavicular line is sometimes chosen for apical pneumothoraces. But this is not recommended due to complications like vascular damage and discomfort.) • Follow strict asepsis. • Local anaesthetic infiltration of skin and rib periosteum. • Make a 2–3 cm horizontal incision over the top of the rib. • Perform blunt dissection of subcutaneous tissue. • The parietal pleura is punctured and finger inserted to avoid organ injury and to clear adhesions. • The proximal end of the thoracostomy tube is clamped and advanced directing it posteriorly in the chest wall. • Connect end of tube to underwater seal. • Suture in place and dress the wound. • Look for bubbling in the underwater seal and fogging of tube. • Order a chest X-ray.
Describe the features of the underwater seal.	• The thoracostomy tube must be wide enough to avoid resistance with its volumetric capacity in excess of half the patient's maximal inspiratory volume. • The volume of water in the underwater seal should be in excess of half the patient's maximal inspiratory volume to avoid water from being drawn in during inspiration. • The drain must be 45 cm below the patient.
Can you connect suction to the tube?	• Routine suction should be avoided. • A persistent air leak with or without incomplete re-expansion of lung is the usual reason. • High-volume, low-pressure suction systems are recommended by the British Thoracic Society.
How would the treatment differ if this were a tension pneumothorax?	• Tension pneumothorax is a medical emergency and is associated with cardiovascular instability. • The treatment is with supplemental oxygen therapy and immediate needle decompression. • A cannula can be introduced in the second anterior intercostal space in the mid-clavicular line on the side of the pneumothorax. • This is then followed by a chest drain.

STEPS	KEY POINTS
What are the treatment options for a simple spontaneous pneumothorax?	According to the British Thoracic Society guidelines: • Breathlessness indicates the need for active intervention and oxygen therapy. • The size of the pneumothorax determines the rate of resolution and is a relative indication for active intervention. • Small pneumothoraces (< 2 cm visible rim between the lung margin and chest wall at the level of hilum) in the absence of breathlessness may be managed with observation alone.
This patient needs a general anaesthetic as he has a dislocated shoulder on the left side. How will you proceed?	• Intubation is the choice if fasting status is not known or with a full stomach. • Trauma, pain, and opiate analgesics are associated with delayed gastric emptying, so this subgroup of patients is at high risk for aspiration of gastric contents. • An intercostal drain with an underwater seal is necessary, prior to intubation, as otherwise a simple pneumothorax can be converted to a tension pneumothorax with positive pressure ventilation. • Nitrous oxide should be avoided as it can rapidly increase the size of the pneumothorax. • Brachial plexus blocks which carry a risk of pneumothorax, and phrenic nerve block which can cause diaphragm dysfunction must be avoided on the other side.

Further reading

1. Macduff A, Arnold A, Harvey J. Management of Spontaneous Pneumothorax. *British Thoracic Society Pleural Disease Guideline 2010*, Section 2.

section 08

BASIC SCIENCE VIVA

08.5
ANATOMY: PITUITARY

Possible questions include:

How do pituitary tumours present, the anatomy and physiology of the pituitary gland, effects of hypo- and hyper-secretion, anaesthetic implications in acromegaly,

… sodium abnormalities post-operatively, diabetes insipidus, syndrome of inappropriate ADH secretion, investigations, diagnosis and treatment

… pituitary hormones, portal circulation, hypothalamo-pituitary axis, Cushing's disease and its anaesthetic implications, hormone replacement

… anatomy and physiology of pituitary gland, pressure effects of tumours, anaesthesia for transsphenoidal hypophysectomy

STEPS	KEY POINTS
How does a patient with pituitary tumour present?	• Hormonal dysfunction—could be over/under secretion of pituitary hormones. • Mass effect—compression of surrounding tissues due to the rapidly growing tumour, increased intracranial pressure. • Incidentalomas—with no hormonal or pressure effect. Diagnosed during imaging for other conditions. • Pituitary apoplexy—emergency situation with signs of acute hormonal imbalance, meningism, visual impairment and other signs of intracranial pathology. This is due to infarction or sudden haemorrhage in an already existing pituitary adenoma.
Describe the anatomy of the pituitary gland.	Pituitary is the 'master gland', secreting hormones that control most of the body functions. It is a pea-sized organ present beneath the hypothalamus in the *sella turcica*—a depression at the base of skull. It is made up of two types of tissues forming the anterior and posterior pituitary gland. *Anterior pituitary gland (adenohypophysis)* is an evagination of the ectodermal Rathke's pouch (nasopharynx) containing **epithelial tissue.**

STEPS	KEY POINTS

- Traditionally, three cell types were distinguished when stained with hematoxylin and eosin.
  - Acidophils stain orange/red and secrete polypeptide hormones—growth hormone (GH) and prolactin (PRL)
  - Basophils stain blue and secrete glycopeptide hormones—thyroid-stimulating hormone (TSH), gonadotrophic hormones (LH/FSH), and adrenocorticotrophic hormone (ACTH).
  - Chromophobes are nonstaining, due to the nonsecretory nature of the cells.

- Currently these cells are classified according to the hormones they produce.
  - Somatotropes make up the majority of the anterior pituitary cells. They produce GH and are responsible for 20% of all pituitary microadenomas.
  - Lactotropes secrete PRL, and prolactinomas are the commonest cause of pituitary adenomas.
  - Thyrotropes—TSH.
  - Gonadotropes—LH/FSH
  - Corticotropes—ACTH

The signal for the secretion by these cells comes from the hypothalamus via individual regulatory hormones. The hypothalamic and the corresponding pituitary hormones, their site of action, and their functions are depicted in Table 8.1.

Posterior pituitary gland (neurohypophysis) is an extension of the brain at the level of the diencephalon and hence contains **neural tissue.**
- Made of pituicytes, which are similar to glial cells.
- It does not produce any hormones but rather stores and releases the hypothalamic hormones (namely, oxytocin and antidiuretic hormone). These hormones are produced by the paraventricular and supraoptic nuclei, respectively (although each nucleus secretes a small proportion of the other hormone), which then pass through the neural axons into the posterior pituitary. The terminal portions of the axons, which store these hormone granules called *Herring bodies,* are closely associated with fenestrated capillaries.

Table 8.1 Hypothalamic and pituitary hormones and their functions

Hypothalamus	Pituitary	Sites of action	Other hormones	Functions
GHRH	Somatotropes—GH	All body cells	–	Protein synthesis, Gluconeogenesis, lipolysis, sodium and water absorption
PIH	Lactotropes—inhibits PRL secretion	Breast	–	Prolactin causes milk production
GnRH	Gonadotropes—LH/FSH	Testes, ovaries	–	Spermatogenesis, ovarian follicular growth
TRH	Thyrotropes—TSH	Thyroid gland	T3 and T4	General growth and metabolism
CRH	Corticotropes—ACTH	Adrenal gland	Glucocorticoids Mineralocorticoids	Gluconeogenesis, lipolysis, sodium and water reabsorption, anti-inflammatory
Oxytocin	–	Breast, kidney	–	Milk secretion and contraction of uterus, water retention
ADH	–	Blood vessel, kidney	–	Arterial vasoconstriction, water reabsorption

STEPS	KEY POINTS

What is the blood supply of the pituitary gland?

Arterial supply

Superior and inferior hypophyseal arteries, which are branches of the internal carotid artery.

- The superior hypophyseal artery ramifies into the *hypthalamo hypophyseal portal circulatory system*. The primary capillary network lies at the pituitary stalk, where the hypothalamic hormones are released. This capillary bed is drained by a set of long portal veins that give rise to the second capillary bed in the anterior pituitary.
- The veins originating in the neurohypophyseal capillary plexus give rise to the short portal veins that will also contribute to the adenohypophyseal capillary plexus and connect the two circulatory systems.
- This hypothalamo-hypophyseal portal system creates a communication between the endocrine and neural cells providing an easy short-loop feedback between the two sets of cells.

Venous drainage

Cavernous sinus → Petrosal sinus → Jugular vein

What is portal circulation, and what are the other examples in the body?

The portal circulation begins and ends in capillaries. Arterial capillaries normally end up forming a vein that enters the right side of the heart. In portal circulation, the primary capillary network drains into a vein known as *portal vein*, which then branches to form the second set of capillaries before draining into a venous system. Other examples of portal circulation in the body are the hepatic portal, placental, renal, ovarian, and testicular circulations.

What are the types of pituitary tumours? What are their clinical manifestations?

Pituitary tumours are responsible for at least three-fourths of all intracranial neoplasms. Considering the size of tumour, they could be divided as:

Microadenomas

- < 10 mm diameter
- Commonly occurring pituitary adenomas
- Clinical effects are mainly due to hormonal hyper-secretion

Macroadenomas

- > 10 mm in size
- Nonsecretory tumours
- Effects are usually due to mass and pressure effects leading to visual disturbances, increased intracranial pressure, and hypopituitarism due to destruction of pituitary tissue.

The pituitary gland is surrounded by structures as shown in Figure 8.6. so the pressure effects relate to the tissues closely related to the tumour.

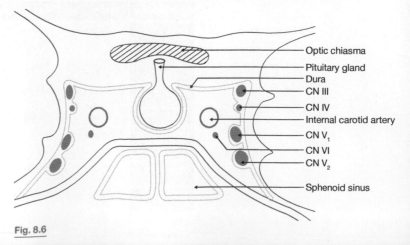

Optic chiasma
Pituitary gland
Dura
CN III
CN IV
Internal carotid artery
CN V$_1$
CN VI
CN V$_2$
Sphenoid sinus

Fig. 8.6

STEPS	KEY POINTS

Floor—sphenoidal air sinus
Roof—diaphragma sella, an invagination of dura, which is traversed by the pituitary stalk, optic chiasm
Lateral walls—cavernous sinus, internal carotid artery, CN III, IV, V$_1$, V$_2$, and VI

Explain the control of GH release.

The stimulation (+) and inhibition (−) of GH secretion is shown schematically in Figure 8.7.

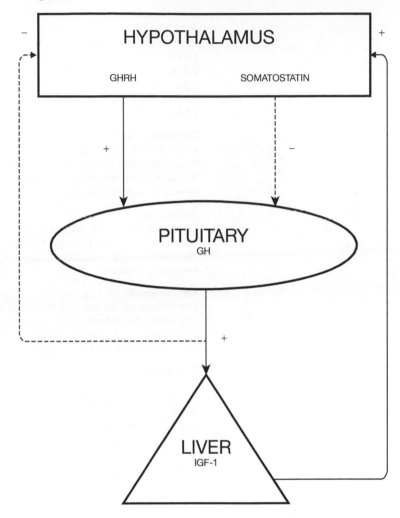

Fig. 8.7

IGF-1 (Somatomedin C) is a hormone that is secreted mainly from the liver upon stimulation by GH. The functions of this hormone are similar to the GH and cause bone and muscle growth along with lipolysis. As the half life of IGF-1 is longer than the GH and does not have a diurnal variation, IGF-1 assay is used to diagnose GH excess or deficiency.

STEPS	KEY POINTS

What is acromegaly and what are its features?

Acromegaly is a condition where there is an increased secretion of the GH in adults. The term gigantism is used when this occurs before epiphyseal fusion. It is a rare condition affecting 6–8 per million.
The main features affecting anaesthesia are discussed.

Airway
Increased size of the skull with prominent lower jaw and malocclusion, macroglossia, thickening of the laryngeal and pharyngeal soft tissues, laryngeal stenosis, hoarse voice due to recurrent laryngeal nerve palsy. In a minority of the patients, there is associated thyroid enlargement leading to tracheal compression. All these features make acromegaly a recognised cause of difficult ventilation and intubation. Careful preassessment, including indirect laryngoscopy, helps with the choice of intubation technique. The mallampati grades can be falsely reassuring and every step is taken to overcome a difficult airway. Awake fibreoptic intubation might be necessary as is awake tracheostomy.

Cardiovascular
About 30% of acromegalic patients have hypertension. Myocardial hypertrophy, interstitial fibrosis, and cardiomegaly leads to ischaemic heart disease and left ventricular dysfunction. ECG and ECHO are mandatory to assess the cardiac function.

Respiratory
Coarsening of features leading to upper airway obstruction, spirometry shows an obstructive picture. The associated obstructive sleep apnoea requires investigation and appropriate treatment to reduce postoperative respiratory morbidity.

Neurological
Compression of surrounding structures leading to visual disturbances, increased ICP, cavernous sinus thrombosis. CN II involvement leads to impaired visual acuity and bitemporal hemianopia. CN III, IV, and VI involvement cause ophthalmoplegia and other visual disturbances.

Endocrine
Impaired glucose tolerance and diabetes mellitus complicates more than 25% of acromegalic patients. This necessitates careful glucose monitoring and treatment with variable rate insulin infusion perioperatively. There is a high likelihood of high PRL secretion contributing to menstrual problems in women and sexual dysfunction in men.

Others
Increased size of hands and feet, arthropathy, myopathy, osteoporosis.

How is acromegaly diagnosed and what are the different modalities of treatment?

Due to the insidious onset of the condition, the diagnosis can be delayed for even a decade.
- Clinical appearance
- Signs and symptoms
- Random GH or IGF-1 concentration
- Failure of suppression of GH after 75 mg glucose administration (GTT)
- MRI to look at the size and extent of tumour

Treatment is aimed at controlling the size and reducing the effects of the tumour. Untreated acromegaly is associated with a 2 to 2.5 times increased mortality compared to healthy adults.

- Surgery
  Is the mainstay of treatment and is currently done by minimally invasive endoscopic procedure through the transsphenoidal route.

STEPS	KEY POINTS

- Drug therapy
  - *Dopamine agonist* —usually Cabergoline.
  - *Somatostatin analogues*—usually octreotide. This helps to reduce the size of tumour before surgery.
  - *Growth hormone receptor antagonist*—expensive but has been shown to normalise the levels of IGF-1.

- Radiotherapy
  Takes longer time to work. But with the invention of the 'gamma-knife' radiosurgery, remission can be achieved in less time.

What are the anaesthetic concerns in a patient undergoing surgery for acromegaly?

Anaesthetic concerns could be divided according to the factors pertaining to:
- Neurosurgical anaesthesia and its implications
  - Haemodynamic stability
  - Maintenance of cerebral oxygenation
  - Prevention of perioperative complications
  - Rapid emergence to facilitate early neurological assessment
  - Adequate postoperative analgesia and antiemesis
  - Anaesthesia for transsphenoidal pituitary surgery is not covered in this question.

- Acromegaly and its implications
  - Effects of acromegaly on various organ functions—airway and other systems as above
  - Intra- and postoperative complications—airway and respiratory compromise, haemorrhage, air embolism, etc.
  - Diabetes insipidus

Explain the physiology of diabetes insipidus after pituitary surgery.

Diabetes insipidus (DI) is due to decreased secretion of (central) or response to (nephrogenic) ADH. Inappropriate water loss leads to *hypernatremia and increased serum osmolality in the context of large volumes of dilute urine.*

Central DI can occur after traumatic brain injury, subarachnoid haemorrhage, infections, brain tumours, and post pituitary surgery. There is *decreased ADH release* characterised by polyuria, polydipsia, and thirst. The treatment aims at replacement of water and ADH. Intranasal (or intravenous) Deamino D arginine Vasopressin (DDAVP) has been the mainstay of treatment.

The criteria for the diagnosis of DI include:
- Increased urine volume > 3 L/day
- Increased serum sodium > 145 mmol/L
- Increased serum osmolality > 300 mOsm/kg
- Decreased urine osmolality < 300 mOsm/kg
- Decreased urine specific gravity < 1.005

Nephrogenic DI occurs due to X-linked recessive mutation or more commonly because of renal dysplasia and drugs such as lithium. *The ADH secretion is normal but the kidneys fail to respond to ADH,* resulting in polyuria. Exogenous ADH has no effect but the treatment is aimed at replacement of water and the use of thiazide diuretics as they allow increased excretion of sodium along with water and hence breaking the polydipsia-polyuria cycle.

STEPS	KEY POINTS
What do you mean by the syndrome of inappropriate ADH secretion (SIADH)?	SIADH is a self-limiting condition where there is increased ADH leading to increased reabsorption of water at the collecting ducts. There is *hyponatremia and decreased serum osmolality in the context of small volumes of concentrated urine.*
	Causes could be manifold but are mainly head injury, meningitis, lung cancer, and infections such as lung and brain abscesses and drugs such as carbamazepine and amitryptilline.
	The diagnostic features include:
	• Decreased serum sodium < 135 mmol/L
	• Decreased serum osmolality < 280 mOsm/kg
	• Increased urine sodium
	• Increased urine osmolality
	• Normal renal and adrenal function
	Treatment is needed only in symptomatic patients and is by electrolyte-free fluid restriction, hypertonic saline and drugs—diuretics (frusemide), demeclocycline (suppresses renal response to ADH), and ADH receptor antagonists.
How does ADH stimulate water reabsorption?	Vasopressin-2 receptors (V_2 or aquaporin-2) are present in the cytoplasm of the principal cells at the collecting duct of the nephron. Stimulation by ADH causes transcription of the aquaporin-2, thereby moving the cytoplasmic aquaporin to the apical membrane. This results in the formation of water conduits through which water reabsorption occurs.

Further reading

1. Anaesthesia and pituitary disease. *Contin Educ Anaesth Crit Care Pain* (2011) **11** (4): 133–137. doi: 10.1093/bjaceaccp/mkr014 First published online: June 21, 2011.

08.6 PHYSIOLOGY: VENTILATOR ASSOCIATED PNEUMONIA

STEPS	KEY POINTS
What do you understand by the term ventilator associated pneumonia (VAP)?	The definition of VAP is the most subjective of the common device-related healthcare-associated infections.
	The National Institute of Clinical Excellence (NICE) 2008 defines VAP as the nosocomial pneumonia that develops 48 hours or more after mechanical ventilation given by means of endotracheal tube or tracheostomy.
	The American Thoracic Society refers to VAP as pneumonia that arises more than 48–72 hours after endotracheal intubation.
	It is the most common nosocomial infection encountered in the intensive care unit (ICU), ranging from 9%–28% of all mechanically ventilated patients with the peak incidence occurring around day 5 of ventilation. Mortality ranges from 24% to 50% and depends on the pathogen and underlying clinical condition of the patient.
What are some other types of pneumonias?	• Hospital-acquired pneumonia (HAP), or nosocomial pneumonia, develops after 48 hours or more after admission to a hospital. Hospitalised patients may have many risk factors for pneumonia, including mechanical ventilation, malnutrition, underlying comorbidities, and immune disturbances. The microorganisms responsible include Methicillin Resistant Staphylococcus Aureus (MRSA), Pseudomonas, Enterobacter, and Serratia.
	• Healthcare-associated pneumonia is the pneumonia that occurs in patients who are hospitalised for at least 2 days in the past 90 days, or are residents of a nursing home or treated with IV antibiotics, received chemotherapy in the last 30 days or haemofiltration in any setting.
	• Community-acquired pneumonia is defined by the British Thoracic Society as comprising symptoms of acute lower respiratory tract illness with new focal chest signs, at least one systemic feature such as fever, sweating, or a temperature $> 38°C$, and no other explanation for the illness. *Streptococcus pneumoniae* is the most common cause of community-acquired pneumonia worldwide.
	• Atypical pneumonia is the pneumonia caused by certain pathogens such as Legionella, Mycoplasma, and Chlamydia. The clinical and radiological features are usually different from commonly occurring pneumonias.

STEPS	KEY POINTS

- Aspiration pneumonia is the inhalation of either oropharyngeal or gastric contents into the lower airways. The resulting lung inflammation is not an infection, but if the aspirated material contains anaerobic bacteria, it can contribute to infection.
- Opportunistic pneumonia includes those that affect immuno-compromised individuals. Main pathogens are Cytomegalovirus, Pneumocystis jiroveci, Mycobacterium avium-intracellulare, and Candida.

What are the clinical and radiological features of VAP?

Accurate diagnosis is usually difficult, and a high index of suspicion is needed. Empirical antibiotic therapy with broad-spectrum antibiotics is started early after appropriate cultures are taken.

The diagnostic criteria include:
a) Clinical: Chest infection with signs such as fever, purulent aspirations, and leucocytosis.
b) Microbiological: bacteriological evidence of pulmonary infection.
c) Radiological: X-ray evidence of lung infection—new or progressive pulmonary infiltrates.

The Clinical Pulmonary Infection Score (CPIS) has been devised to increase the accuracy of diagnosis. The CPIS takes into account clinical (temperature, presence of tracheal secretions), physiological (leucocytosis and worsening gas exchange), microbiological (positive culture of tracheal aspirate), and radiographic evidence to assign a numerical value. Scores can range from 0 to 12 with a score of ≥ 6 showing good correlation with the presence of VAP although both the sensitivity (77%) and specificity (42%) of the score is low.

The appearance of new infiltrates on CXR plus two or more signs of pulmonary infection, such as new purulent secretions, worsening gas exchange, leucocytosis, or pyrexia, increases the likelihood of VAP.

What are the common pathogens associated with VAP?

Mainly caused by gram-negative organisms, but gram-positive bacteria such as MRSA are not uncommon.
Typically, bacteria causing *early onset VAP* include Streptococcus pneumoniae, Haemophilus influenzae, methicillin-sensitive Staphylococcus aureus (MSSA), Gram-negative bacilli, Escherichia coli, Klebsiella pneumonia, Enterobacter and Proteus species, and Serratia marcescens.

Culprits of *late VAP* are drug-resistant organisms such as MRSA, Acinetobacter, Pseudomonas aeruginosa, and extended-spectrum beta-lactamase producing bacteria (ESBL).

What are the risk factors for VAP?

Patient factors: advanced age, low serum albumin, ARDS, COPD and other lung diseases, impaired consciousness, trauma and burns, multiple organ failure, large volume gastric aspirates, and upper respiratory tract colonisation.

Interventional factors: prolonged ventilation, level of sedation, use of neuromuscular blocking agents, antacids, proton pump inhibitors (PPI) and H_2 blockers, nasogastric tube, supine position, frequent circuit changes, and transfer outside ICU.

STEPS	KEY POINTS
What is the pathological process of VAP?	It is thought to be caused by entry of infected secretions into distal bronchi. Patients are usually immunosuppressed, and their oropharynx becomes colonised with organisms, especially gram-negative bacteria. Oral and nasal tubes cause trauma, leading to infections such as sinusitis.
	The natural protections like cough reflex, tracheobronchial secretions, mucociliary linings, saliva, and nasal mucosa are less effective in these patients.
	The pathogens enter the lower lung through mechanical routes such as around the endotracheal tube cuff, suction catheter, and ventilation tubings.
How do you prevent VAP?	General measures: Use of sterile equipment, regular hand washing, using barrier nursing such as gloves and an apron, and minimal contact with patient usually reduce the incidence of any infection in ICU.
	Specific measures: This include reducing the load of pathogens and their entry into lower respiratory tract.

- *Reducing aero-digestive colonisation*
  - Oral decontamination using topical antiseptics such as chlorhexidine mouthwash
  - Selective decontamination of digestive tract (SDD) using nonabsorbable antimicrobials such as polymyxin E and amphotericin B has been tried with variable success. Although studies suggest that SDD is effective in reducing the incidence of VAP, this intervention is not commonly used in the UK because of fears of encouraging Clostridium difficile, antimicrobial resistance, and the emergence of multi-drug resistant pathogens.

- *Reducing aspiration*
  - Nursing the patient in semi-recumbent position is crucial and proven to reduce VAP significantly.
  - Colonisation and leak around the tracheal cuff is a cause for migration of pathogens to lungs. Secretions should be cleared from top of the cuff regularly by subglottic suctioning, and cuff pressures are maintained at acceptable levels (> 20 cms H_2O) to prevent micro-aspiration.

- *Minimising duration of ventilation*
  - This is achieved by early tracheostomy, which has proven to lower the incidence of VAP. Periodic 'sedative interruptions' and daily assessment of readiness to extubate may reduce the duration of mechanical ventilation.

- *Choice of drugs to change pH of gastric contents*
  - Reducing the acidity of stomach in stress ulcer prophylaxis is claimed to increase the incidence of VAP by increasing the proliferation of gram-negative bacteria. Use of H_2 blockers or sucralfate, instead of PPIs, are suggested to reduce the risk.
  - Enteral feeding can increase the risk of VAP by altering the gastric acidity and risk of aspiration, but benefits of enteral feeding usually outweigh this small risk.

Further reading

1. Technical patient safety solutions for prevention of ventilator-associated pneumonia in adults: understanding NICE guidance. http://guidance.nice.org.uk/PSG002

08.7 PHARMACOLOGY: ANTICHOLINESTERASES

STEPS	KEY POINTS
How do anticholinesterases exert their effects?	They inhibit the action of acetylcholinesterase (AChE) by occupying its active site, thus preventing it from breaking down acetylcholine (ACh). However, the actions of anticholinesterases are not specific to the neuromuscular junction (NMJ); therefore, autonomic cholinergic effects are also seen (bradycardia, salivation). Thus, anticholinesterases are often given with an anticholinergic (e.g. glycopyrrolate).
What are the indications for anticholinesterases?	<ul><li>Reverse effects of nondepolarising neuromuscular blocking drugs by increasing the amount of ACh available to compete with the neuromuscular blocking drugs at the neuromuscular junction</li><li>Diagnosis of myasthenia gravis (Tensilon test)</li><li>Treatment of myasthenia gravis</li><li>Active ingredient in pesticides and nerve gases</li><li>Treatment for urinary retention</li><li>Treatment for paralytic ileus</li><li>Treatment for glaucoma</li></ul>
How do you classify anticholinesterases?	There are three groups of anticholinesterases based on their mechanisms of action:

Easily reversible inhibition
- Only example is edrophonium.
- Phenolic quaternary amine.
- Used to distinguish between a myasthenic crisis (muscle power improved) and cholinergic crisis (clinical symptoms worsened).
- The amine group is attracted to the anionic site of AChE, whilst its hydroxyl group forms a hydrogen bond at the esteratic site, stabilising the complex.
- ACh is therefore unable to reach the active site of AChE.
- This complex is easily reversible; therefore, ACh can compete with edrophonium for AChE.

Formation of a carbamylated enzyme complex
- e.g. neostigmine, pyridostigmine, physostigmine
- Carbamate esters
- Produce a carbamylated enzyme when reacting with AChE
- This complex has a slower rate of hydrolysis than ACh and AChE complex; therefore, it stops AChE hydrolysing Ach

STEPS	KEY POINTS

Irreversible inactivation by organophosphorous compounds
- Organophosphate compounds are highly toxic.
- They are the main ingredients in insecticides (e.g. tetraethylpyrophosphate [TEPP]) or nerve gases (e.g. Sarin).
- Esteratic site of AChE is phosphorylated by organophosphorous compounds, resulting in enzyme inhibition.
- The complex formed is very stable and is resistant to hydrolysis or reactivation.
- Plama cholinesterases are also inhibited.

How does organophosphate poisoning present?

Organophosphates are highly lipid soluble and therefore rapidly absorbed across the skin.

Toxic manifestations include nicotinic and muscarinic effects, autonomic instability, and CNS effects.

Mild
- Miosis, blurred vision
- Excess salivation
- Headache
- Nausea
- Mild muscle weakness and muscle twitching
- Mild agitation

Moderate
- Pinpoint pupils, conjunctival injection
- Disorientation
- Coughing, wheezing, sneezing, drooling
- Bronchospasm and difficulty in breathing

Severe
- Confusion and agitation
- Convulsions
- Cardiac arrhythmias
- Respiratory depression and arrest
- Coma and death

How do you treat organophosphate poisoning?

General
- Ensure person protective equipment is worn and that patient has been decontaminated.
- Remove patient's clothing if not already done and place in double bag, seal, and store securely.
- Shower, wash down, or rinse with liquid soap and water.
- Irrigate eyes with lukewarm water/normal saline solution.
- If ingestion of organophosphates within previous 2 hours, activated charcoal may be used.

Specific
- Airway: Intubate and ventilate if required, use suction on secretions. Avoid suxamethonium.
- Breathing: 100% oxygen.
- Circulation: Large bore access, ABG, U&E, glucose, monitor ECG, and treat arrhythmias.
- Alert local health protection team and seek expert advice (e.g. Toxbase).

STEPS	KEY POINTS
	Drugs

- Atropine: For moderate and severe symptoms, give atropine 0.6–4 mg IV (child 20 mcg/kg IV), every 10–20 minutes until secretions dry up.
- Pralidoxime: 2 g or 30 mg/kg IV for adult over 4 minutes. Continue every 4–6 hours or commence infusion. May be continued for 7 days until atropine is not required.
- Diazepam: 5–10 mg iv adult, 1–5 mg iv child.

08.8 PHYSICS: HUMIDITY/TEMPERATURE

STEPS	KEY POINTS
Why is humidification important?	**Respiratory tract effects** Without humidification, gases can dry and keratinise part of the bronchial tree, reducing ciliary activity and impairing mucociliary clearance. Over time, inflammatory changes can occur in the pulmonary epithelium, causing mucus plugging, atelectasis, and superimposed chest infection. All of the above will impair gas exchange. Patients undergoing prolonged anaesthesia, those with pre-existing pulmonary diseases, and those at extremes of ages are particularly at risk. **Degree of humidification** High humidity is uncomfortable. Low humidity increases the risk of static sparks.
How is humidity expressed?	**Absolute humidity** Mass of water vapour that is present per unit volume of gas SI unit g/m^3 or g/L Temperature dependent: At 20°C, it is 17 g/m^3; at 37°C, it is 44 g/m^3. **Relative humidity** Ratio of the mass of water in a given volume of air to the mass of water in the same volume were it to be fully saturated. Expressed as percentage.
What are the methods of humidification?	**Passive** Heat and moisture exchange filter **Active** Hot water bath humidifier Cascade humidifier Nebulisers—gas-driven or ultrasonic
How can humidity be measured?	*Relative:* **Hair hygrometer** • Mounted on wall of operating theatre • Direct reading of relative humidity • Hair gets longer as humidity increases • Hair length controls pointer moving over a scale • Accurate for relative humidity between 30%–90%

STEPS	KEY POINTS

Wet and dry bulb hygrometer
- Consists of two thermometers, one in air and the other submerged in water.
- Temperature of mercury in bulb on thermometer in the air is in equilibrium with its surrounding—read true ambient temperature.
- Thermometer submerged in water reads lower temperature due to cooling effect from evaporation and loss of latent heat of vapourisation.
- Difference between temperatures is related to rate of evaporation of water, which depends on ambient humidity.

Regnault's hygrometer
- Consists of silver tubing containing ether.
- Air is blown through the ether, thereby cooling it.
- This initiates condensation on the shiny outside surface.
- Temperature at which condensation occurs is known as the dew point (i.e. temperature at which the ambient air is fully saturated).
- Relative humidity = $\dfrac{\text{saturated vapour pressure (SVP) at dew point}}{\text{SVP at ambient temperature}}$

Absolute:

Transducers
- Depends on change in electrical resistance or capacitance of a substance when it absorbs water vapour from the atmosphere.

Mass spectrometry
- Humidity can be measured by light absorption technique based upon the reduction of ultraviolet light transmitted when water vapour is present.

What is heat?

State of energy an object has in relation to the kinetic energy of its molecules or atoms.
Heat will transfer down a temperature gradient from a warm object to a cooler one.
Heat energy is measured in Joules (J).

What is temperature?

Measure of the thermal state of a substance. It is a property of a system and determines whether heat can be transferred to or from an object.

Standard international (SI) unit for temperature measurement is Kelvin (K). It is based on the tripe point of water (the temperature at a specific pressure at which water exists in all three phases).
1 unit Kelvin = 1/273.16 of thermodynamic triple point of water.
Change in temperature of 1 K is equivalent to change in temperature of 1°C.

How is hypothermia graded?

Hypothermia is defined as body temperature below normal (36.7–37.0°C).
Mild hypothermia: 34–36.5°C
Moderate: 27–34°C
Profound: < 17°C

What are the consequences of hypothermia?

Cardiovascular
- Increased myocardial oxygen demand and consumption due to shivering
- Arrhythmias, sinus bradycardia
- Vasoconstriction, poor peripheral perfusion, increased systemic vascular resistance
- ECG: J waves in lead II if < 32°C, AV block, fibrillation

STEPS	KEY POINTS

Neurological
- Decreased cerebral blood flow
- Reduction in cerebral metabolic consumption by 7% per °C
- Neuroprotection via decreased neurotransmitter release
- Impaired conscious state at 33°C
- Coma at 30°C
- Decreased train of four ratio

Respiratory
- Increased VO_2 with shivering (up to 300%)
- Increased PVR, V/Q mismatch, impaired hypoxic vasoconstriction
- Decreased ventilatory drive, decreased bronchial tone, increased dead space
- Increased gas solubility

Renal
- Decreased renal blood flow and glomerular filtration rate due to decreased cardiac output

Gastrointestinal tract
- Decreased blood flow, metabolic and excretory functions
- Decreased gut motility

Haematological
- Decreased platelet function
- Coagulopathy as clotting enzymes are temperature dependent
- Increased fibrinolysis
- Increased haematocrit
- Left shift of Hb-O_2 dissociation curve

Endocrine and metabolic
- Decreased basal metabolic rate by 5%–7% per °C if not shivering
- Metabolic acidosis
- Acute rise in potassium with rewarming
- Decreased insulin, causing hyperglycaemia

How is heat lost in the operating theatre?	Vasomotor tone is reduced during general anesthesia causing vasodilatation, which increases heat loss. Factors related to surgery and anaesthesia (e.g. exposure of body cavity, irrigation and infusion of cold fluids, operating room temperature) will contribute to hypothermia.

Radiation 40%
- Heat loss by infrared radiation from exposed portions of the body to neighbouring objects that are not in direct contact.

Convection 30%
- Air layer adjacent to the body becomes less dense and rises as it becomes warmed. This produces a convection current carrying heat away from the subject.
- Laminar flow ventilation in operating theatre exacerbates the convection current.

Evaporation 20%
- Evaporation of sweat from skin or body fluids from mucosal or tissue surfaces results in heat loss due to latent heat of vapourisation.

Respiration 10%
- Via inspiring dry gases

STEPS	KEY POINTS
How can heat loss be reduced?	Radiation: By increasing the room temperature and covering exposed surfaces with warm blankets Convection: By forced air warming devices and fluid warmers Evaporation: By covering the patient Respiration: By humidifying the inspired gases; intravenous fluids should be warmed during infusion
How is temperature measured?	**Nonelectrical** • Gas expansion thermometers (e.g. Bourdon gauge dial) • Liquid expansion thermometers (e.g. mercury, alcohol) • Bimetallic strip dial thermometer • Chemical thermometer **Electrical** • Thermocouple—Seebeck effect • Resistance thermometer (e.g. platinum wire) • Thermistor **Infrared** Tympanic membrane thermometer

CLINICAL VIVA

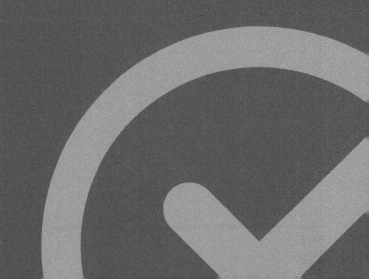

09.1 LONG CASE: ACUTE CERVICAL SPINE SUBLUXATION

HISTORY *A 65–year-old male awaiting a lobectomy for lung malignancy presents with acute neck pain following a fall. His past medical history consists of diet-controlled diabetes mellitus, hypertension, and a hiatus hernia. His medications include candesartan, bendroflumethiazide, enoxaparin, simvastatin, and lansoprazole.*

STEPS	KEY POINTS	
On Examination	Heart rate	80/min
	BP	140/80 mmHg
	Saturation	95% on room air
	On auscultation he has some rhonchi at the right lower base and a harsh ejection systolic murmur loudest at the left sternal edge in the second intercostal space.	
Blood Results	Awaited	
	Arterial blood gas	
	FiO_2	0.21
	pH	7.32
	pCO_2	5.1 kPa
	pO_2	9.5 kPa
	HCO_3	23
	BE	1.2
	Hb	9.8 g/dL
ECG		

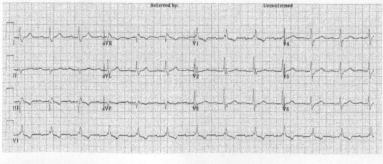

Fig. 9.1

STEPS	KEY POINTS
Echocardiogram	LA: dilated LV: thickened RA: normal size and function RV: normal size and function Aortic valve: thickened and calcified Valve area: 1.7 cm^2 Peak gradient: 27 mmHg Mitral valve: minimal mitral regurgitation Tricuspid valve/Pulmonary valve: normal Ejection fraction: 70%
Lateral C spine XR: current	See Figure 9.2.

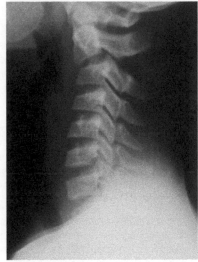

Fig. 9.2

Chest X-ray	Done 1 week ago See Figure 9.3.

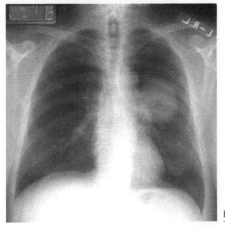

Fig. 9.3

STEPS	KEY POINTS

Lung function tests

Measurement	Lower limit of normal	Patient's value	% of predicted
Forced vital capacity (FVC)	2.07 L	2.63 L	96%
Forced expiratory volume in one second (FEV1)	1.56 L	2.15 L	101%
FEV1/FVC ratio	68.3%	81.7%	
Residual volume (RV)	1.30 L	1.77 L	85%
Total lung capacity (TLC)	3.77 L	4.01 L	83%
Diffusing capacity (DLCO) (mL/min/mm Hg)	16.4	9.29	43%
Adjusted diffusing capacity (mL/min/mm Hg/L)	3.34	2.65	59%

Summarise the case.

This 65-year-old patient presents with an acute neck pain due to cervical spine subluxation. He has multiple comorbidities including diet-controlled diabetes, hypertension on dual therapy, lung cancer awaiting resection, aortic stenosis, and a hiatus hernia for which he is on PPI therapy. He is also anticoagulated.

Following anaesthetic and surgical assessment, he may need urgent surgery requiring optimisation of comorbidities where possible and plans for managing his difficult airway and anaesthesia with experienced personnel. A cardiology assessment is important as his ECG shows a trifascicular heart block.

What is the significance of the aortic stenosis? What are your concerns for anaesthetising him?

My concerns relate to the possibility of a fixed cardiac output and inability to compensate for hypotension with increased contractility. I would ask about symptoms of angina, syncope and breathlessness, palpitations and peripheral oedema, and an idea of his exercise tolerance. According to the information given, he has mild-moderate aortic stenosis without any evidence of LV dysfunction.

Under Goldman's risk criteria, it marks a risk factor for perioperative cardiac complications. Severity depends on presence of symptoms, development of conduction abnormalities, and presence of left ventricular dysfunction although these are difficult to correlate.

Invasive monitoring is recommended for aortic valve area < 1 cm^2 and mean gradient > 30 mmHg.

When anaesthetising him, I would take care to treat hypotension, arrhythmias, and electrolyte imbalances early, place invasive monitoring with arterial line for continuous monitoring of BP and central line so that vasoconstrictors can be given if needed. In this way I hope to prevent both spinal cord and myocardial hypoperfusion in the first instance.

What abnormalities does the ECG show?

Trifascicular block (incomplete)
- Right bundle branch block
- Left axis deviation (= left anterior fascicular block)
- First-degree AV block

What are the causes of trifascicular block?

- Ischaemic heart disease
- Hypertension
- Aortic stenosis
- Congenital heart disease
- Hyperkalaemia (resolves with treatment)
- Digoxin toxicity

STEPS	KEY POINTS
Why is it a concern?	Incomplete trifascicular block may progress to complete heart block, although the overall risk is low. Patients who present with syncope and have an ECG showing trifascicular block usually need to be admitted for a cardiology workup, and these patients will require insertion of a permanent pacemaker.
	Asymptomatic bifascicular block with first-degree AV block is not an indication for pacing.
Comment on the radiographs.	Chest X-ray done 1 week ago Mass in the left lung in the perihilar region. This patient is known to have and is awaiting lung resection for cancer. The current chest signs indicate the presence of chest infection, and I would like to repeat the chest X-ray.
	C spine—lateral radiograph The X-ray is not labeled. It shows bilateral facet fracture-dislocation at C4-C5
How can you interpret the lung function tests?	The FEV1/FVC ratio is normal, leaving us with either a restrictive or a normal pattern. As both the FVC and total lung capacity are normal, we conclude that the spirometry and lung volumes are normal. This suggests that the airways and lung parenchyma are functioning normally. But the diffusing capacity is significantly reduced and remains low even when corrected for lung volumes.
	Differential diagnosis • Anaemia—the number of haemoglobin molecules to which carbon monoxide can bind is reduced, decreasing the ability of the lungs to transfer carbon monoxide to the blood, thus lowering the diffusing capacity without affecting any of the lung volumes or capacities. • Pulmonary arterial hypertension.
Tell me about lung cancer, some types, and its systemic complications.	Lung cancer can be subdivided into non-small cell lung cancer (NSCLC—85%) and small cell lung cancer (SCLC—15%). NSCLC is further subdivided into adenocarcinoma, squamous cell carcinoma, and large cell carcinoma. SCLC often presents late and is more rapid in progression.
	I would take a history and note any weight loss/cachexia. I would be interested in any investigations he may have had to date, any imaging/ mass effects of the tumour itself, any metastasis, evidence of paraneoplastic syndromes (Cushing's, SIADH, Eaton-Lambert), and any related medications including chemotherapy or radiotherapy. I would also note any anaemia and that he has increased thrombotic risk, which may be why he is anticoagulated.
What is your initial management of the patient?	I would take an ABC approach to managing this patient and would ensure his airway is patent and his C spine stabilised and that his breathing and circulation are not compromised.
	My history would concentrate on the duration of symptoms and any associated trauma or injuries. My concerns relate to a pathological fracture/ degenerative disease or trauma, and management should ensure that a full primary and secondary survey have been completed via ATLS protocols if appropriate.
	More extensive history would include a full anaesthetic assessment including airway, fasting status, social history, allergies, and previous anaesthetics. Specific to him I would like to know about any active reflux, reasons for and timing of anticoagulation, and steroid therapy. I would be interested in breathlessness/cough/signs of heart failure/palpitations/syncope/angina and, most importantly, acute or chronic neurology.
	A full and complete examination and documentation should occur.

STEPS	KEY POINTS

Additional investigations would include:

Blood tests
- Full blood count to exclude any anaemia/thrombocytopenia/infection
- Coagulation screen
- Renal function (as a baseline in view of diabetes)
- Electrolytes including Ca/Mg/PO$_4$/Na/K
- HbA$_1$C and glucose
- Liver function tests
- Group and screen should also be sent.

CXR

A recent Chest radiograph to exclude chest infection in view of findings on auscultation.

CT/MRI

It is likely to be indicated and beneficial presurgery, and if associated trauma, a full body CT may be indicated.

He is listed for urgent cervical spine fixation. How would you manage his airway? Talk me through your technique.

Manipulation of his airway could result in significant cord compromise; hence, due care should be given to technique.

I feel the most stable way to manage would be via an awake fibreoptic intubation (AFOI). I would like to do this in a safe environment with other experienced personnel and senior support. Alternatives would be to perform an asleep FOI or to do standard laryngoscopy with a manual in-line stabilisation technique. AFOI will mean there is less neck movement, will require less mouth opening on the part of the patient, and allows a continuous monitor of neurology even after the endotracheal tube has been placed. Asleep methods can be considered with fasted patients with good airway assessment.

In order to perform the AFOI, I would need to explain the procedure to the patient, alleviating any anxiety, and assess suitability and prepare medication and equipment. I would ensure good intravenous access and supplementary oxygen via nasal sponge and establish full monitoring. I would treat with an antisialogogue such as glycopyrrolate and low-dose midazolam.

Procedure

Sedation: Remifentanil target-controlled infusion and/or midazolam to obtund anxiety.

Nose and throat: Check nostril patency and choose best side. Apply topical vasoconstrictors and local anaesthetic in the form of 10% lignocaine to the chosen nostril and back of throat.

Larynx and trachea: Various methods have been followed in anaesthetising the larynx and trachea such as the cricothyroid puncture, internal laryngeal nerve block at the hyoid bone, etc. I am used to the spraying of the local anaesthetic using an epidural catheter via the side port of the fibreoptic scope.

Prepare the tube: Railroad the reinforced nasal tube on the fibreoptic scope with copious lubricant.

Intubation: Once position is confirmed (auscultation/EtCO$_2$ trace), check neurology once more and then anaesthetise with either propofol or volatile agent.

I would have the difficult airway trolley to hand with a laryngeal mask available for rescue. I would secure with tape, avoiding ties (and also compression of neck veins), and recheck tube position with fibreoptic scope once secured

The surgeon tells you that the cervical spine fixation is done with the patient in the prone position.

STEPS	KEY POINTS

What are the implications of the prone position?

These relate to personnel required, monitoring and line displacement, pressure-related problems, and physiological implications. In this case it should be discussed whether the surgeons would be using Mayfield pins as an alternative for head placement.

Appropriate numbers of trained staff should be available in theatre for both proning and reversal at the end of the procedure. Lines and monitoring should be rationalised for transfer of patient and should be well secured to avoid displacement. Care should be taken to use special mattresses and head supports to avoid pressure to organs, abdomen, and nerves overlying joints (e.g. hips, elbows, and thighs). Whilst rotating arms during positioning, care should be taken to prevent brachial plexus injuries. Eyes should be lubricated, taped, and padded and checked at regular intervals to avoid complications of abrasions and ischaemic retinopathy. Abdominal pressure may cause IVC compression, reduced venous return, poor cardiac output, regurgitation of stomach contents, and reduced thoracic compliance. Oxygenation may, however, improve in the prone position due to improved ventilation/perfusion matching. Once patient is in position, a systematic final check should occur from head to toe to ensure the following are checked: tube not kinked, air entry adequate, no pressure on face/eyes/brachial plexus/breasts/abdomen/anterior superior iliac spines/genitalia/knees and feet.

What are the main principles for perioperative management of this patient aside from those mentioned already?

These relate to the surgery itself and the patient's comorbidities and prevention of complications. Through use of invasive monitoring and perhaps cardiac output monitoring if available, I would aim for optimal cardiac output and avoid excessive fluids; this may require the use of low-dose infusion of vasopressors. A remifentanil-based technique with volatile agent will help control tachycardia and hypertension through easy adjustment for periods of higher stimulation (placement of pins/bony manipulation). Care should be taken with assessing blood loss and use of cell salvage if considered appropriate.

This patient will require regular assessment of blood sugars and may require a sliding scale perioperatively. Normal care with temperature, warming measures, and prevention of thromboembolism should be taken (e.g. TED stockings and intermittent pneumatic compression devices).

Will you extubate this patient? When will you decide that it is safe to do so?

I would ideally like to wake and extubate this patient early for prompt assessment of their neurology but in a careful and controlled manner to avoid coughing. Use of lignocaine spray on cuff and using a remifentanil-based technique can aid a smooth extubation. I would ensure that temperature, pO_2, $EtCO_2$, and reversal of neuromuscular blockade have been corrected. I would ensure that the patient has adequate pain relief with possible long-acting local anaesthetic infiltrated by the surgeon at the end, a multimodal technique, and avoidance of large doses of opiates that may compromise wakefulness at the end. A guedel may be helpful to prevent biting on the tube.
After a period in recovery, a high-dependency bed should be made available.

In this patient my concerns are of a superadded chest infection, making laryngospasm and coughing more likely; hence, the importance of adequate suctioning and use of adjuncts such as remifentanil/pre-intubation lignocaine spray.

Further reading

1. Brown et al. Aortic stenosis and noncardiac surgery. *CEACCP*. 2005; **5**(1).
2. www.Lung cancer.org
3. Knight et al. Patient positioning in anaesthesia. *CEACCP*. 2004; **4**(5): 160–3.
4. Kamarkar et al. Tracheal Extubation. *CEACCP*. 2008; **8**(6): 214–220.

09.2 SHORT CASE: DISEASES OF RED CELL MORPHOLOGY

HISTORY *A 19-year-old Afro-Caribbean man is booked on the emergency list for an open appendicectomy. He is noted to be Sickledex test positive.*

STEPS	KEY POINTS
What is a Sickledex test?	A qualitative solubility test in which a sample of the patient's blood is mixed with a deoxygenating agent and a solubility buffer to determine the presence of > 10% of haemoglobin S (HbS) in the sample. It determines the presence of HbS but does not diagnose sickle cell disease.
What test is used to diagnose sickle disease? What genetic variants may be diagnosed using this test?	**Haemoglobin electrophoresis** • Quantifies the amount of HbS to determine hetero/homozygous genotyping (sickle trait versus sickle disease) • Also measures other abnormal haemoglobins including HbC and thalassaemia
What is the underlying defect in HbS?	• Inherited haemoglobinopathy resulting from mutation on chromosome 11, causing substitution of Glutamine by Valine in the 6th amino acid of β chains resulting in the formation of haemoglobin S. • Haemoglobin S is biochemically unstable and can precipitate out of solution when in the deoxygenated state, forming the pointed, slightly curved 'sickle cells'.
What are the different types of sickling crises?	• Vaso-occlusive crisis Sickle-shaped red blood cells obstruct capillaries and restrict blood flow to an organ, resulting in ischaemia, pain, necrosis, and often organ damage. • Aplastic crisis Acute worsening of the patient's baseline anaemia. This crisis is normally triggered by parvovirus B19, which directly affects erythropoiesis by invading the red cell precursors and multiplying in them and destroying them. • Splenic sequestration crisis Spleen is affected in the process of clearing defective red blood cells. It is usually infarcted before the end of childhood in patients with sickle-cell anaemia.

STEPS	KEY POINTS
	• Haemolytic crisis Accelerated drops in haemoglobin. Common with co-existent G6PD deficiency.
What other system manifestations or comorbidities might the patient present with, related to sickle cell disease?	**Respiratory** • Acute chest syndrome • Pulmonary hypertension **Neurological** • Acute brain syndrome • Recurrent infarcts **Haematology** • Anaemia **Musculoskeletal** • Bone marrow dysplasia **Renal** • Renal failure **Gastro-intestinal** • Asplenism, may require antibiotic prophylaxis • Gallstones • Jaundice **Genitourinary** • Priapism
What is acute chest syndrome?	• Dyspnoea, cough, haemoptysis, and pleuritic chest pain caused by recurrent pulmonary infarctions • Radiological finding of a new infiltrate on X-ray • Management—broad-spectrum antibiotics, fluid management, oxygenation, chest physiotherapy, bronchodilators, and intermittent incentive spirometry
What are your clinical priorities in managing patients with sickle cell disease undergoing surgery?	**Careful, well-balanced anaesthesia** • Avoid hypoxia. • Ensure adequate hydration. • Maintain normothermia. • Optimal analgesia. • Avoid oxidant drugs such as prilocaine, nitroprusside, vitamin K, aspirin, and penicillin, as they may precipitate haemolysis. Consider regional anaesthetic techniques where likely to be beneficial. Avoid venostasis—caution with tourniquets.
At what PaO_2 does sickling occur? What is the mechanism behind the process?	• Homozygous (SS) cells begin to sickle at much higher oxygen saturation, typically 85% (PaO_2 5–5.5 kPa). • Heterozygous (AS) cells may deform below the saturation 40% (PaO_2 2.5–4.0 kPa). (Sickling with sickle cell trait is therefore rarely a problem without concomitant stasis.) • Desaturation of Hb S results in the polymerisation of haemoglobin, forming large aggregates called tactoids, which deform the red cells into the typical sickle shape.

STEPS	KEY POINTS
When is exchange transfusion used?	• Traditionally, an aggressive transfusion policy targeting an Hb S concentration of < 30% was suggested. Now a simple transfusion policy to a haemoglobin of 10 g d/L is recommended. • In high-risk cases, a more aggressive approach may be required. This must be discussed in advance with a haematologist, as the risk of transfusion-related complications such as iron overload, alloimmunisation, transfusion-related acute lung injury, and allergic reactions are all increased.
What happens to the oxygen dissociation curve in sickle cell disease?	Rightward shift due to increased 2, 3–DPG in response to chronic anaemia [This question ideally starts with structure of red cell, and subsequent questions are directed at sickle cell disease, G6PD deficiency, hereditary spherocytosis, or thalassemia.]
Describe the structure of RBC. How is it different from other body cells?	Red blood cells are biconcave discs (7 microns in diameter); this structure gives it a higher surface area to volume ratio for diffusion of oxygen and allows it to negotiate tight passages in the vasculature. RBC contain large amounts of protein but do not have a nucleus, mitochondria, or ribosomes.
What are the diseases of the red cell membrane?	Red cell membrane disorders are inherited diseases due to mutations in membrane or skeletal proteins, resulting in decreased red cell deformability, life span, and premature death of the erythrocytes. The red cell membrane disorders include hereditary spherocytosis, elliptocytosis, ovalocytosis, and stomatocytosis.
What is hereditary spherocytosis? Describe the pathogenesis and issues.	Hereditary spherocytosis is the most common congenital haemolytic anaemia, with an autosomal dominant inheritance. **Pathogenesis** The molecular defect involves the genes encoding for proteins (spectrin, ankyrin, band 3, and protein 4.2) that are involved in the attachment of the cytoskeleton to the red cell membrane. This results in loss of surface area and leads to spherical, osmotically fragile cells that get trapped in the spleen. **Diagnostic test** • Blood film • Osmotic fragility test • Electrophoresis **Clinical features** • Haemolytic anaemia sometimes requiring exchange transfusion • Jaundice, splenomegaly, and cholelithiasis. **Treatment** • Folate therapy in mild forms; red cell transfusions in severe forms. • Splenectomy, with appropriate counseling about the risk of infections and post-splenectomy antibiotic and vaccinations.
What are the other disorders of red cells?	**Red cell destruction** • Haemoglobinopathy • Enzymopathy (G6PD deficiency) • Autoimmune • Membrane disorder (already discussed) **Disorders in red cell production** • Thalassemias • Myelodysplasia • Aplastic anaemia

STEPS	KEY POINTS

Explain thalassemia.

Thalassemia is the genetic defect in haemoglobin synthesis resulting in decreased or absent synthesis of one of the two globin chains (α or β).

- Imbalance of globin chain synthesis leads to decreased haemoglobin production and precipitation of excess globin (toxic).
- Found in people of African, Asian, and Mediterranean heritage.

β thalassemia

It is an autosomal recessive disorder. In the homozygous state (i.e. thalassemia major) it causes severe, transfusion-dependent anaemia. In the heterozygous state or β thalassemia trait (i.e. thalassemia minor), it causes mild to moderate microcytic anaemia.

Clinical features

- Anaemia
- Extramedullary haematopoiesis
- Complications of long-term transfusion
- Increased risk for infections
- Cholelithiasis

Diagnostic test

- Blood smear: microcytic/hypochromic anaemia
- Hb electrophoresis (HbA_2, HbF)
- Iron stores usually elevated

Treatment

- Definitive treatments are stem cell transplant and simple transfusion.
- Chelation therapy to avoid iron overload has to be started early.

The major causes of morbidity and mortality in β thalassemia are anaemia and iron overload.

Discuss G6PD deficiency.

Glucose-6-phosphate dehydrogenase (G6PD) deficiency is inherited as an X-linked disorder (G6PD locus at Xq28), which primarily affects men.

The G6PD enzyme catalyses the oxidation of glucose-6-phosphate to 6-phosphogluconate while concomitantly reducing the oxidized form of nicotinamide adenine dinucleotide phosphate ($NADP^+$) to reduced nicotinamide adenine dinucleotide phosphate (NADPH). NADPH, a required cofactor in many biosynthetic reactions, maintains glutathione in its reduced form. See Figure 9.4. GSH and GSSG – reduced and oxidised form of glutathione

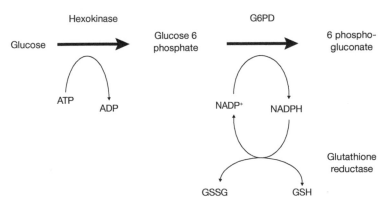

Fig. 9.4

STEPS	KEY POINTS
	Reduced glutathione acts as a scavenger for dangerous oxidative metabolites in the cells. Red blood cells rely heavily upon glucose-6-phosphate dehydrogenase (G6PD) activity because it is the only source of NADPH that protects the cells against oxidative stresses.

Haemolysis is triggered by:
- Infections
- Ingestion of fava beans
- Oxidant drugs such as sulfa, dapsone, antimalarial drugs, and chloramphenicol
- Surgery

Clinical features
- Asymptomatic
- History of neonatal jaundice, requiring exchange transfusion
- Haemolysis
- Gallstones and splenomegaly

Treatment
- Avoid oxidant drugs
- During acute crisis, stop the offending factor
- Folic acid supplementation
- Blood transfusion is rarely necessary

09.3 SHORT CASE: PERMANENT PACEMAKER

HISTORY *You are asked to review a 70-year-old man in preassessment clinic who is scheduled for bilateral inguinal hernia. He has a permanent pacemaker (PPM), which was inserted 6 years ago.*

STEPS	KEY POINTS
What are your key preoperative concerns when anaesthetising patients with PPMs?	**Patient factors** • Indication for pacemaker • Comorbid cardiac disease • Underlying cardiac function • Patients' long-term use of anticoagulants (e.g. warfarin) **Pacemaker factors** • Age and type of pacemaker or ICD, manufacturer, device, and serial number • Date pacemaker was last checked • Details provided with the registration card or 'PPM passport' **Surgical factors** • Use of diathermy • Surgical site proximity to the pacemaker
What are the different types of PPM?	**NASPE/BPEG revised classification of pacemakers** (North American Society of Pacing and Electrophysiology/British Pacing and Electrophysiology Group)

I (chamber paced)	II (chamber paced)	III (response to sensing)	IV (rate modulation)	V (multisite pacing)
0 = none	0 = none	0 = none	0 = none	0 = none
A = atrium	A = atrium	T = triggered	R = rate modulation	A = atrium
V = ventricle	V = ventricle	I = inhibited		V = ventricle
D = dual	D = dual	D = dual		D = dual

STEPS	KEY POINTS
How does the 'rate modulation' function?	An accelerometer or other means of measuring physical activity is incorporated into the pacemaker, usually increasing the paced rate to match physiological demand.
If surgical diathermy is required intra-operatively, how can risk of pacemaker malfunction be minimised? (MHRA guidelines)	The use of surgical diathermy can give rise to electrical interference, and this can present additional risks when used in patients with pacemakers. Also, the energy induced into the heart lead system causes tissue heating.

STEPS	KEY POINTS

Preoperative
- Check correct functioning of the pacemaker.
- Programme parameters to avoid inappropriate inhibition.

Intraoperative
Wherever possible, avoid surgical diathermy in these patients. But if it is deemed necessary, bipolar use is safer than monopolar diathermy.
- Monopolar, where necessary, should be used in short bursts at as low an energy as possible.
- Return plate should be placed as far away from the PPM as possible.
- Cables from diathermy equipment should be kept well away from PPM.
- In patients where the ICD is deactivated and where access to the anterior chest wall will interfere with surgery due to sterility, connect external defibrillator using remote pads.

Postoperative
Confirm device functionality on completion of surgery.

How would your management change if the patient had an implantable cardiac defibrillator (ICD)?

PPMs and ICDs have a magnetic switch that will respond to a magnet when positioned over the device.

Elective procedures
The ICD is programmed to 'monitor only' mode by the cardiac physiologist to prevent unnecessary shock in the event of accidental sensing of electrical interference. External pads placed on the patient with external defibrillator ready to attach if required.

Emergency procedure
Consider positioning a clinical magnet over the implant (done for whole duration of surgery) to inhibit inappropriate shock delivery (if the device has been programmed to respond this way). Any tachyarrhythmias during this time warrant use of external defibrillation equipment.

In patients with pacemakers, securing a magnet over the pacemaker implant site will not necessarily guarantee asynchronous (non-sensing) pacing. Magnet response may vary between manufacturers' models and according to particular programmed settings.

Postoperatively, the patient should be managed on a high-dependency or coronary care unit until the ICD has been checked and reactivated.

Further reading

1. Guidelines for the perioperative management of patients with implantable pacemakers or implantable cardioverter defibrillators, where the use of surgical diathermy/electrocautery is anticipated. Medicine and Healthcare products Regulatory Agency. MHRA.gov.uk

09.4 SHORT CASE: BLEEDING TONSIL

HISTORY *You have been called to see a 5-year-old child who had a tonsillectomy 6 hours previously. The child is bleeding and needs to go back to theatre for haemostasis. When you arrive on the ward, the child is agitated and says he feels sick. The postoperative blood loss is reported to be minimal by the nursing staff.*

STEPS	KEY POINTS
On examination	Looks pale Pulse: 125/min Respiratory rate: 25/min Blood pressure: 70/30 mmHg Capillary refill time: 4 seconds
What are the specific problems in this case?	• Hypovolaemia/hypotension • Risk of aspiration due to swallowing of blood • Difficult intubation secondary to laryngeal oedema and bleeding • A second general anaesthetic • Management of an anxious child and parents • Bleeding diathesis
What are the types of post-tonsillectomy bleeding?	The incidence of bleeding following tonsillectomy is 0.5%–2% depending upon the surgical technique. • Primary—this may occur within 24 hours of surgery. • Secondary—this may occur up to 28 days post-surgery and is associated with sloughing of the eschar (dead tissue) overlying the tonsillar bed, loosened vessel ties, or infection from underlying chronic tonsillitis.

STEPS	KEY POINTS
How would you preoperatively assess this child and commence resuscitation?	• The presenting signs relate to the quantity of blood loss. • Blood loss is secondary to venous or capillary ooze from the tonsillar bed. It may be difficult to measure, as bleeding may occur over several hours and large amounts of blood may be swallowed. Brisk bleeding may lead to the child spitting blood. The child may be hypovolaemic with low haemoglobin. • Tachycardia, tachypnoea, delayed capillary refill, and decreased urine output are early indicators of hypovolaemic shock, whereas hypotension and altered sensorium are late signs of hypovolaemia, with decompensated shock. • The cardiovascular status is assessed by considering cardiovascular parameters as well as perfusion of other organs:

Heart rate—this child may be tachycardic due to anxiety, but this may also be due to catecholamine release to maintain cardiac output in the presence of hypovolaemia. Bradycardia is caused by acidosis and hypoxia and is a preterminal sign.

Capillary refill time—hypovolaemia leads to a poor skin perfusion and prolonged capillary refill time (> 2 seconds). Mottling, pallor, and peripheral cyanosis are also indicators of poor skin perfusion.

Blood pressure is difficult to measure, especially in younger children. Hypotension is a late sign of hypovolaemic shock.

Tachypnoea may be due to anxiety but also occurs in response to acidosis secondary to poor tissue perfusion and severe anaemia.

Core/skin temperature difference of more than 2°C is an important sign of shock.

Decreased or absent urine output—Poor urine output (< 1 mL/kg/h in children, and < 2 mL/kg/h in infants) indicates inadequate renal perfusion.

• Resuscitation should be with isotonic crystalloid (0.9% Saline or Hartmann's solution), colloid, or blood; intravenous boluses of fluid, 20 mL/kg stat, repeated if necessary after reassessment of the cardiovascular system. Large volumes of fluid may be required (40–60 mL/kg). Hypotonic fluids such as 5% dextrose, 0.18% saline, and 2.5% dextrose or 0.45% saline and 5% dextrose must not be used in the acute resuscitation of hypovolaemic children.

How would you anaesthetise this child?

There is some debate about the safest technique of anaesthesia for a bleeding tonsil. The two common choices are:
1. Inhalational induction in the head down, lateral position.
2. Modified intravenous rapid sequence induction with cricoid pressure.

The pros and cons of each technique are discussed below.

Inhalational induction
Pros: Inhalational induction is a technique that is familiar to anaesthetists, and oxygenation is well maintained during spontaneous ventilation. Inhalational induction in the lateral position helps drain blood from the airway by means of gravity, and clots can be gently suctioned from the airway once an adequate depth of anaesthesia is achieved. Suxamethonium may be given prior to intubation, either with the child remaining on his or her side or turned into the supine position and cricoid pressure applied.

STEPS	KEY POINTS
	Cons: Inhalational induction with a volatile agent in an anxious child who is bleeding can be difficult. Deep anaesthesia may be induced inadvertently, particularly in a child recovering from anaesthesia a few hours earlier. Deep anaesthesia is a risk factor for cardiac arrest in a child who may still be hypovolaemic. Intubating in the lateral position is unfamiliar to most anaesthetists, and many would turn the child into the supine position prior to intubation.

Intravenous rapid sequence induction

Pros: Anaesthesia can be induced in the supine position with the application of cricoid pressure to reduce the risk of aspiration. The use of muscle relaxants helps produce ideal conditions for intubation. Intravenous induction is less stressful for the child who should already have an intravenous cannula in situ.

Cons: A modified rapid sequence induction is required as it is impossible to adequately preoxygenate an anxious child who is bleeding; facemask ventilation will be required after the administration of suxamethonium. Care must be taken not to inflate the stomach during facemask ventilation, as this will encourage regurgitation and aspiration. There is a risk of hypoxia if intubation is difficult and spontaneous respiration has been lost.

What steps should be taken intraoperatively?

During the operation, further fluid and blood should be given as guided by clinical monitoring—heart rate, capillary refill, core-peripheral temperature difference, and blood pressure. Near patient testing using a Hemocue® or the WHO haemoglobin scale, if available, can guide transfusion requirements.

The child may become cold during surgery due to large volume transfusion. The child should be kept well covered to maintain body temperature and, if possible, a warming blanket used with temperature monitoring. Hypothermia may exacerbate coagulopathy.

Once haemostasis is achieved, a large-bore gastric tube should be passed under direct vision to empty the stomach. Nondepolarising neuromuscular blockade should be reversed. The trachea should be extubated with the child fully awake in the left lateral, head-down position. Alternatively, particularly in the absence of a tipping trolley, the 'tonsil' position may be used, where a bolster is placed under the child's chest in the lateral position so that the head is below the level of the chest and fluids drain from the mouth.

What postoperative care should be taken?

Postoperatively it is important to monitor the child closely in a well-lit area (do not return them to a dark ward area at night), with regular observation of vital parameters. Blood transfusion may need to be continued in recovery. The haemoglobin should be measured and coagulation screen sent if possible. Minimum haemoglobin of 8 g/dL is acceptable provided there is no further bleeding. The child will require iron supplements for the next 6 weeks if this is the case.

section 09

BASIC SCIENCE VIVA

09.5 ANATOMY: PARAVERTEBRAL BLOCK

Indications, benefits over epidural, anatomy and contents, technique, complications...

STEPS	KEY POINTS
Comment on the X-ray in Figure 9.5.	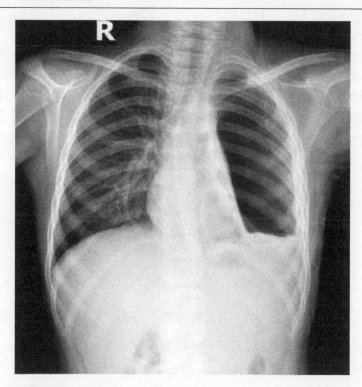

Fig. 9.5

CXR – PA view
No bronchovascular markings on left hemithorax Air with fluid level on the left side
Mediastinal shift to right
Diagnosis – Hydropneumothorax.

STEPS	KEY POINTS
What is bronchopleural fistula (BPF)?	Bronchopleural fistula is the abnormal communication between pleural cavity and the bronchial tree. It is defined as persistent air leak for greater than 24 hours after the development of pneumothorax or failure to inflate the lung despite chest drainage for 24 hours.

STEPS	KEY POINTS
How is BPF diagnosed?	**Clinical presentation—as above** **CXR:** Radiological features that are suggestive of diagnosis include: • Steady increase in intrapleural air space • Appearance of a new air fluid level • Changes in an already present air fluid level • Development of tension pneumothorax **CT** • Pneumothorax, pneumomediastinum • Underlying lung pathology • Presence of actual fistulous communication

What are the causes of BPF?	The most common cause of BPF is positive pressure ventilation after thoracotomy leading to dehiscence of the bronchial stump, which presents at 3–10 days post surgery.
	
	Other causes are listed below.
	• Infection
	  o Necrotising infection—lung abscess, empyema, tuberculosis
	
	• Trauma
	  o Bullae rupture
	  o Thoracic trauma
	
	• Iatrogenic/postsurgical
	  o Post-thoracotomy
	  o Post-chemo/radio therapy
	  o Boerhaave's syndrome
	
	• Neoplastic
	  o Tumour invasion of bronchus from oesophagus or lung
	
	• Diffuse lung disease
	  o Pneumocystis carinii pneumonia
	  o ARDS
	
	• Miscellaneous
	  o Spontaneous pneumothorax

What are the presenting features of a persistent broncho pleural leak?	It depends on the onset and size of air leak and the underlying pathology and can have an acute, subacute, or delayed presentation. The symptoms and signs can vary from simple productive cough to full-blown sepsis, dyspnoea, and acute tension pneumothorax.
What are the problems encountered in ventilating patients with BPF?	Large BPF leads to inadequate ventilation due to the following: • V/Q mismatch causing hypoxia and hypercapnia. • Failure to expand the collapsed lung. • Need for *flow limitation* to aid healing: use of small tidal volume, less PEEP, short inspiratory time, and reduced respiratory rate—all these manoeuvres reduce the airway pressure and fistula flow but impair ventilation at the same time. • Need for *selective ventilation* of the unaffected lung; differential, or independent ventilation with the use of double lumen tubes. • *High-frequency ventilation* (HFV) had been successful in patients with normal lung parenchyma and proximal BPF compared to patients with lung disease. • Associated with high mortality.

STEPS	KEY POINTS
How do you treat BPF surgically?	Large BPFs not amenable to conservative management need intervention. The technique of treatment depends on the size and position of the fistula and the underlying pathology.
	Bronchoscopic application of sealants or sclerosing agents is suitable for distal and small BPFs less than 5 mm.
	Video-assisted thoracoscopic surgery (VATS) is a less invasive technique that gives access to a wide range of therapeutic procedures.
	Surgical closure of the bronchial stump with muscle flap, additional lobectomy, or decortication might be needed.
What are the principles in anaesthetising a patient for corrective BPF surgery?	• Not a case for an occasional thoracic anaesthetist; need experience in thoracic anaesthesia and BPF management, as this procedure carries a high mortality.

	• **Preassessment**
	  o Airway exam
	  o Chest drains
	  o Antibiotics if infectious cause is suspected

	• **Protection of healthy lung**
	  o Chest drain before intubation
	  o Anaesthetise in lateral position with healthy lung in the nondependent position
	  o Prevent cross-contamination
	  o Avoid ventilation until the good side is isolated

	• **Anaesthesia**
	  o Rapid IV induction with prompt endobronchial intubation into good side (or)
	  o Inhalational induction with spontaneous ventilation until lung isolation is achieved (or)
	  o Awake fibreoptic intubation and lung isolation techniques
	  o Maintain anaesthesia preferably with TIVA to avoid volatile leak into the BPF

	• **Analgesia**
	  o Very important to aid coughing and clearing secretions and prevent atelectasis
	  o Needed for adequate incentive spirometry, physiotherapy, and early mobilisation
	  o To prevent DVT, PE, and cardiorespiratory complications

	• **Postoperative**
	  o Prompt discontinuation of positive pressure ventilation postoperatively (negative pressure ventilation preferable)
	  o Optimal analgesia with the use of short-acting anaesthetic drugs to help with enhanced recovery

What are the various options for postoperative analgesia?	• Multimodal analgesia o Paracetamol, NSAIDS, Tramadol, gabapentin, etc. • IV opioids, preferably as PCA • Intrathecal opioid • Thoracic epidural block • Thoracic paravertebral block • Intercostal block • Intrapleural catheters

STEPS	KEY POINTS
What are the causes of pain after thoracotomy?	• *Incisional pain*: skin and muscles—intercostal nerves, nerves supplying serratus anterior and latissimus dorsi • *Visceral pain*: vagus nerve • *Referred pain*: ipsilateral shoulder pain due to pain referred from pericardium and diaphragm • *Neuropathic pain*: intercostal neuritis or damage to other peripheral nerves • *Chest drain pain*: corresponding intercostal nerves
Explain the anatomy of paravertebral space.	*[You might be given an unlabeled diagram of the spine and then expected to discuss the anatomy with the picture provided. See Figure 9.6.]*

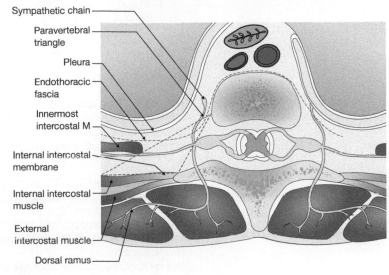

Sympathetic chain
Paravertebral triangle
Pleura
Endothoracic fascia
Innermost intercostal M
Internal intercostal membrane
Internal intercostal muscle
External intercostal muscle
Dorsal ramus

Fig. 9.6

Boundaries
The space is bounded by the following structures.
Apex (laterally): posterior intercostal membrane and intercostal space
Base (medially): vertebral body, intervertebral disc, and the vertebral foramen with its corresponding spinal nerve
Anterior: parietal and visceral pleura and lung parenchyma
Posterior: transverse processes of the vertebrae, heads of ribs and costotransverse ligament

The PVS communicates with epidural space medially through the intervertebral foramina and intercostal spaces laterally.

Contents
The division of the PVS into anterior subserous compartment and posterior subendothoracic compartment by the endothoracic fascia is of no significant importance.

The contents include neural tissue surrounded loosely by areolar and adipose tissue.

Spinal nerves: with white and grey rami communicantes within the medial aspect of the PVS.
Sympathetic chain: lies at the neck of the rib anterior to the intercostal neurovascular bundle.

STEPS	KEY POINTS

What are the indications of paravertebral block (PVB)?

- Acute pain
  - o Surgical pain
    - - Unilateral thoracic surgery—open thoracotomy, video-assisted thoracoscopic surgery (VATS), cardiac and breast surgery
    - - Unilateral abdominal surgery—renal surgery and open cholecystectomy
  - o Nonsurgical pain
    - - Rib fracture

- Chronic pain
  - o Post-herpetic neuralgia
  - o Post-surgical chronic pain
  - o Relief of cancer pain (e.g. mesothelioma or deposits)

- Therapeutic
  - o Control of hyperhidrosis

The contraindications are similar to any other central neuraxial blockade.

How would you perform a thoracic paravertebral block for open thoracotomy?

Knowing the incision

Ascertain the extent of surgical procedure to know the dermatomal distribution of the incision after discussion with the surgeon about the planned approach and extent of surgery.

As a rough guide:
For VATS procedure: T3 to T8, depending on the site of operation.
For muscle-sparing thoracotomy: The incision is about 5–7 cm long extending vertically from T2 to T9.
For posterolateral thoracotomy: Incision spans over at least six dermatomal levels—T3 posteriorly to T8 anteriorly, with chest drains placed at 8th/9th intercostal space.
(Total mastectomy requires blockade extending from T1 to T6 level.)

Choosing the type of block

Single or multiple injections: If anaesthesia of several dermatomes is required a small volume, multiple injection technique is recommended. For example, to block T3 to T8, three injections at T3, T5, and T7 are done with 8–10 mL of local anaesthetic at each level.

Prerequisites

Consent, intravenous access, noninvasive monitoring, presence of full resuscitation facilities, and trained assistant.

Approach and technique

The experience and local policy guides the choice of technique—landmarks or nerve stimulator or ultrasound guided blocks.

The patient is positioned in the sitting or lateral decubitus position (with the side to be blocked uppermost) and supported by an attendant.
To block T3 to T8, the skin is marked at tips of the spinous processes and at points 2.5 cm lateral to these. The parasagittal points correspond with appropriate transverse processes.

Following strict aseptic precautions, the site of injection is infiltrated with 2% lignocaine. An 18 G graduated epidural needle is advanced perpendicular to the skin, until contact with the transverse process is established. Loss of resistance (LOR) syringe with saline is attached to the needle, and while continuously testing for LOR, the needle is 'walked off' the structure in a caudad and lateral direction and advanced approximately 1 cm (a maximum of 1.5 cm).

STEPS	KEY POINTS

As the costotransverse ligament is penetrated, a 'pop' is felt as the needle enters the PVS. This is aptly called a 'change of resistance' rather than LOR, as the complete LOR is experienced when the needle punctures the pleura and goes intrapleural.

After careful aspiration to confirm that the needle tip is not intravascular or intrathecal, the predetermined dose of local anaesthetic should be administered.

What are the advantages of PVB over epidural block?

Procedure
- Easy to teach, learn, and perform
- Can be done in anaesthetised patients

Side effects
- Decreased neurological complications: PDPH, radicular pain, paraplegia, and peripheral nerve lesions.
- Decreased side effects: less sedation, nausea, and vomiting, as PVB is dependent on the use of local anaesthetics only. Systemic opioid might be used; thus, opioid-related risks are minimised but not absent.
- Decreased cardiovascular side effects: severe hypotension is rare because of the unilateral blockade.
- Decreased or no incidence of urinary retention.
- Lack of motor blockade of the lower extremities.
- Better preservation of pulmonary function.

Effects
PVB provides analgesia comparable to an epidural without its side effects. The block is equivalent to epidural in terms of success rate, postoperative pain scores, and analgesic efficacy.
(Better analgesia compared to intrapleural block.)

Effects similar to epidural block
- Inhibition of chronic pain by preventing sensitisation of the CNS by blocking the 'sensory flow'
- Prevention of cardiopulmonary complications and decreased perioperative morbidity

What are the complications of PVB?

Adequacy of the block
- Failure up to 5%

Damage to surrounding structures
- Parietal pleural puncture—intrapleural block
- Parietal and visceral pleural puncture—pneumothorax
- Vascular puncture—bleeding, haemothorax, local anaesthetic toxicity
- Epidural placement
- Dural puncture—high spinal, PDPH

Extension of the block
- Bilateral block—10%
- Stellate ganglion block (hoarseness) in high-thoracic PVB

Further reading
1. Tighe SQM, Greene MD, Rajadurai N. Paravertebral block *Contin Educ Anaesth Crit Care Pain* (2010) **10** (5): 133–137.

09.6 PHYSIOLOGY: PULMONARY HYPERTENSION

STEPS	KEY POINTS
Define pulmonary hypertension (PHT).	Pulmonary hypertension is defined as a mean pulmonary artery pressure (PAP) > 25 mmHg at rest or with a pulmonary capillary wedge pressure (PCWP) < 15 mmHg. Pulmonary hypertension is considered moderately severe when mean PAP > 35 mmHg. PAP > 50 mmHg can be associated with right ventricular failure.
How can you classify PHT?	**WHO classification** **Group 1. Pulmonary arterial hypertension (PAH)** • Idiopathic (BMPR2 gene mutation) • Drug- and toxin-induced • Associated with connective tissue diseases • Congenital heart disease **Group 2. Pulmonary venous hypertension due to left heart diseases** • Systolic dysfunction • Diastolic dysfunction • Valvular disease **Group 3. Pulmonary hypertension due to lung diseases and/or hypoxemia** • Chronic obstructive pulmonary disease • Interstitial lung disease • Sleep-disordered breathing **Group 4. Chronic thromboembolic pulmonary hypertension** **Group 5. PH with unclear multifactorial mechanisms** • Haematological disorders: myeloproliferative disorders, splenectomy • Systemic disorders: sarcoidosis, neurofibromatosis, vasculitis • Metabolic disorders: glycogen storage disease, thyroid disorders
Explain the pathophysiology of PHT.	• Pulmonary vasculature Any of the above causes result in medial hypertrophy and intimal fibrosis of the pulmonary vasculature thereby narrowing the vessels. The endothelin, nitric oxide, and prostacyclin pathway also have a role in the development of PHT. The end result is an increase in pulmonary vascular pressures. • Right ventricle As the right heart has to pump against an increased afterload, it hypertrophies and fails when the PAP is > 50 mmHg.

STEPS	KEY POINTS

- Left ventricle
  Left ventricular failure can then ensue, due to both reduced volume reaching the left heart and interventricular septal interdependence.

- Coronary perfusion
  The coronary circulation to the right heart is dependent on perfusion pressure at the aortic root, which in turn is dependent on systemic vascular resistance (SVR).
  SVR must be aggressively defended in order to maintain coronary perfusion to the right heart. Ischaemia to the right ventricle can put in place a downward spiral of right heart failure, with ensuing cardiovascular collapse.

What are the symptoms and signs of PHT?

Symptoms
- Dyspnoea (60% of patients)
- Weakness (19%)
- Recurrent syncope (13%)

Signs
- Fixed or paradoxical splitting of second heart sound in the presence of severe right ventricular dysfunction.
- Pulmonary and tricuspid valve regurgitation murmur.
- Elevated jugular venous pressure (JVP) in the presence of volume overload and right ventricular failure. Large 'v' waves are present in associated severe tricuspid regurgitation.
- Hepatomegaly and ascites.
- Dependent pitting edema of varying degrees.

How would you diagnose PHT?

Clinical findings
- As above

Investigations
- CXR
- ECG: right atrial enlargement, right axis deviation, right ventricular hypertrophy, and characteristic ST depression and T-wave inversions in the anterior leads
- Echocardiography: useful for assessing right and left ventricular function, pulmonary systolic arterial pressure and excluding congenital anomalies and valvular disease
- V/Q scanning: excludes interstitial lung disease and thromboembolic disease
- Pulmonary angiography: excludes thromboembolic disease
- Cardiac catheterisation: assesses pressures and determines pulmonary vasoreactivity
- Cardio pulmonary exercise testing: 6-minute walk testing commonly used as a surrogate test for aerobic capacity and severity

What is the finding on the chest radiography?

Right heart
- Right atrial enlargement may be present if significant tricuspid regurgitation is present, which is shown as a widened right heart border.
- Right ventricular enlargement is seen as a decrease in the retrosternal space on the lateral image.

Pulmonary vasculature
- Enlarged central pulmonary arteries that taper distally.
- Increase in the transverse diameter of the right interlobar artery is indicative of pulmonary hypertension.

STEPS	KEY POINTS

- Peripheral vessel opacity—oligaemic lung fields.
- Kerley B lines may be present. These indicate the presence of pulmonary venous hypertension.

What are the treatment options?

Dilators
- Calcium channel blockers—dilate the pulmonary resistance vessels and lower the pulmonary artery pressure.
- Epoprostenol—intravenous, parenteral prostacyclin analogue
- Bosentan—oral, endothelin receptor antagonist
- Sildenafil—oral phosphodiesterase type 5 (PDE-5) inhibitor

Ancillary treatment
- Oxygen
- Digoxin
- Diuretics

Surgical
- Atrial septostomy—palliative
- Lung transplant

What are the anaesthetic implications?

Induction
- All IV induction drugs have been safely used, although Ketamine can increase PVR.
- Nondepolarising and depolarising muscle relaxants can be used safely.

Maintenance
- All volatile agents can be safely used in PHT except nitrous oxide.

Monitoring
- Invasive blood pressure and cardiac output monitoring.
- Pulmonary artery catheter is indicated in severe cases and in major surgery.

Specific drugs
RV failure and raised PVR can be targeted with inhaled selective pulmonary vasodilators such as nitric oxide and prostacyclin.

Neuraxial blocks
No direct effect on PVR but can cause decreased SVR and coronary perfusion pressure. It can also lead to bradycardia due to inhibition of cardioaccelerator fibres. Decreased preload and bradycardia can be detrimental.

Avoid
- Increased PVR
- Decreased venous return
- Marked decreases in SVR
- Myocardial depression
- Tachy/brady arrthymias

Treat high PVR with
Hyperventilation, nitric oxide, morphine, glyceryl trinitrate, sodium nitroprusside, tolazoline, prostacyclin (PGI_2), isoprenaline, and aminophylline

What increases PVR?

Nitrous oxide, adrenaline, dopamine, protamine, serotonin, thromboxane A2, prostaglandins such as $PGF_2\,\alpha$ and PGE_2, hypoxia, hypercarbia, acidosis, PEEP and lung hyperinflation, cold, anxiety and stress

Further reading

1. ATOTW 228. *Anaesthesia for the Patient with Pulmonary Hypertension*.
2. Guidelines for the diagnosis and treatment of pulmonary hypertension. *European Heart Journal* (2009) **30**, 2493–2537 doi:10.1093/eurheartj/ehp297.

09.7 PHARMACOLOGY: TARGET CONTROLLED INFUSION

STEPS	KEY POINTS
What are the indications of total intravenous anaesthesia (TIVA)?	• During intra- and inter-hospital transfer of patients • When inhalational agents cannot be used (e.g. bronchoscopy) • When inhalational agent is contraindicated (e.g. malignant hyperthermia) • To reduce postoperative nausea and vomiting • To reduce pollution • As another mode of maintenance of anaesthesia
What properties make propofol an ideal agent for TIVA?	**Physical properties** • Cheap • Stable • Safe • Long shelf life **Pharmacokinetic properties** • Rapid onset and offset • Small volume of distribution • Rapid metabolism • No excitation or emergence phenomenon **Pharmacodynamic properties** • Antiemetic effect • No comparative toxic effect A drug with a smaller Vd, rapid metabolism, high clearance, and short context sensitive half-life is ideal for TIVA/TCI.
What is TCI?	TCI means 'Target Controlled Infusion' in which a microprocessor-controlled syringe pump automatically and variably controls the rate of infusion of a drug to attain a user-defined target level in an effect site (brain) in the patient. A pharmacokinetic model is a mathematical model that can be used to predict the blood concentration profile of a drug after a bolus dose or after an infusion of varying duration. These models are typically derived from measuring arterial or venous plasma concentrations after a bolus or infusion in a group of volunteers, using standardised statistical approaches and computer software models.

STEPS	KEY POINTS

Basically, the components of the system are:
- User interface, which allows the user to enter data such as the patient's details and target drug concentration and displays useful numeric and graphic information regarding the infusion rates
- Computer or microprocessor, which implements the pharmacokinetic model, accepts data and instructions from the user, performs the necessary calculations, and controls and monitors the infusion device
- Infusion device, which is capable of infusing rates up to 1200 mL/hr with a precision of 0.1 mL/hr

Define volume of distribution and clearance and describe how these could affect the pharmacokinetics of intravenous anaesthetic agents.

Volume of distribution (Vd)
This is the apparent volume in which the drug is distributed.
Vd = dose/concentration of drug.

Clearance
Clearance represents the volume of plasma (Vp) from which the drug is eliminated per unit time to account for its elimination from the body. Clearance can also be used to describe how quickly the drug moves between compartments.

Clearance = Elimination × Vp.

From these parameters it is possible to derive three main calculations.

1. Loading dose
The drug is initially distributed into the central compartment before distribution to peripheral compartments. If the initial volume of distribution (Vc) and the desired plasma concentration for therapeutic effect (Cp) are known, it is possible to calculate the loading dose to achieve that concentration.

Loading dose = Cp × Vc

2. Bolus dose to achieve a new concentration
It can also be used to calculate the bolus dose required to rapidly increase the concentration during a continuous infusion.

Bolus dose = $[C_{new} - C_{actual}]$ × Vc

3. Rate of infusion to maintain a steady state concentration
Rate of infusion to maintain steady state = Cp × Clearance

Which compartment model better explains the working of a TCI?

A 2- or 3-compartment model can be used to mathematically describe the behaviour of anaesthetic drugs with considerable accuracy.

Conventionally the compartment into which the drug is injected is known as the central compartment (1) and its volume of distribution is the initial volume of distribution (V_1).

From the central compartment, drug transfers rapidly to the second compartment (2) due to its abundance in vessels and lastly into the third compartment (3), which is the slower, vessel-poor compartment.

The sum of all these compartments is known as 'volume of distribution at steady state'.

STEPS	KEY POINTS

Define context sensitive half time (CSHT).

Time for the plasma concentration to fall to half after stopping an infusion at steady state.

It is a comparison between the distribution and elimination clearances. For example, a high distribution clearance and a low elimination clearance increase the CSHT.

After 4 hours of infusion, the ratio of distribution clearance to elimination clearance for fentanyl is 5:1 and that of propofol is 1:1, accounting to the CSHT of 250 min and 20 min, respectively. As remifentanil is degraded by plasma esterases, distribution clearance is less than elimination clearance, so CSHT is very short.

Drug	Distribution Clearance: Elimination clearance	CSHT at 2 hours	CSHT at 4 hours
Fentanyl	5:1	48	250
Propofol	1:1	16	20
Remifentanil	<1	4.5	6

Define rate constant.

A coefficient of proportionality relating the rate of a chemical reaction at a given temperature to the concentration of reactant or to the product of the concentrations of reactants. It is measured in units of reciprocal time (time^{-1})

The rate of drug elimination (k) is assumed to be proportional to the amount of drug in the compartment at any time, while the concentration (C) decreases with time (t) in a monoexponential manner.

$Ct = C_0e^{-kt}$, where e = 2.718

K10 is the symbol used to denote the rate constant for metabolism or elimination, whereas K12, K21, K13, K31 symbolise the rate constants for drug transfer between respective compartments.

Define half-life.

Half-life is the time required to reduce the plasma concentration to half of its initial value.

What is time constant?

Time constant is the time taken for the plasma concentration to reach '0' if the initial rate of decline had continued.

What are the working principles of Marsh and Schnider models?

These models are used for propofol TCI (Minto for remifentanil)

Marsh Model
The Marsh model assumes that the central compartment volume is directly proportional to weight only. The age is entered but not used in the calculations (however, the pump will not function if age < 16 is entered).

Schnider Model
The Schnider model is incorporated into the 'newer generation' TCI pumps. It is a 3-compartment model for propofol where age, height, and weight are entered into the system. The lean body mass for the patient is calculated, and this is used to calculate doses and infusion rates. The central compartment is fixed (i.e. the same for every patient).

STEPS	KEY POINTS
Differences between the Marsh and the Schnider models	• Size of the central compartment Schnider uses a fixed central compartment volume that is smaller (4.27 L in a 70 kg patient) than that used in the Marsh model (15.9 L). Because of this, the estimated concentrations after a bolus will vary markedly. • Age The Schnider model is considered better for the elderly as it takes age into account and allows for the reduced rate of clearance. • Dose of propofol Differences in infusion rates that occur during the first few minutes after an increase in target concentrations decreases with time. Overall, less propofol is used with the Schnider model. • Body weight The Marsh model uses total body weight instead of lean body mass in its calculations, and there is a risk of overdosing obese patients if their actual body weight is entered. Therefore, it is proposed that the ideal body weight of a patient is entered if the patient is obese.

09.8 PHYSICS: CARDIAC OUTPUT MONITORING

STEPS	KEY POINTS
What do you mean by dynamic fluid responsiveness?	In a spontaneously ventilating patient, systolic blood pressure fluctuates with ventilation by 5–10 mmHg. This is known as the respiratory swing. Pulsus paradoxus is when the difference in systolic blood pressure between inspiration and expiration is greater than 10 mmHg.
	In patients undergoing positive pressure ventilation, reverse pulsus paradoxus occurs. During inspiration, stroke volume (SV) from the right ventricle decreases and that from the left ventricle increases due to the increased intrathoracic pressure. This causes an increase in blood pressure during inspiration and decrease during expiration.
	Stroke volume variation (SVV) is one method of measuring patient's dynamic fluid responsiveness. It is defined by:
	$$\frac{SV_{max} - SV_{min}}{SV\ mean}$$
	It is represented as a percentage and reflects the change in SV during the respiratory cycle and can be assessed continuously by any beat-to-beat cardiac output monitor. SVV of greater than 10% suggests that patient is fluid-responsive as it indicates that SV is sensitive to fluctuations in preload caused by the respiratory cycle.
What are the specific causes of central venous pressure (CVP) inaccuracies?	**Patient factors** • Altered in ventilated patients due to increase in intrathoracic pressure • Tricuspid valve disease (e.g. tricuspid regurgitation can cause discrepancy between digital display and end diastolic, end expiratory pressure) **Equipment related** • Transducer height • Damping/resonance • Pressured bag—sufficient pressure?

STEPS	KEY POINTS

Draw an arterial line trace and explain what information can be obtained from it. See Figure 9.7

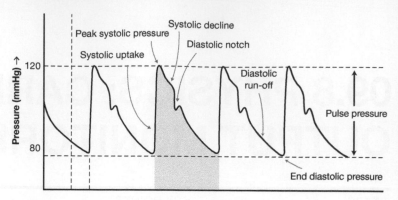

Fig. 9.7

Upstroke
- dP/dT
- Marks the stage of ventricular ejection
- Represents contractility
- Slope can be slurred in aortic stenosis

Dicrotic notch
- Closing of aortic valve
- Represents systemic vascular resistance (SVR)
- If very low, suspect low SVR (e.g. septic shock)

Area under the curve
- Up to dicrotic notch represents SV

Pulse pressure
- Widened pulse pressure suggests aortic regurgitation (in diastole, the arterial pressure drops to fill the left ventricle through the regurgitating aortic valve)
- Narrow pulse pressure suggests cardiac tamponade or low-output state (e.g. aortic stenosis, severe cardiogenic shock, massive pulmonary embolism, or tension pneumothorax)

How can cardiac output be monitored?

- Pulmonary artery catheter—still the gold standard
- Pulse pressure analysis (e.g. PiCCO™, LiDCO™, FloTrac™/Vigileo™)
- Oesophageal Doppler
- Applied Fick's principle (e.g. NICO™ system)
- Bioimpedance

What are the properties of an ideal cardiac output monitor?

- Accurate
- Easily reproducible results
- Quick and easy to use—minimal setup and interpretation of information
- Operator-independent—skill of operator should not affect information
- Continuous measurement
- Minimal drift
- Safe to staff and patients
- Noninvasive
- Cost-effective
- Fast response time

STEPS	KEY POINTS
Discuss LiDCO™ and how it works.	LiDCO™ uses pulse pressure analysis to track continuous changes in stroke volume. It follows an algorithm that is based on the assumption that the net power change in the system in a heartbeat is the difference between the amount of blood entering the system (SV) and the amount of blood flowing out peripherally.
	It uses the principle of conservation of mass (power) and assumes that, following correction for compliance, there is a linear relationship between net power and net flow. Some studies describe LiDCO™ as a pulse *power* analysis.
	LiDCO™*plus* requires calibration using lithium indicator dilution technique (performed via a peripheral cannula).
	LiDCO™*rapid* uses nomograms for cardiac output monitoring and does not require lithium calibration.
Explain the working of oesophageal Doppler.	When sound waves are reflected from a moving object, their frequency is altered. This is the Doppler effect. By using an ultrasound probe to visualise directional blood flow, the change in frequency before and after reflection of moving red blood cells can be determined. This, together with the cross-sectional area of the blood vessel being observed, can be used to determine flow using the formula:
	Flow = Area × Velocity
	Aortic area is not measured using this method; it is estimated using an algorithm based on body surface area.
	The Doppler probe is passed into the oesophagus and rotated until the transducer faces the descending aorta (the oesophagus and descending aorta run close and parallel to each other) and the resultant characteristic waveform is studied.
	The Doppler shift (Fd) produced by moving blood flow is calculated by the ultrasound system using the following equation:
	$Fd = 2FtVCos\,\theta\,/\,C$
	Ft is the transmitted Doppler frequency, V is the speed of blood flow, Cos θ is the Cosine of the blood flow to beam angle, and C is the speed of sound in tissue
What haemodynamic parameters can be deduced using the Doppler? See Figure 9.8.	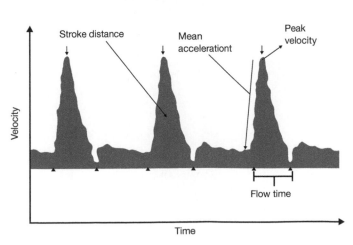

Fig. 9.8 Image of Descending Aortic Waveform (from Deltex Medical CardioQ manual)

STEPS	KEY POINTS

Cardiac output (Q = SV × HR)
- Q is estimated by minute distance.

Stroke volume
- The area under the systolic part of the waveform is defined as Stroke Distance (SD). The Stroke Volume is calculated from the measured SD and the nomogram derived constant.

Corrected (systolic) flow time (FTc) indicates preload.
- Normal = 0.33–0.36s

Peak velocity (PV)
- Indicates contractility.
- Interpretation of FTc and PV indicates afterload.

Heart rate

Further reading

1. Deltex Medical CardioQ manual.
2. Mezger V, Habicher M, Sander M. Update on perioperative hemodynamic monitoring and goal-directed optimization concepts. Annual update in *Intensive Care and Emergency Medicine 2014*.

CLINICAL
VIVA

10.1 LONG CASE: MEDIASTINAL MASS

HISTORY *A 16-year-old-girl with 6 weeks' history of cervical lymphadenopathy has been added to the end of your list for cervical lymph node biopsy to aid diagnosis.*
She complains of increasing face and neck swelling, exertional dyspnoea, shortness of breath, and coughing while lying flat. She also has been complaining of noises when breathing.

STEPS	KEY POINTS					
Past Medical History	She has no other medical condition.					
Drugs	Nil					
On Examination	Anxious Comfortable at rest Chest: Clear					
Investigations	Hb	13.3 g/dL	(12–15)	APPT	22 sec	(21–34 sec)
	WCC	17.4 × 10⁹/L	(4–11)	PT	12 sec	(11–13.6 sec)
	Neutrophils	4.5 × 10⁹/L	(2–7.5)	INR	1.0	(0.9–1.2)
	Lymphocytes	12.2 × 10⁹/L	(1.5–3.5)			
	Eosinophils	0.1 × 10⁹/L	(0.04–0.44)	Na	138 mmol/L	(137–145)
	Basophils	0.1 × 10⁹/L	(0.0–0.1)	K	4.4 mmol/L	(3.6–5.0)
	Monocytes	0.5 × 10⁹/L	(0.2–0.8)	Urea	6 mmol/L	(1.7–8.3)
	Platelet count	300 × 10⁹/L	(150–400)	Creat	80 umol/L	(62–124)
CXR	See Figure 10.1.					

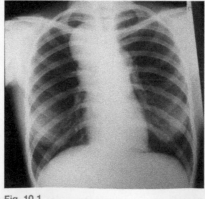

Fig. 10.1

STEPS	KEY POINTS
CT Chest	See Figure 10.2.

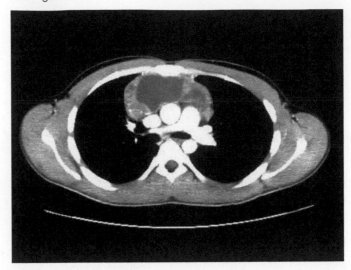

Fig. 10.2

Summarise the case.	This is a paediatric patient with no previous medical illness presenting with possible haematological malignancy for an urgent procedure. There is also a risk with her airway due to the presence of neck swelling and a mediastinal mass.
What are the main issues?	• Paediatric case with consent issues • Potential difficult airway due to facial and neck swelling • Potential difficult airway due to tracheal compression • Possible haematological malignancy and its implications • Haemodynamic instability due to compression of great vessels • Urgent procedure
Can you talk through the investigations?	**Bloods** Lymphocytic leucocytosis Otherwise normal **Chest X-ray** Asymmetric hilar lymphadenopathy Lobulated mediastinal widening **CT chest** No level indicated Large anterior mediastinal mass is seen with hypodense areas representing necrotic component in the middle. Trachea seems slightly pushed to the right and is flattened.
What are the causes of lymphocytosis?	Lymphocytes make up 20%–40% of leucocytes. Causes of increased lymphocyte count can be classified as: **Absolute** • Acute—Cytomegalovirus (CMV) and Epstein-Barr virus (EBV), pertussis, hepatitis, toxoplasmosis • Chronic—tuberculosis, brucellosis • Lympho proliferative malignancy (CLL, ALL, lymphoma)

STEPS	KEY POINTS

Relative
- Age < 2 yrs
- Connective tissue diseases
- Hormonal imbalance—Addison's disease and thyrotoxicosis

What is the differential diagnosis for hilar and generalised lymphadenopathy?

Bilateral hilar lymphadenopathy
- Sarcoidosis
- Tuberculosis
- Lymphoma
- Silicosis

Generalised Lymphadenopathy
- Malignant
  - Lympho proliferative malignancy
  - Myelo proliferative malignancy

- Nonmalignant
  - Infective
    - Infectious mononucleosis
    - Toxoplasmosis
    - HIV
    - Tuberculosis
  - Autoimmune connective tissue disorders
    - Rheumatoid arthritis
    - SLE
  - Drug-induced
    - Allopurinol
    - Atenolol
    - Penicillin
    - Gold

How would you assess the patient preoperatively?

History
- Severity of dyspnoea: factors worsening dyspnoea, positional changes, functional assessment, etc.
- Presence of added noises: time of onset, quality and timing with regards to respiratory cycle, positional changes
- Past medical history
- Anaesthetic history: whether the child has had any anaesthetics in the past, previous grade of intubation, history of reflux and allergies

Examination
- General assessment of extent of facial and neck swelling
- Airway assessment
- Signs of Superior Vena Cava Obstruction (SVCO)

Investigations
- Imaging: All patients with an anterior mediastinal mass should have a chest radiograph and a CT scan prior to any surgical procedure to plan the airway management. The CT scan will show the site, severity, and extent of the airway compromise to assess the level and degree of obstruction.
- Nasal endoscopy to assess the cord function.
- Lung function tests to look for the extent of intrathoracic or extrathoracic obstruction.
- ECHO to rule out pericardial effusion and cardiac compression.

STEPS	KEY POINTS

Are you concerned about the noise when breathing? What is its importance?

Yes. The added noise here is called stridor.

Stridor occurs due to turbulence caused by the passage of air through narrowed airway. The timing of the stridor with respect to the respiratory cycle indicates the location of the narrowing.
- Inspiratory stridor (laryngeal)—obstruction above the level of glottis
- Expiratory stridor (tracheobronchial)—obstruction in the intrathoracic airways
- Biphasic stridor—obstruction between glottis and subglottis or a critical obstruction at any level

What are the complications due to mass effect of the mediastinal tumour?

- Vascular compromise—SVCO and pulmonary vessel obstruction
- Laryngeal nerve palsy
- Dysphagia
- Stridor and airway compromise

What is superior vena cava obstruction (SVCO) and what are its features?

The thin-walled SVC gets easily compressed by the mediastinal mass and results in obstructive damage of venous flow from the upper half of the body.

The disease is characterised by facial and neck swelling, head fullness, nasal stuffiness, orthopnoea, dysphagia, stridor, and positive Pemberton's sign (facial plethora and respiratory distress when both arms are elevated, demonstrating the presence of thoracic inlet obstruction).

Causes of SVCO
- Intrinsic: thrombus
- Extrinsic: tumours

Challenges during anaesthesia
- Need for supplemental oxygen
- Orthopnoea—induction in the sitting-up position
- IV cannula in the lower extremity
- Airway oedema
- Mucosal bleeding
- Laryngeal nerve palsy
- Haemodynamic instability due to decreased venous return

How would you proceed with this case?

Preoperative
- History, examination, and investigations, as discussed earlier
- Optimisation: This is an urgent surgery to aid diagnosis, so procedure cannot be delayed.
- Explain to the child and her parents about her journey in theatre and give reassurance.
- Discussion with patient and family regarding the choice of anaesthetic— LA versus GA.
- Premedication with benzodiazepine in an anxious patient but generally avoided if there is risk of airway compromise.

STEPS	KEY POINTS

Intraoperative
- Involving senior surgeon, anaesthetist, and ODP
- Emergency drugs and equipment

Emergency drugs—atropine, suxamethonium (controversial), fluids and vasopressors.

Airway equipment—rigid bronchoscopy and difficult airway trolley, jet ventilation, cardiopulmonary bypass (CPB) on standby. Femoro femoral bypass is the most common setup.

Monitoring
- AAGBI monitoring
- Arterial line in case of vascular compromise
- Femoral access for CPB

Anaesthetic choice
- Local anaesthetic infiltration alone
- Superficial and deep cervical plexus blocks
- General anaesthesia

LA versus GA

Local anaesthesia	General anaesthesia
Indication - Symptomatic patients with definite airway obstruction on CT/MRI - Tracheal cross-sectional area of ≤ 50% predicted - PEFR ≤ 50% predicted	**Indication** - Patient refusal - Contraindication to LA (or a paediatric patient as in this case)
Choice - Superficial cervical plexus block - Deep cervical plexus block	**Choice** - Ketamine - Spontaneously breathing patient with LMA

Avoid
- General anaesthesia, as it can cause loss of intrinsic muscle tone, decreased lung volumes, and decreased transpleural pressure gradient
- Muscle relaxants
- Positive pressure ventilation, which can precipitate severe hypotension and also increases intrathoracic tracheal compression
- Coughing, as it can cause complete airway obstruction by positive pleural pressure, increasing intrathoracic tracheal compression

Explain the technique of superficial cervical plexus block. Is it easier to perform in this patient?

Superficial and deep cervical plexus blocks are done for superficial neck surgery such as carotid endarterectomy and cervical lymph node excision. Both types of blocks have a similar pattern of sensory distribution, but deep block is associated with greater risk for complications such as vertebral artery puncture, systemic toxicity, and nerve root injury. So, there is a trend towards favouring the superficial approach.

Preparation
- Explaining the risks and obtaining informed consent
- Intravenous access
- AAGBI monitoring
- Emergency drugs and equipment

Anatomy
The cervical plexus is formed from the anterior primary rami of the first four cervical spinal nerves, C 1–4. It lies deep to the internal jugular vein and the sternocleidomastoid muscle and superficial to the transverse process of cervical vertebrae and the scalene muscles and spreads into four cutaneous branches: the greater auricular nerve, lesser occipital nerve, supraclavicular nerve, and the transverse cervical nerve.

STEPS	KEY POINTS

Position

Supine or semi-sitting position with the head facing away from the side to be blocked

Landmarks

Neck and facial swelling can make the procedure difficult and risky and can potentiate airway and vascular compromise. Ultrasound guidance may be helpful in this case.

Technique

- Sterile technique
- Skin infiltration with local anaesthetic solution
- 25 G needle with flexible tubing attached to a 20 mL syringe of marcaine—0.25% to 0.5%
- Needle insertion site behind the posterior border of the sternocleidomastoid muscle at its midpoint between the mastoid and the clavicle
- Injection made in a fan-wise fashion at a depth of approximately 1 cm

The anxious patient has refused to have surgery under local infiltration or nerve blocks. How would you proceed with general anaesthetic?

Aim to prevent cardiac compression, airway occlusion, and SVC obstruction.

Induction

- IV cannula in the lower extremity
- Induction in sitting position (semi Fowler's position)
- Inhalational (preferred choice) or IV induction agent titrated to effect
- Choose spontaneous ventilation with LMA
- Awake fibreoptic technique if intubation is necessary with a reinforced smaller calibre and longer endotracheal tube

Maintenance

- Maintenance with gas in spontaneously breathing patient
- TIVA with short-acting drugs for quick emergence

Emergence

Postoperative airway obstruction due to airway oedema, tracheomalacia, and bleeding warrant the need for awake extubation in ITU. The following steps would aid in an uneventful extubation:

- Test for leak around the endotracheal tube cuff.
- Administer dexamethasone or chemo radiotherapy in sensitive tumours to shrink size of tumour.
- Use adrenaline nebulisers.
- Extubate over airway exchange catheters.

Following gas induction, the patient stops breathing and you are unable to ventilate her. What would you do now?

Follow difficult or failed intubation guidelines. But cricoid puncture and emergency tracheostomy are futile if the level of airway obstruction is at the intrathoracic tracheobronchial tree.

Simple measures

- Change in position—lateral, sitting up, or prone—to decrease the mechanical effect of the tumour.
- Avoid positive pressure ventilation for fear of luminal closure.
- Administer high-dose steroids for tumour shrinkage.
- Direct laryngoscopy and endobronchial intubation down the least obstructed lumen.
- Awake fibreoptic intubation with difficult airway.

STEPS	KEY POINTS

Other measures
- Rigid bronchoscopy—dilatation of stenosis, laser, and electro cautery to debulk the tumour and stenting to bypass
- Low-frequency jet ventilation with Sander's injector or high-frequency translaryngeal jet ventilation with Hunsaker's catheter
- CPB bypass and ECMO to restore oxygenation when other measures fail

You have managed to intubate the patient with a 6 mm microlaryngoscopy tube (MLT). You have transferred the patient after biopsy to ITU for monitoring and extubation when ready.

How can you reduce the tumour size in the postoperative setting?
- High-dose steroids—dexamethasone
- Chemotherapy or radiotherapy depending upon the type of tumour
- Endoscopic debulking of the tumour

What is the chemotherapy choice for lymphoma?

Non-Hodgkin's Lymphoma
- CHOP: Cyclophosphamide, Hydroxydaunomycin (Doxorubicin), Oncovin (Vincristine), Prednisone
- COPP: Cyclophosphamide, Oncovin, Procarbazine, Prednisone

Hodgkin's Lymphoma
- ABVD: Adriamycin, Bleomycin, Vinblastine, Dacarbazine
- BEACOPP: Bleomycin, Etoposide, Adriamycin, Cyclophosphamide, Oncovin, Procarbazine, Prednisone

Following chemotherapy in ITU, the blood test showed serum potassium of 6.9 mmol/L. What are the possible causes?

Normal serum potassium	3.5–5.5 mmol/L
Mild hyperkalemia	5.5–6.0 mmol/L
Moderate hyperkalemia	6.1–7.0 mmol/L
Severe hyperkalemia	> 7.0 mmol/L

Causes of hyperkalemia in this case
- Decreased excretion—renal failure
- Redistribution—metabolic acidosis, tumour lysis syndrome secondary to chemotherapy or the tumour itself

What is tumour lysis syndrome?

Discussed elsewhere.

How do you treat high K?

Treatment is necessary if K^+ is > 7 mmol/L or if patient is symptomatic with ECG changes

1. Stop further accumulation of potassium.
   - Stopping drugs that increase potassium
   - Low-potassium diet
2. Protect cardiac cells
   - 10% Calcium gluconate—10 mL intravenously over 2 min. Repeat as necessary.
3. Redistribution
   - Salbutamol nebulisers: 2.5–5 mg
   - Insulin infusion: 10 U actrapid + 50 mL 50% glucose as an IV infusion
4. Removal of potassium from the body
   - Haemodialysis
   - Calcium resonium enema

10.2 SHORT CASE: PREOPERATIVE ANAEMIA

HISTORY *A 58-year-old female is listed for elective hemicolectomy for colon carcinoma. Her blood results are shown below.*

Hb	8.4 g/dL (13–16)
PCV	0.35 (0.38–0.56)
MCV	71 fL (80–100)
MCH	20 pg (26–34)
Platelets	218 (140–400)
U's & E's normal	

STEPS	KEY POINTS
Comment on these blood results and suggest possible causes of her anaemia.	Her FBC shows a microcytic, hypochromic anaemia. Possible causes include: • Chronic blood loss (e.g. from GI tract in association with her colon cancer) • 'Anaemia of chronic disease' (resulting in reduced production and lifespan of red cells) • Bone marrow failure (due to recent chemotherapy, metastatic infiltration, or a concurrent haematological malignancy) • Dietary iron deficiency • Chronic kidney disease is unlikely given her normal U's & E's
What could you do about the anaemia, and what are the general principles of managing preoperative anaemia?	In general, management should involve balancing the benefits of correcting the anaemia against the risks of delaying surgery. This is an elective case, but the cancer diagnosis lends it a degree of urgency. However, anaemia increases her risk of postoperative morbidity (particularly 'MACE'—major adverse cardiovascular events—such as MI or stroke) and overall mortality. In this case, the options are: • Do nothing and proceed with surgery (not advisable as it increases her perioperative risk). • Correct the cause (will require further investigation and may take weeks, or even months; most likely cause is her cancer). • Red cell transfusion causes rapid correction of Hb, but concerns exist regarding allogeneic blood transfusion and long-term survival/cancer recurrence rates. The current evidence on this is inconclusive, however. Cautious transfusion should also be practised in patients at risk of fluid overload.

STEPS	KEY POINTS
	• Initiate oral iron therapy (may take several weeks to correct Hb, depending on degree of deficiency).
	• Deliver intravenous iron therapy (emerging evidence that this is a cost-effective means of reducing perioperative transfusion requirements).

The urgency of correcting the Hb depends not only on the urgency of surgery but also whether she has evidence of cardiovascular compromise (shortness of breath/chest pain/heart failure), in which case urgent transfusion would be warranted.

What role does 2,3 DPG (diphosphoglycerate) play in oxygen delivery to tissues?

Oxygen delivery is determined by cardiac output (CO) and arterial O_2 content (CaO_2).

$$DO_2 = CO \times CaO_2$$

• Arterial O_2 content depends on Hb and O_2 saturation (plus a tiny contribution from dissolved O_2, unless you are in a hyperbaric chamber).
• In chronic anaemia, a low Hb is partly compensated by increasing CO.
• Increased levels of 2,3 DPG in RBCs improves oxygen delivery to tissues by shifting the Hb O_2 dissociation curve to the right.

Would you transfuse this patient, and if so, when?

This would depend on urgency of surgery and whether the anaemia is symptomatic. In general, I would try to avoid transfusing unless I felt she was sufficiently anaemic to place her at risk of an adverse cardiac event—in which case I would transfuse her urgently—or if surgery was deemed urgent.

Are there concerns regarding transfusion in cancer patients [already mentioned above]?

Concerns exist that blood transfusion may increase the risk of disease recurrence and/or decrease long-term survival.

• A 1993 study of 475 patients with colorectal cancer found no difference in survival between patients who received allogenic transfusions and those who had an autologous transfusion. Furthermore, a 20-year follow-up of these patients showed significantly better survival in those who received allogenic transfusions.
• A retrospective American study from 2013 of 27,000 patients with colorectal cancer found a significantly higher 30-day mortality and rate of postoperative complications in those who received blood transfusions.

What do you know about fast-track surgery?

Fast-track surgery, also known as enhanced recovery, means a targeted approach to perioperative care of minimising disruption to the patient's usual activities and returning them to normal function as soon as possible after surgery. The theoretical advantages include quicker patient discharge and reducing the per-patient cost of treatment.
• Preoperative preparation aims to minimise fasting times, avoid bowel preparation, and optimise nutrition/hydration.
• Intraoperative management, in particular the anaesthetic management, involves goal-directed fluid therapy guided by cardiac output monitoring to maximise oxygen delivery, and multimodal analgesia to minimise postoperative pain.
• Postoperative management aims to restore oral intake and mobility as soon as possible and to minimise invasive lines/catheters.

The overall aim is to improve surgical outcomes by reducing avoidable postoperative complications (e.g. DVT/PE, chest infections, ileus).

STEPS	KEY POINTS
The patient is also a smoker and reports shortness of breath on exertion. How else might you investigate her?	Her exertional shortness of breath may be due to anaemia or an underlying respiratory or cardiac disease.
	• History and examination: Is she known to have COPD? If so, how severe? How much exertion precipitates shortness of breath? Does she have signs of respiratory/cardiac failure?
	• CXR and ABG on air would be mandatory in this instance. Lung function tests may also be indicated.
	• Formal testing of functional capacity would be useful. An exercise test or stress echo would be good; best would be cardiopulmonary exercise testing (CPET). CPET involves the patient performing ramped exercise on an exercise bike, while recording ECG, HR, BP, and expired gases. It correlates well with risk of postoperative adverse events, because it reflects the patient's degree of cardiorespiratory reserve, and thus their ability to increase oxygen delivery in the face of the postoperative stress response to surgery. The most useful measurements obtained are VO_2 max (the patient's maximum oxygen delivery) and anaerobic threshold (AT is the point at which the demands of cellular metabolism exceed the oxygen supply to tissues). A VO_2max < 15, and AT < 11 are strong predictors of postoperative complications following major surgery.
Other potential questions for this short case:	Transfusion thresholds; oxygen delivery and flux equation; methods to minimise perioperative blood transfusion; classification/investigation of anaemia.

10.3 SHORT CASE: CHOLESTEATOMA

HISTORY *You are doing ENT list and a 12–year-old boy has been listed for mastoidectomy for cholesteatoma.*

STEPS	KEY POINTS
What are the issues with this case?	• Paediatric age group • Prolonged operation and redo operations • Need for hypotensive anaesthesia • Need for facial nerve monitoring • High incidence of PONV • Operation near the airway—difficult to get to the airway
What is cholesteatoma?	• Squamous epithelium trapped in the skull base affecting middle ear, temporal bone, and mastoid. • It is a fatal destructive lesion, as it erodes and destroys the structures within the temporal bone.
What is the significance of cholesteatoma? What happens if it is left untreated?	• It grows and expands at the expense of the bones and structures surrounding it. • It causes bony erosion due to pressure effects and also enzymatic osteoclastic activity. • It causes pressure effects and CNS complications.
What symptoms might this child have?	• Painless otorrhoea • Dizziness • Sensorineural deafness • Other symptoms due to pressure effects and invasion of surrounding structures—brain abscess, sigmoid sinus thrombosis, epidural abscess, meningitis, and facial nerve palsy
How would you manage the airway?	• GA with reinforced LMA or • ET Tube
If you plan to intubate this child, what is the problem you would encounter? How would you overcome this?	Need for facial nerve monitoring calls for no muscle relaxant on board. If we have used muscle relaxant for intubation, then it might be difficult to use the facial nerve monitoring. It can be overcome by: • Use a short-acting muscle relaxant, which would have worn off by the time facial nerve monitoring, is needed. • Avoid muscle relaxants altogether and use a potent opiate for intubation.
What are the advantages and disadvantages of using a reinforced LMA?	Advantages: Less stormy emergence, less airway stimulation Disadvantages: Need for controlled ventilation to control CO_2, chance of aspiration as it is not a definitive airway

STEPS	KEY POINTS
Which nerve is at risk of being damaged during this procedure? How would you treat it?	The facial nerve, near its exit from the skull base through the stylomastoid foramen, is very close to the ossicles at this level. • Immediate decompression if nerve injury is suspected. • Evidence for steroid use is unconvincing.
How would you achieve hypotensive anaesthesia in this patient?	• 15° head tilt to prevent venous ooze • Adrenaline infiltration by surgeons • Controlled ventilation to decrease $PaCO_2$ • Drugs—sevoflurane and remifentanil, propofol and remifentanil, labetalol infusion, etc
What would be your choice of analgesia and antiemesis?	**Analgesia** • Intraoperative: WHO ladder —simple analgesics, NSAIDS, LA by surgeons, great auricular nerve block by anaesthetist, opioids if necessary • Postoperative: WHO ladder **Antiemesis** • Good hydration and balanced analgesia • Use of TIVA, avoiding N_2O • Avoidance of prolonged starvation times • Drugs—dexamethasone, ondansetron, cyclizine, and droperidol

10.4 SHORT CASE: CARDIAC RISK STRATIFICATION

HISTORY *You are asked to see a 65-year-old patient with a known history of hypertension, ischaemic heart disease, and congestive cardiac failure who had been booked for urgent below knee amputation due to acute ischaemia and gangrenous limb. He is on ramipril, aspirin, and warfarin. ECG shows irregular ventricular response around 125–140/min.*

STEPS	KEY POINTS
What are the issues presented to you?	• Elderly patient with significant comorbidities • Emergency surgery • Need for assessment of cardiac condition • Rate control of atrial fibrillation • INR optimised if abnormal • High chance of sepsis, which needs to be treated
Why would you need to assess the cardiac status?	The purpose of preoperative cardiac risk assessment is to • Identify patients at increased risk of an adverse perioperative cardiac event. • Assess the medical status of these patients and the cardiac risks posed by the planned noncardiac surgery. • Recommend appropriate strategies to reduce the risk of cardiac problems over the entire perioperative period and to improve long-term cardiac outcomes.
How would you assess this patient's cardiac status?	<u>History and physical examination</u>—to help to identify markers of cardiac risk and assess the patient's cardiac status. High-risk cardiac conditions include recent MI, decompensated heart failure, unstable angina, symptomatic arrhythmias, and symptomatic valvular heart disease. Patients with severe aortic stenosis, elevated jugular venous pressure, pulmonary oedema, and/or third heart sound on examination are at high surgical risk. <u>Evaluation of functional status</u>—The metabolic equivalent of a task (MET) is a physiological concept expressing the energy cost of a physical activity. • 1 MET: Eat, dress, use the toilet, and walk indoors around the house • 4 METs: Climb a flight of stairs (usually 18–21 steps) or run short distances • > 10 METs: Participate in strenuous sports such as swimming and skiing. On assessment, patients with < 4 METs are considered to have poor functional capacity and are at relatively high risk of a perioperative event, while patients with > 10 METs have excellent functional capacity and are at very low risk of perioperative events, even if they have known CAD. Patients with a functional capacity of 4–10 METs are considered to have fair functional capacity and are generally considered at low risk of developing perioperative events.

STEPS	KEY POINTS

Cardiac risk stratification using clinical predictors—assessment of clinical predictors of increased perioperative risk for MI, heart failure, and cardiac death.

High risk:
Recent MI or severe angina
Decompensated heart failure
Severe valvular heart disease
Significant arrhythmias

Intermediate risk:
History of ischaemic heart disease
Compensated heart failure
Diabetes mellitus
Renal insufficiency (preop creatinine > 177 mmol/L)
Cerebrovascular disease

Investigations

- Preoperative resting 12-lead ECG can show arrhythmias, ventricular hypertrophy, and ischaemic changes.
- Preoperative noninvasive evaluation of ventricular and valvular function with echocardiography.
- Stress testing: Exercise ECG and stress imaging (Dobutamine stress echo and dipyridamole thallium scan) provides an estimate of functional capacity, detects myocardial ischaemia, and assesses haemodynamic performance during stress.
- Coronary angiography: Indicated in patients with evidence of high cardiac risk; identifies specific blood vessels with perfusion problems.
- Brain natriuretic peptide (BNP): BNP appears to independently predict major adverse cardiac events in the first 30 days after vascular surgery and can significantly improve the predictive performance of the revised cardiac risk index.
- Assessment of both cardiac and respiratory elements of exercise is done with cardiopulmonary exercise testing (CPEX).

Discuss the cardiac risk scoring systems in anaesthesia.

- New York Heart Association (NYHA) functional classification of heart disease
  I: No symptoms and no limitation of ordinary physical activity
  II: Mild symptoms and slight limitation during ordinary activity
  III: Symptoms and limitation in less than ordinary activity
  IV: Symptoms even at rest

- Goldman cardiac risk index – nine multifactorial index of cardiac risk in the noncardiac surgery setting

Risk factors	Points
Elevated JVP	11
Third heart sound	11
Myocardial Infarction in past 6 months	10
ECG: premature arterial contractions or any rhythm other than sinus	7
ECG: > 5 ventricular ectopics	7
Age > 70	5
Emergency procedure	4
Intra-thoracic, intra-abdominal or aortic surgery	3
Poor general health status	3

STEPS	KEY POINTS

The incidence of complications related to the score achieved is shown in the table below.

Class	Score	Incidence of severe cardiovascular complications
I	0–5	1%
II	6–12	7%
III	13–25	14%
IV	> 26	78%

- Lee's revised cardiac risk index: Six independent variables and each assigned one point.
  - High-risk surgical procedure
  - History of ischaemic heart disease
  - History of congestive heart failure
  - History of cerebrovascular disease
  - Preoperative treatment with insulin
  - Preop serum creatinine > 2 mg/dL (177 mmol/L)

Class	Points	Risk
I	0	0.4%
II	1	0.9%
III	2	6.6%
IV	> 3	11%

STEPS	KEY POINTS
How will you anaesthetise this patient?	• Thorough preoperative assessment and preoptimisation as much as possible. • Choice of anaesthetic: Regional techniques are not advisable due to coagulopathy and sepsis. General anaesthesia with titrated doses of anaesthetics to avoid hypotension. • Invasive monitoring, optimal analgesia, and treatment of arrhythmias are important. • Assess the chances for postoperative complications, and admission to a high-dependency or intensive care unit would be ideal.
What are the analgesic options?	• Simple analgesics like paracetamol followed by opioid analgesics. • Anti-inflammatory drugs are relatively contraindicated due to sepsis, severe heart disease, and probable acute kidney injury. • Nerve blocks can be given if coagulation is controlled. Femoral and sciatic nerve block gives pain relief for 12 to 24 hours. • Local anaesthetic infiltration by surgeons especially to the cut ends of nerves reduces incidence of phantom limb pain. • Catheter infiltration of local anaesthetic through a pump is another option.

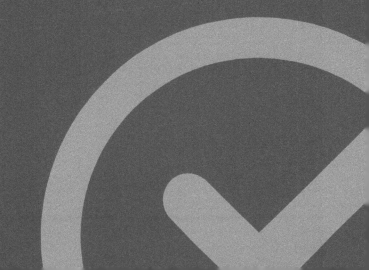

section 10

BASIC SCIENCE VIVA

10.5 ANATOMY: INTRAOSSEOUS ANATOMY

HISTORY *A 10-year-old child has been brought to A&E with a history of diarrhoea and vomiting for the past 3 days.*

STEPS	KEY POINTS
How would you assess dehydration in children?	**Parental observation** Parental report of vomiting, diarrhoea, or decreased oral intake is sensitive in identifying dehydration in children. **Physical examination** Weight loss, capillary filling time, pulse, respiration, blood pressure, sunken eyes, lethargy, and dry mucous membranes. **Laboratory assessment** Serum bicarbonate < 17 mmol/L may improve sensitivity of identifying children with moderate to severe hypovolemia. Severity of dehydration is classified according to these clinical parameters into mild, moderate, and severe. Combination of physical examination findings are the most specific and sensitive tool for accurately diagnosing dehydration in children and categorising its severity. Overdiagnosis of dehydration may lead to unnecessary tests and treatment, whereas underdiagnosis may lead to increased morbidity. *Attempts at cannulation by medical personnel have failed.*
What else could you do?	European resuscitation council (ERC) recommends the use of intraosseous (IO) route if establishing peripheral venous access is delayed.
What are the sites of insertion?	• Tibial—anterior surface, 2–3 cm below the tibial tuberosity • Femoral—anterolateral surface, 3 cm above lateral condyle • Humeral—posterolateral surface • Iliac crest—in older children
Describe the procedure of inserting an IO needle in the tibia.	**Identify site and landmarks** • Identify the tibial tuberosity, just below the knee, by palpation. • Locate a consistent flat area of bone 2 cm distal and slightly medial to the tibial tuberosity.

STEPS	KEY POINTS
	Asepsis **Procedure** • Insert needle at 90 degrees to skin. • Advance until a 'give' is felt as cortex penetrated. • Attach the syringe and aspirate for sample. • Flush to confirm positioning. • Attach 20 mL syringe and push infusion in boluses.
What do you do after insertion of the IO needle?	Once inserted, correct placement is confirmed before delivery of drugs by aspirating from the needle; presence of IO blood indicates correct placement, but absence of aspirate does not necessarily imply a failed attempt. 1. Aspiration of contents (not always possible) 2. Flushing without subcutaneous swelling
What drugs can be given?	All drugs but should be flushed by 5–10 mL of saline to reach circulation.
How can you infuse fluids?	The following methods are used to overcome venous resistance. • Use of pressure bag • 20 mL syringe and a 3-way tap for easy and rapid aspiration and infusion
List some common complications associated with intraosseous route.	• Extravasation • Fracture and growth plate injuries • Osteomyelitis • Compartment syndrome • Local haematoma • Fat emboli
Is there an age limit for the insertion of an IO needle?	Intraosseous insertion is typically recommended for use in children younger than 6 years; however, it is now recognised to be both safe and effective in older children and adults.
What are the contraindications for IO access?	**Absolute** • Fracture of that particular bone **Relative** • Cellulitis overlying the insertion site • Previous attempt on the same bone • Osteogenesis imperfecta because of a higher likelihood of fractures • Osteoporosis
What are the different needle sizes available?	Different-sized needles are available for adult and paediatric use. The newer EZ-IO type has three types of needles: 15 mm 3–39 kg 25 mm > 39 kg 45 mm > 39 kg, for those having excessive tissue over the targeted insertion site
What structures do you pass through as you insert the intraosseous needle?	• Skin • Subcutaneous tissue • Periosteum • Cortical bone • Cancellous bone • Medullary cavity

STEPS	KEY POINTS
What can be given through the IO needle?	All resuscitation fluids, drugs, and blood products can be given via the IO route. Studies have shown the administration of ceftriaxone, chloramphenicol, phenytoin, tobramycin, and vancomycin may result in lower peak serum concentrations.
What are the parts of a long bone?	• *Epiphysis*: filled with cancellous bone and covered by the cortex, a hard thin casing. • *Diaphysis*: shaft of the bone composed of a thick, hard cortex with a hollow interior space (the medullary cavity). • *Epiphyseal plate*: the junction between the epiphysis and the diaphysis where bone growth occurs.

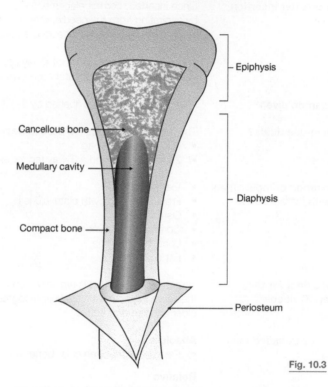

Fig. 10.3

The image shows the structures on longitudinal section of tibia.

STEPS	KEY POINTS
Describe the vascular supply of bone to explain the passage of fluids and drugs when given through the intraosseous route.	• The vessels of the IO space connect to the central circulation by a series of longitudinal canals (Haversian canals) that contain a tiny artery and vein.

Describe the vascular supply of bone to explain the passage of fluids and drugs when given through the intraosseous route.

- The vessels of the IO space connect to the central circulation by a series of longitudinal canals (Haversian canals) that contain a tiny artery and vein.
- The Haversian canals are cross-connected by a series of Volkmann canals, which penetrate through the hard cortex of the bone to connect the IO vasculature with the major arteries and veins of the central circulation.
- Red marrow is found in cancellous bone and contains a high concentration of blood, and yellow marrow is found in the medullary cavity of the long bones of adults. Fluids and medications infused into either the red or yellow marrow quickly reach the central circulation.

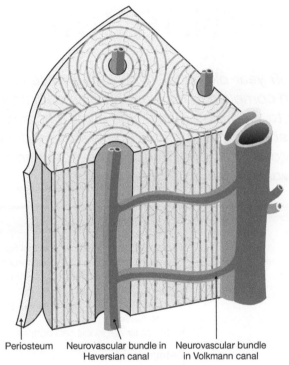

Periosteum   Neurovascular bundle in Haversian canal   Neurovascular bundle in Volkmann canal   Fig. 10.4

Figure shows the intricate connection of the intraosseous vascular channels.

10.6 PHYSIOLOGY: CHRONIC REGIONAL PAIN SYNDROME

HISTORY *A 59-year-old female who is otherwise fit and well comes to the pain clinic with complaints of severe burning pain and intermittent swelling from the right palm to the mid-forearm. She gives a history of fall onto her right arm while at work about 6 months ago. She feels very depressed, as she is unable to continue work due to inability to use the affected arm. On examination the right arm looked swollen and was tender to touch.*

STEPS	KEY POINTS
What is the definition of complex regional pain syndrome (CRPS)?	The diagnosis of CRPS by clinical assessment is a diagnosis of exclusion. Diagnostic criteria for CRPS according to 'Budapest criteria' 2007: • Patient has continuing pain which is disproportionate to the inciting event. • Patient has at least one sign in two or more of the categories (see below). • Patient reports at least one symptom in three or more of the categories (see below). • No other diagnosis can better explain the signs and symptoms. **Categories** **Sensory** Allodynia (to light touch and/or temperature sensation and/or deep somatic pressure and/or joint movement) and/or hyperalgesia (to pinprick) **Vasomotor** Temperature asymmetry (more than 1 degree) and/or skin colour changes and/or skin colour asymmetry **Sudomotor/oedema** Oedema and/or sweating changes and/or sweating asymmetry **Motor/trophic** Decreased range of motion and/or motor dysfunction (weakness, tremor, dystonia) and/or trophic changes (hair/nail/skin)
What is allodynia?	Allodynia is pain due to a stimulus that does not normally provoke pain.

STEPS	KEY POINTS
What is hyperalgesia?	Hyperalgesia is an increased response to a stimulus that is normally painful.

What are the differences between CRPS I and II?	**Type 1** • Formerly known as reflex sympathetic dystrophy/Sudek's atrophy. • Associated with injury to tissue (e.g. bones, joints, connective tissue but not necessarily to nerves). • Trauma may be relatively trivial, most commonly precipitated by an orthopaedic injury to distal extremity (e.g. lower leg or wrist). **Type 2** • Formerly known as 'causalgia'. • Characterised with actual significant nerve injury without transection. • More commonly associated with proximal nerves in upper leg and upper limb. • Most frequently affected areas are sciatic, tibial, median, and ulnar nerves.
What are the treatment options for CRPS?	**Multidisciplinary approach** **Engagement** • Education and information for the patient and their family **Medical management** • Simple analgesia (e.g. paracetamol, NSAIDS) • Opioids • Antidepressants, anticonvulsants • Free radical scavengers (e.g. vitamin C, intravenous N-acetylcysteine) **Psychosocial and behavioural management** • Cognitive behavioural therapy • Psychotherapy **Physical management** • Physiotherapy • TENS machine: noninvasive neuromodulation • Functional restoration **Regional techniques** • Intrathecal drug administration (e.g. opioids, clonidine) • Preemptive regional anaesthesia preoperatively • Regional nerve blockade (e.g. brachial or lumbar plexus block) • Sympathetic blockade including intravenous local anaesthetics (Bier's block), Stellate ganglion block **Surgical techniques** • Thoracic or lumbar sympathectomy • Spinal cord stimulation: implanted epidural electrode system (invasive neuromodulation). Low-frequency pulsed stimulation appears to be a successful method. • Limb amputation as last resort for irreversible infection or ischaemia

STEPS	KEY POINTS

Other proposed treatments
- NMDA antagonists: ketamine at low dose subcutaneously or infusion
- Capsaicin: topical capsaicin depletes peptide neurotransmitters from primary afferent pain pathways
- Glucocorticoids: may help with acute inflammatory stages of disease process
- Calcium-modulating drugs: calcitonin and bisphosphonates (both reduce bone resorption) help reduce symptoms in early CRPS
- One trial shows low dose intravenous immunoglobulin reduced pain intensity in a small group of patients who did not respond well to other treatments. A larger study involving individuals with acute phase of CRPS is underway.
- Hyperbaric oxygen: proposed benefit is a reduction in swelling and pain and improved range of motion

10.7 PHARMACOLOGY: ANTICOAGULANTS AND BRIDGING

HISTORY *You are asked to anaesthetise an 84-year-old patient with a fractured neck of femur, who is normally on warfarin, and has an INR of 3.5.*

STEPS	KEY POINTS
What are your main concerns regarding perioperative anticoagulation?	• Indication for warfarin: AF? heart valve? recurrent thromboembolic disease? • Correct of coagulopathy prior to surgery – consider prothrombin complex concentrate, fresh frozen plasma, vitamin K • Not emergent surgery although should avoid prolonged delay • May permit neuraxial anaesthesia techniques • Bridging therapy will depend on indication for warfarin and patient assessment • Other fall-related complications, especially head injury, should be excluded
What is warfarin? How does it work?	• Synthetic coumarin derivative • Antagonises vitamin K metabolism to deplete active vitamin K, inhibiting the vitamin K-dependent synthesis of clotting factors II, VII, IX, and X
What is unfractionated heparin? How does it work?	• A mixture of sulphated glycosaminoglycans of variable lengths and molecular weights (3,000 to 30,000 Daltons) • Activates antithrombin III (AT) to inhibit clotting factors IIa, IXa, Xa, XIa, and XIIa
What is the difference between unfractionated and fractionated heparin? Why would you choose one over the other?	• Fractionated or low-molecular-weight heparin (LMWH) is a mixture of heparin salts with an average molecular weight of less than 8,000 Daltons • AT activated by LMWH selectively inhibits factor XIa **Advantages of LMWH** • For prophylactic doses, less frequent subcutaneous dosing • For treatment doses, no requirement for continuous intravenous infusion and regular APTT monitoring • Lower risk of heparin-induced thrombocytopaenia (HIT)

STEPS	KEY POINTS

Advantages of heparin
- As an intravenous infusion, therapeutic levels can be rapidly attained
- Ability to monitor effect using APTT
- Rapid elimination once infusion stopped
- May be reversed with protamine (less effective for LMWHs)

What other drugs for thromboprophylaxis are available?

- Fondaparinux—synthetic analogue of the pentasaccaride fragment of heparin
- Danaparoid—heparinoid
- Lepirudin—direct thrombin inhibitor
- Dabigatran—direct thrombin inhibitor
- Rivaroxaban—direct factor Xa inhibitor

How will you reverse the effect of warfarin?

Target INR for regional anaesthesia is 1.5, but higher INR might be acceptable for GA and surgery.
- Stop warfarin. The effect of warfarin will reverse over a period of 2 to 4 days.
- Vitamin K is a specific antidote for warfarin. Oral or intravenous administration of vitamin K can be expected to reverse warfarin –4 to 6 hours after administration.
  - Oral vitamin K is the treatment of choice unless very rapid reversal of anticoagulation is required. For most patients, 1–2 mg of oral vitamin K is sufficient, but if the INR is particularly high, 5 mg orally may be required.
  - A sustained response is achieved with intravenous vitamin K 5–10 mg. Initial effect may appear in 2 to 4 hours, and multiple doses may be needed.
- Prothrombin Complex Concentrate (PCC) (e.g. Octaplex/Beriplex) is derived from virally irradiated human plasma, thus reducing the risk of viral transmission, and contains the clotting factors II, VII, IX, and X. PCCs provide immediate reversal of warfarin, but the effect will begin to wear off after 6–12 hours.

Earlier PCCs were associated with a significant thrombotic risk due to the presence of phospholipids and activated clotting factor VII, as well as protein C & S, but the newer products carry a very low risk.

The combination of vitamin K and a prothrombin complex concentrate is the treatment of choice for rapid reversal of warfarin.
Note: Fresh frozen plasma (FFP) is not recommended according to the British Committee for Standards in Haematology (BCSH). The BCSH guidelines state that FFP has only a partial effect and is not the optimal treatment for reversal of warfarin anticoagulation in the absence of severe bleeding. (Grade B recommendation, level IIa evidence).

[Further questions may include timings of epidural catheter insertion and removal related to thrombopropyhlactic treatment, and recent evidence for use of rivaroxaban in elective joint replacement (i.e. RECORD trials).]

10.8 PHYSICS: PERIPHERAL NERVE MONITORING

STEPS	KEY POINTS
How can neuromuscular function be monitored?	**Clinical** • Grip strength • Ability to sustain head lift for at least 5 seconds • Ability to produce vital capacity of at least 10 mL/kg **Neuromuscular stimulation equipment** • Peripheral nerve stimulator • Mechanomyography: uses force transducer to quantitatively measure contractile response • Acceleromyography: measures movement of joints caused by muscle movement • Electromyography: measures electrical activity associated with action potential propagation in a muscle cell (research use)
What are the important characteristics of the peripheral nerve stimulator?	Portable, battery-powered, and easy to use Able to deliver different impulses: • Supramaximal current output of 50–60 mA at all frequencies to ensure all nerve fibres are depolarised • Monophasic square waveform • Single twitch at 0.1 Hz • Train of four (TOF) at 2 Hz • Tetanic stimulation at 50 Hz
What is supramaximal stimulus?	If a nerve is stimulated with sufficient intensity, all fibres supplied by the nerve contract and a maximum response is triggered which depends on the number of muscle fibres activated. This stimulus should be truly maximal throughout the test period to maintain accuracy; hence the electrical current applied is at least 20% to 25% above that necessary for a maximal response.

STEPS	KEY POINTS

What do you mean by train of four (TOF)?

- The pattern involves stimulating the ulnar nerve with a TOF supramaximal twitch stimuli.
- Four stimuli are given at 0.5 s intervals, at frequency of 2 Hz.
- TOF is more sensitive than single twitches in monitoring neuromuscular blockade.
- Observer can compare T1 (first twitch of the TOF) to T0 (control).
- TOF ratio can be calculated by comparing T4 twitch height to T1.
- The extent of block can be deduced from number of TOF counts:

TOF count		Extent of block
1–2–3	T4 lost	75%
1–2	T3–T4 lost	80%
1	T2–T3–T4 lost	90%
0	T1–T2–T3–T4 lost	100%

Explain the observation following nondepolarising and depolarising neuromuscular blocking agents.

Nondepolarising neuromuscular blocking agents (NDMB): repetitive stimulation (TOF or tetanus) is associated with fade (reduction in amplitude of evoked responses with T4 affected first, then T3, followed by T2, then finally T1) and post-tetanic facilitation.

Depolarising neuromuscular blocking agents (DMB): no fade or post-tetanic facilitation observed. Repeated dose of suxamethonium can give characteristics of NDMB—phase II block).

Normal Responses (No drugs present)	Nondepolararizing Block	Depolarizing Block (Succinylcholine)	
		Phase I	Phase II

Train of four at (2 HZ)

$\frac{4}{1}$ = TOF ratio

Fade

Constant but diminished

TOF < 0.3

Fade

TOF ratio of 0.15 – 0.25: indicates adequate surgical relaxation
TOF ratio of > 0.9: essential for safe extubation and recovery post surgery

What is double burst stimulation?

- Used when a profound block is present.
- Two bursts of tetanic stimulation at 50 Hz, separated by 750 msec are given.
- The duration of each square wave impulse in the burst is 0.2 msec.
- DBS was developed with the specific aim of allowing manual (tactile) detection of small amounts of residual blockade under clinical conditions.

STEPS	KEY POINTS

Which nerves are normally used for stimulation?

- Ulnar nerve (adductor pollicis—adducts thumb)
- Zygomatic branch of facial nerve—orbicularis oculi muscle
- Peroneal nerve—dorsiflexion of foot
- Posterior tibial nerve—plantar flexion of big toe

The diaphragm is the most resistant (but with shorter onset times) of all muscles to both depolarising and non-depolarising relaxants requiring 1.5 to 2 times as much drug as the adductor pollicis muscle for an identical degree of blockade.

What are the differences between phase I and phase II blocks?

	Phase I	Phase II
Cause	Single dose of depolarising neuromuscular blocking agent	Repeated doses of depolarising neuromuscular blocking agent
Nature of block	Partial depolarising	Partial nondepolarising
Single twitch	Decreased	Decreased
T4:T1	> 0.7	< 0.7
1 Hz twitch	Sustained, no fade	Fade demonstrated
Post-tetanic potentiation	None	Present
Effect of anticholinesterases	Block augmented	Block antagonised

Radiology for the Final FRCA

B Krishnachetty

Special thanks to
Dr Sidath Liyanage, Consultant Radiologist
Dr Ali Zaman, Specialist registrar, Clinical Radiology
Southend University Hospital
For proof-reading and providing the images.

The radiological images frequently appearing in the Final FRCA are the radiographs of the chest and neck and computed scans of head and chest.

This section will cover most of the exam images and their interpretation in a methodical approach with 'pearls and mnemonics' where possible.

| Chest Radiograph | It is customary to follow a systematic approach in the study of a chest X-ray to ensure thoroughness and accuracy. This task is based on careful observation, sound anatomical principles, and good pathophysiological knowledge. |

| Identify patient details and date of exam |
| Please Rest In Peace (**P RIP**) |
| **ABCDE – BIT** |

P – Projection

This is written on the film. The different projections of importance to us are Postero Anterior (PA), Antero Posterior (AP), Lateral, Supine, and Lateral decubitus.

PA	AP
Cassette is near the anterior chest Rays from behind Standing position Hands on hip and elbow forwarded	Cassette near the back Rays from front Sitting or supine position Hands by side
Fig. 1 PA view	**Fig. 2** AP view
Less magnification of mediastinal structures Scapula is rotated out so the lung fields are clear	All anterior structures appear magnified—heart, mediastinum, sternum, clavicles, and ribs.

Lateral—helpful in viewing retrosternal and chest wall lesions
Lateral decubitus—used in diagnosing very small collection of air or fluid in the pleural space.

R – Rotation

An image is not rotated if the clavicular heads are equidistant to the corresponding thoracic spine.

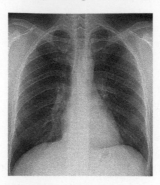

Fig. 3 Non-rotated film

I – Inspiration

An inspiratory picture shows a 'lot of lung'. In inspiratory films the level of the diaphragm is at the level of ribs 5/6 anteriorly and 8/10 posteriorly. (AR_6PR_{10})

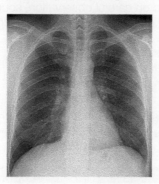 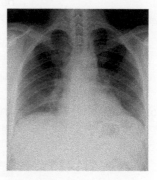

Fig. 4 Inspiration   **Fig. 5** Expiration

P – Penetration

A film is adequately penetrated if the vertebral bodies can be visualised against the cardiac silhouette.

ABCDE – BIT approach
A: Airway (trachea, bronchi, and hila)
B: Breathing (lungs and pleura)
C: Circulation (heart and mediastinum)
D: Diaphragm
E: Everything else! Bone, Intervention, Tissue

Satisfaction of search is a common problem. Do not abandon search prematurely!

Tudedenham WJ. Radiology 1962.

A—Trace the trachea down to the hila looking for shifts, foreign bodies, and abnormalities.

B—Lung and pleura
Lung—Scrutinise the lung margin clearly and then scan both lungs starting at the apices and working down, comparing left with the right at each level.
Pleura—Normally invisible but become visible in fluid collections, and pleural plaques and pleurally based masses.

C—Heart and mediastinum
Heart—Trace the borders of the heart. (See picture 30)
Right heart border is formed predominantly by the right atrium along with the lower part of SVC, whilst the left border is formed by the aortic arch, pulmonary artery, left atrium, and ventricle. The right and left ventricle forms the inferior border.
Cardiothoracic ratio (CT ratio)—The width of the heart should be no greater than 50% of the width of the rib cage.

Do not forget to look behind the heart!
Mediastinum—Look for superior, anterior, and posterior mediastinal masses.

D—Diaphragm
The right diaphragm is normally higher than the left due to the liver. Trace the hemidiaphragms and compare them for symmetry and sharpness and then the costo- and cardio-phrenic angles for obliteration or radiolucency.

Do not fail to look below the diaphragm!

E—Everything else
- **B**ones—ribs, sternum, scapula, clavicle, spine, and humerus for deposits and fracture
- **I**ntervention—tubes and lines, chest drains, pacemakers, and metallic valves
- **T**issue—skin and chest wall for surgical emphysema; breast and axilla for previous operations

A normal chest radiograph can be summarised as
'...the trachea is central and the hila are normal. Lung fields are clear with no air or fluid collection. Heart and mediastinum appear normal and not displaced. There is no free air under the diaphragm, and the angles are clear. Also, the bones and soft tissues appear normal...'
Before diagnosing a CXR as normal, look at the areas where pathology is commonly missed.

Commonly missed areas/review areas
Apices (including behind the 1st rib and clavicle)—small pneumothoraces and masses
Hila—masses and lymph nodes; left hilum is 1–2 cm higher than right
Behind the heart—left lower lobar collapse and hiatus hernia
Below the diaphragm—free gas
Soft tissues—breast shadow or absence (look for lung and bone metastasis)

Some terms before we discuss different pathology. Silhouette sign

Explains the loss of the silhouette or lung-tissue interface due to any pathology that replaces the normal air-filled lung.

Normally, if an intrathoracic opacity is in anatomical contact with the heart border, then the opacity will obscure that border.

e.g. Heart, aorta, and diaphragm.

If an intrathoracic opacity is in the posterior pleural cavity so not in direct anatomical contact with the heart border, this causes an overlap but not an obliteration of that border.

e.g. Heart border is obscured in RML collapse but not obscured in LLL collapse.

Air bronchogram

On a normal CXR, the wall of the bronchi are not normally visible unless seen end on. When the alveoli no longer contain air and opacify, the air-filled bronchi passing through the alveoli may be visible as branching linear lucencies.

Air bronchograms can be seen in consolidation, collapse, pulmonary oedema, and severe interstitial lung disease.

Kerley lines

A lines—linear opacities measuring 1–6 cm extending from periphery to the hila caused by distension of anastomotic channels between peripheral and central lymphatics.

B lines—short horizontal lines, due to oedema of the interlobular septae, situated perpendicularly to the pleural surface at the lung base.

C lines—reticular opacities at the lung base. Most frequently thought of as Kerley B 'en-face'.

Mediastinal masses

The mediastinal masses can be identified on the PA views but lateral films and/or CT scans are required to confirm further diagnosis.

Anterior mediastinum: mass anterior to trachea and bronchi, blurring the silhouette of the ascending aorta and heart border.

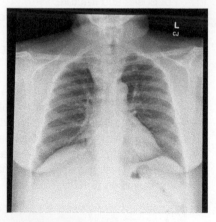

Fig. 6 Anterior mediastinal mass

Causes (4 T's)
Thymic tumour
Teratoma
Thyroid enlargement
Terrible lymph nodes
Ascending aortic aneurysm

<u>Middle mediastinum:</u> mass anterior to the heart, causing an abnormal lung hilum.
Causes
Bronchogenic cyst
Aortic arch aneurysm
Lymph nodes

<u>Posterior mediastinum:</u> mass posterior to heart, causing a loss of thoracic spine contour and descending thoracic aorta.

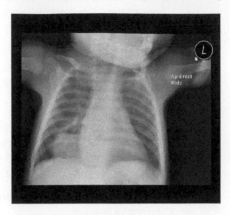

Fig. 7 Posterior mediastinal mass

Causes
Neurogenic mass
Spinal metastases
Hiatus hernia
Aortic aneurysm
Lymph nodes

Remember specific causes for each. Lymph nodes and aortic aneurysm are common causes for all mediastinal masses.

Hilar mass

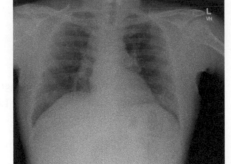

Fig. 8 Hilar mass

Sarcoidosis
Silicosis
Lymphadenopathy
TB
Neoplasm—primary and secondary carcinoma, lymphoma

Lungs

Pulmonary opacification

The causes of lung opacity are classified as follows:

Air space opacification
- Consolidation
- Atelectasis

Interstitial opacification
- Fine reticular pattern—interstitial pneumonia
- Course reticular pattern—honeycomb, pulmonary fibrosis
- Reticulonodular pattern—sarcoidosis
- Linear pattern—pulmonary oedema

Nodular opacification
- < 3 mm: miliary TB
- < 30 mm: nodular—lung metastasis, granuloma
- > 30 mm: mass—bronchogenic carcinoma

Lung collapse or atelectasis

Characteristics of lung collapse
- Triangular opacity caused by the collapsed lobe
- Loss of lung volume with fissure displacement and rib crowding
- Hilar, mediastinal, tracheal, and diaphragmatic displacement
- Compensatory hyperinflation of other lobes

The specific diagnostic features are due to the presence of oblique and horizontal fissures.

RUL

Lung collapses against the apex and the mediastinum.
Horizontal fissure is pulled upwards.

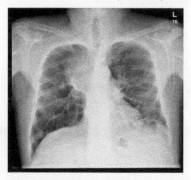

Fig. 9 Right upper lobe collapse

RML

Lung collapses against the mediastinum.
Loss of visualisation of right heart border.
Depression of horizontal fissure.

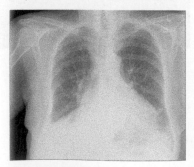

Fig. 10 Right middle lobe collapse

RLL

Lung collapses downward, medially, and posteriorly.
Persistence of the heart border but silhouetting of the right hemidiaphragms.
Postero inferior movement of oblique fissure.

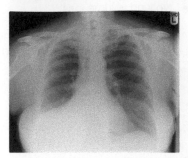

Fig. 11 Right lower lobe collapse

LUL

Lung collapses anteriorly against the anterior chest wall.
Left hilum is elevated
Luftsichel sign may be present – crescentic lucency aound the left side of the aortic knuckle. This is caused by the overexpanded apical segment of the LLL positioning itself between the collapsed upper lobe and aortc arch.
Oblique fissure is pulled forward.

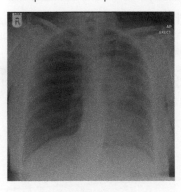

Fig. 12 Left upper lobe collapse

LLL

Lung collapses medially, inferiorly, and posteriorly.
Triangular opacity projected behind the left heart.
Loss of visualisation of the left hemidiaphragms behind the heart (Silhouette sign).

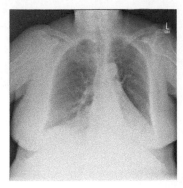

Fig. 13 Left lower lobe collapse

Consolidation

Characteristic features
- Confluent ill-defined fluffy appearance
- Bat-wing distribution
- Presence of air bronchograms and air alveolograms
- No lung volume loss

RUL

Air space opacification abutting the horizontal fissure.
Loss of outline of upper right heart border.

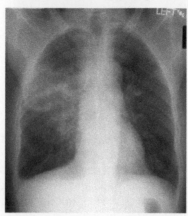

Fig. 14 Right upper lobe consolidation

RML

The fluffy opacity close to the horizontal fissure.
Indistinct right heart border and loss of medial aspect of right hemidiaphragm.

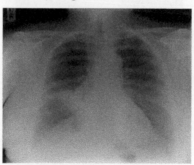

Fig. 15 Right middle lobe consolidation

RLL

Air space shadowing that abuts the right hemidiaphragm.

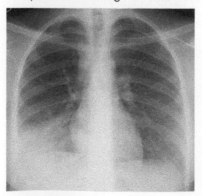

Fig. 16 Right lower lobe consolidation

LUL

Shadowing in the left upper lobe with loss of upper mediastinal contour.

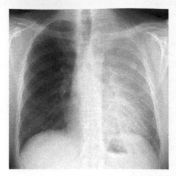

Fig. 17 Left upper lobe consolidation

LLL

Consolidation silhouetting the left hemidiaphragm.
Positive lateral spine sign—density of lower thoracic spine is increased on lateral X-ray.

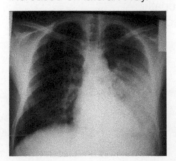

Fig. 18 Lower lobe consolidation

Understanding right and left lobar consolidation

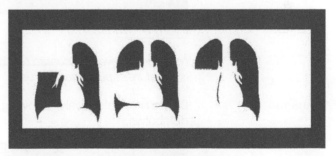

Fig. 19 Right upper, middle and lower lobe consolidation

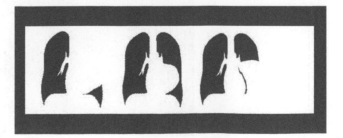

Fig. 20 Left upper, lingual and lower lobe consolidation

Features comparing collapse and consolidation

Feature	Collapse	Consolidation
Shape of opacity	Smooth, wedge-shaped opacity with apex at hilum	Confluent and ill-defined
Lung volume	Lost	No
Fissure	Displaced	Not displaced
Loss of aeration	Yes	Yes
Compensatory hyperinflation	Yes	Yes
Air bronchogram	Yes	Yes

Interstitial lung disease

Thickening of tissue surrounding alveoli and capillaries
Causes (SAD CHIN)
Sarcoidosis
Asbestosis
Drugs—fibrosis
Collagen vascular disease
Histiocytosis X
Idiopathic
Neoplasm

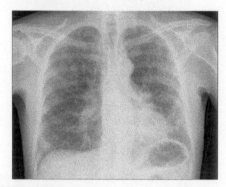

Fig. 21 Pulmonary fibrosis

Note the honeycomb coarse reticular interstitial opacification, which is a feature of pulmonary fibrosis.

Pulmonary oedema

Diffuse linear interstitial shadowing in a typical bilateral perihilar distribution.

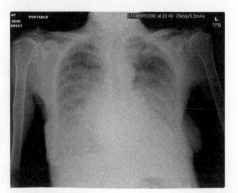

Fig. 22 Pulmonary oedema

Causes and characteristics of cardiogenic and noncardiogenic oedema are listed below.

	Cardiogenic	Noncardiogenic
Cause	All causes of cardiac dysfunction	Trauma, ARDS, renal cause, transfusion, aspiration, and post resuscitation (TARTAR)
Position	Central perihilar area	Uniform
Cardiomegaly	Yes	No
Cephalisation of pulmonary vessels	Yes	No
Kerley A, B, C lines	Yes	No
Pleural effusion	Yes	No
Course	Clears rapidly No long-term lung problem	Clears slowly Can lead to pulmonary fibrosis

Pneumothorax

Air in the pleural space with or without mediastinal shift depending on the volume of air.

The margin of the lung can be traced as a white pleural line with no lung markings beyond.

In supine position, diagnosis can be difficult as air tracks up anteriorly and medially, giving a sharper heart border.

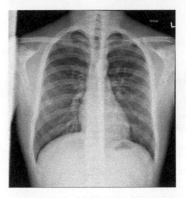

Fig. 23 Right apical simple pneumothorax

Note the hyperlucency and lung border at the right apex. There are no lung markings beyond the lung margin.

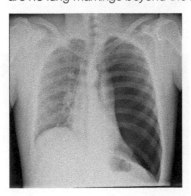

Fig. 24 Left tension pneumothorax

Note the mediastinal shift to the right side and collapsed lung at the hilum.

Pneumomediastinum

Air outlines the structures that are not normally visible, giving lucency around great vessels, heart border, etc.

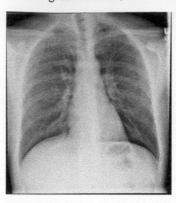

Fig. 25 Pneumomediastinum

Pneumopericardium

Lucent area around heart extending up to pulmonary arteries.
Lucent strip on inferior border of heart—continuous diaphragm sign.

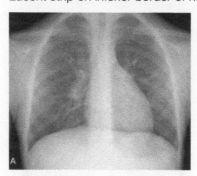

Fig. 26 Pneumopericardium

Note the lucent strip on inferior border of heart.

Pleural effusion

Fluid in the pleural space.
Around 150–200 mL of fluid is necessary for the diagnosis of effusion in the erect frontal view and 75 mL in lateral decubitus view.

Erect: obliteration of the costo- and cardio-phrenic angles and opacity with meniscus
Supine: graded haze giving a ground glass opacity

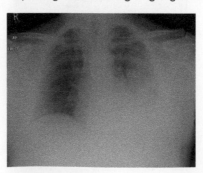

Fig. 27 Pleural effusion

Obliteration of left costo and cardiophrenic angles and a generalised opacity with meniscus on the left hemithorax.

Pericardial effusion   Fluid in the pericardial cavity associated with cardiomegaly.
                            X-ray shows an enlarged globular heart.

Emphysema   Signs of hyperinflation and air trapping
                            - Decreased lung markings
                            - Flat diaphragm and hyperexpanded lung
                            - Presence of bullae and peribronchial thickening

                            Signs of Cor Pulmonale
                            - Right ventricular enlargement
                            - Pulmonary hypertension—enlargement of the central pulmonary
                              arteries with oligaemic peripheral lung fields

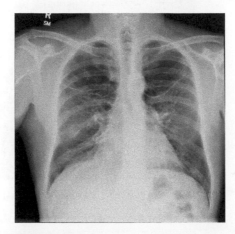

Fig. 28 Emphysema

Decreased lung markings with the presence of bullae.

Pulmonary tuberculosis Primary TB—initial infection with mycobacterium tuberculosis
                            - Area of consolidation in mid/lower zones
                            - Perihilar, paratracheal lymphadenopathy

                            Post-primary tuberculosis—reactivation of a primary focus
                            - Focal patchy air space disease with upper lobe fibrosis
                            - Cavitation and lymph node calcification

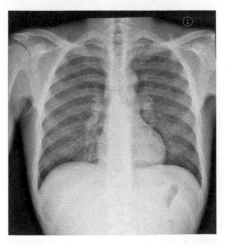

Fig. 29 Miliary TB

Heart
Cardiomegaly

CXR features
- Increased CT ratio
- Signs of cause and effect can be seen, such as signs of failure, etc.

Causes
- Ischaemic heart disease
- Valvular heart disease
- Congenital heart disease
- Dilated cardiomyopathy
- Pericardial effusions

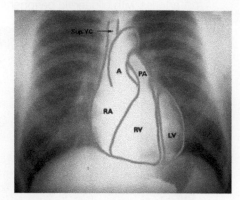

Fig. 30

The picture shows the formation of heart borders by various chambers.

Right atrial enlargement

CXR features
- Prominence of right heart border
- Filling of the retrosternal clear space on lateral view

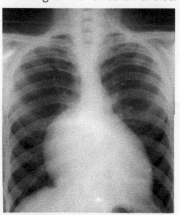

Fig. 31 Right atrial enlargement

Causes
- Any cause of pulmonary hypertension
- Pulmonary and tricuspid valvular disease

Right ventricular enlargement

CXR features
- Rounded left heart border and uplifted apex on PA projection
- Filling of the retrosternal space and rotation of the heart posteriorly in lateral X-ray

Causes
- Pulmonary stenosis
- Pulmonary artery hypertension
- Atrial septal defect
- Tricuspid regurgitation
- Dilated cardiomyopathy

Left atrial enlargement

CXR features
- Double right heart border
- Abnormal elevation (splaying) of left main bronchus
- Posterior displacement of the oesophagus which is seen on the barium swallow

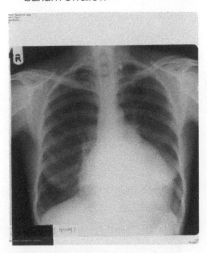

Fig. 32 Left atrial enlargement

Causes
- Mitral valvular disease

Left ventricular enlargement

CXR feature
- Posterior displacement of the heart
- Rounding of cardiac apex

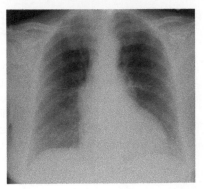

Fig. 33 Left ventricular hypertrophy

Causes
- Pressure overload—hypertension, aortic stenosis
- Volume overload—aortic regurgitation, mitral regurgitation
- Wall abnormalities—left ventricular aneurysm, hypertrophic cardiomyopathy

Pulmonary embolism

CXR features
- Can be normal
- Nonspecific signs—atelectasis, consolidation, pleural effusion, cardiomegaly
- Specific signs—prominent pulmonary artery, wedge-shaped opacity depicting haemorrhagic infarction of the lung

Prosthetic valves

The figure below shows the valve topography and the position of the two commonly replaced valves: aortic and mitral.

		Aortic valve	Mitral valve
PA view	Fig. 34	Horizontal to the ascending aorta Above and in the middle of the heart	Below the aortic valve
Lateral view	Fig. 35	Anterior and centre	Posterior and inferior to the aortic valve

Pacemakers

- Single chamber—one lead that terminates in the right ventricle
- Dual chamber—two leads terminating in right atrium and right ventricle
- Biventricular—three leads terminating in the right atrium, right ventricle, and left ventricle. So biventricular pacemaker is a dual chamber pacemaker with an extra lead in the left ventricle
- Implantable cardioverter defibrillator—ICD lead contains one or two coils to enable delivery of energy to myocardium. Proximal coil typically resides within the SVC, and the tip is preferably located in the apex of right ventricle

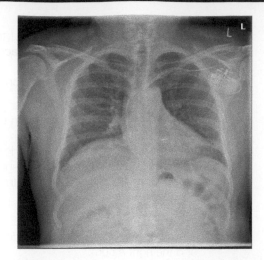

Fig. 36 Pacemaker

Dual chamber pacemaker containing two leads terminating in right atrium and right ventricle

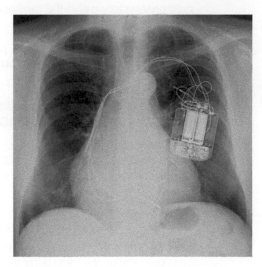

Fig. 37 Implantable cardioverter defibrillator.

The ICD lead containing thickened coils.
The pulse generator and lead wires can be seen with electrodes for contact with the endocardium and myocardium. Look for integrity of the leads along the whole length to assess for lead fracture, thinning, or dislodgement.

Tubes and lines

Endotracheal tube
The tip should ideally lie in the mid-tracheal region about 5 cm from carina (in adults) or T4/T5 interspace with neutral head position. The minimum safe distance is 2 cm.
Look for malposition and endobronchial intubation.

Chest drains
Thoracostomy tubes are placed in the pleural space to evacuate air or fluid.
Look for position of the tip—anterior for air and posterior for fluid.
Look for fenestrations—all holes should be inside the pleural cavity.
Check for injury to adjacent structures—surgical emphysema, pneumothorax, etc.

Central line
The tip of the invasive line is positioned at the junction of the SVC and the right atrium.
Look for injury—haemothorax, pneumothorax, etc.

Pulmonary floatation catheter
Follow the course as the catheter passes from the right atrium to the pulmonary artery. The tip is positioned in the proximal interlobar pulmonary artery within the mediastinal shadow.

Nasogastric tube
…NG tube passed down midline, past level of diaphragm, and deviates to left with tip seen in stomach…
Look at NPSA for more details

Cervical Spine

Again, follow a systematic approach in the interpretation of the Lateral C-Spine radiograph. (**AABCDS**)

A—Adequacy
An adequate film should include all seven cervical vertebrae and C7/T1 junction with optimum density so that the soft tissue shadow is visible clearly.

A—Alignment
a. Atlanto occipital alignment
   The anterior and posterior margins of the foramen magnum should line up with the dens and the C1 spinolaminar line.

b. Vertebral alignment
   The following four lines should be traced along to look for any incongruity, which should be considered as evidence of ligamentous injury or occult fracture.

   1. Anterior vertebral line—joining the anterior margin of vertebral bodies
   2. Posterior vertebral line—joining the posterior margin of vertebral bodies
   3. Spinolaminar line—joining the posterior margin of spinal canal
   4. Interspinous line—joining the tips of the spinous processes

B—Bony landmarks
Trace the outline of each vertebra.
The vertebral bodies should be rectangular and roughly equal in size. The pedicles, laminae, and the facet joints are inspected for any abnormality.

C—Cartilaginous space

The most important cartilaginous space to remember is the 'predental space or the Atlanto-Dental Interval' (ADI), which is the distance from dens to the body of C_1.

ADI should be < 3 mm in adults and < 5 mm in children.

An increase in ADI depicts a fracture of the odontoid process or disruption of the transverse ligament.

D—Disc space

Disc spaces should be roughly equal in height and symmetrical. Loss of disc height can happen in older patients with degenerative diseases.

S—Soft tissue

Prevertebral soft tissue space thickness can help in the diagnosis of retropharyngeal haemorrhage, which can be secondary to vertebral fractures.

Maximum allowable distance is as follows
Nasopharyngeal space (C1): 10 mm
Retropharyngeal space (C2–C4): 5–7 mm
Retrotracheal space (C5–C7): 14 mm in children and 22 mm in adults

Cervical spondylosis

Nonspecific degenerative process of spine and is characterised by joint space narrowing, osteophyte formation leading to spinal stenosis.

Rheumatoid arthritis

Progressive chronic systemic inflammatory condition affecting mainly the hands, C spine, and temperomandibular joints.

Common C spine characteristics are
a. Erosion of the odontoid process and loosening of the attachment of the transverse ligament of the atlas leads to the anterior subluxation of the atlas on the axis. Flexion in such a neck causes an increased ADI and spinal cord compression.
b. Cranial migration of the odontoid peg can also lead to compression of pons and medulla.

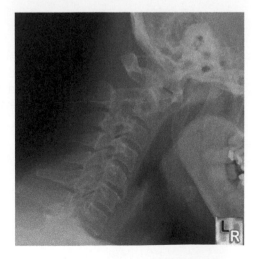

Fig. 38 Rheumatoid arthritis

Lateral radiograph of the neck with the head in flexion shows an increased distance between the anterior border of the dens and the posterior border of the anterior tubercle of C1 (black line).

Ankylosing spondylitis

Degenerative disease involving synovial joints of spine, hips, knees, shoulders, and sacroiliac joints. This causes atlantoaxial subluxation, fractures, squaring of the lower thoracic vertebrae, formation of vertically oriented desmophytes, and joint fusion, giving a classic 'bamboo spine'.

These degenerative diseases can make endotracheal intubation difficult. Careful assessment with flexion and extension views and MRI is advisable in severe cases. Awake fibreoptic intubation is often the choice of airway control in these scenarios. Also the associated pulmonary fibrosis can lead to a poorly compliant respiratory system.

CT head

Acoustic neuroma

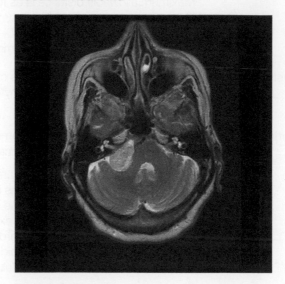

Fig. 39 Acoustic neuroma

T2-weighted scan (CSF bright).
Hyperintense mass in the right cerebello-pontine angle (CPA), which is displacing and compressing the pons, middle cerebellar peduncle, and cerebellar hemisphere. Fourth ventricle is also slightly effaced. Appearances in keeping with an extra-cannicular acoustic neuroma.

Differential for CPA mass includes meningioma.

Cholesteatoma

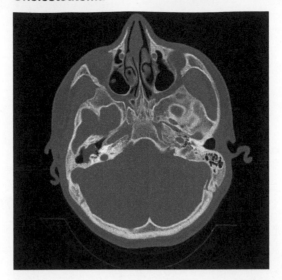

Fig. 40 Cholesteatoma

CT of the temporal bones showing nondependent soft opacification of the inferior right middle ear cavity. Look for ossicular chain and mastoid air cell destruction with cholesteatoma.

Pituitary adenoma

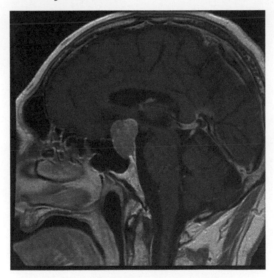

Fig. 41 Pituitary adenoma

Sagittal Post contrast T1-weighted scan shows an enhancing sellar and suprasellar mass. The pituitary gland is not seen, and the optic chiasm is compressed. Appearances in keeping with a pituitary macroadenoma.

ECGs for Anaesthetists

Author

Dr Parminder S Chaggar

Senior Registrar in Cardiology

Email: pchaggar@doctors.org.uk

Introduction

The electrocardiogram (ECG) is an electrical representation of the heart and a common source of anxiety for medical professionals when attempting interpretation. However, the ECG is constructed in a systematic fashion, and understanding some basic principles greatly aids interpretation. As with many aspects of medicine, understanding 'normality' forms the basis for detecting abnormalities and repeated ECG interpretation aids pattern recognition. Even once adequately experienced to routinely use pattern recognition during ECG interpretation, applying a logical, stepwise approach can be a useful tool when reading particularly challenging ECGs. This will also reduce the risk of missing important findings when distracted by an obvious abnormality.

The ECG is a versatile tool in patient management and can provide valuable information on heart rate (HR), rhythm, conduction disorders, cardiac chamber sizes, and clues to the cause of symptoms such as chest pain, breathlessness, palpitation or dizziness, including both cardiac and extra-cardiac diagnoses. However, ECG findings have to be interpreted in the clinical context. It is important to understand why the ECG was performed and if there is a specific clinical question that requires answering. For example, 2 mm of anterior ST-segment elevation may hold very different significance in an elderly patient with crushing central chest pain, who is suffering an acute myocardial infarction (MI), compared to an asymptomatic teenager, in whom it may be normal; or right axis deviation which may be physiological in a tall, thin individual but a marker of more significant conduction tissue disease in a patient with dizzy spells.

This chapter is not the *tour de force* in ECG interpretation and is not completely exhaustive but is intended to provide the reader with some basic tools to understand how an ECG is composed and therefore aid interpretation of the findings within their clinical context. Some previous knowledge in ECGs and experience in ECG interpretation is assumed. The reader is encouraged to apply a logical and stepwise approach to interpreting even straightforward ECGs, as this is valuable practice for more difficult traces and this method should be applied to your day-to-day clinical work where opportunities for reading ECGs are abundant. As with many things in life, practice makes perfect....

**The basics
ECG construction**

The ECG is a graphical representation of cardiac electrical activity and constructed from a number of surface electrodes that all 'look' at the heart from different angles in two orthogonal planes. As there are numerous other electrical currents in the body, it is important the patient is as relaxed, still, and comfortable as possible to reduce interference from skeletal muscle activity. Any current traveling towards the electrode is represented by a positive deflection above an isoelectric line, and conversely, a current traveling away from the electrode will cause a negative deflection. A current tangential to the electrode will result in a biphasic deflection with the ratio of positive to negative determined by the degree to which the vector points towards or away from the electrode.

A standard 12-lead ECG is composed of six limb leads and six chest leads. The limb leads (I, II, III, aVL, aVR, and aVF) look at the heart in a vertical or coronal plane, while the chest leads (V1–6) look at the heart in a horizontal or transverse plane (Figure 1). Since the shape of the ECG trace in any given lead is determined by the relative vector of the cardiac impulse, the surface position of the electrodes will impact on the trace recorded. In most circumstances this may be of minor significance but can become important when interpreting cardiac axis, for example. Therefore, understanding how the ECG was recorded may be relevant to the clinical context. Optimal electrode positioning is described in Table 1.

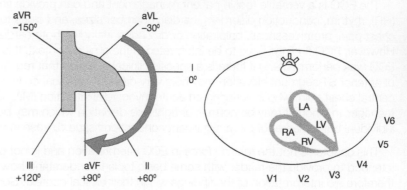

Fig. 1 ECG lead positions in relation to the heart. The limb leads are shown in the left panel and "look" at the heart in a vertical plane. Normal cardiac axis is between −30° and +90°. The chest leads are in the right panel and look at the heart in a horizontal plane.

Table 1. Optimal ECG electrode positioning in a standard 12-lead ECG recording

ECG Electrode	Positioning
RA	Outer aspect of right wrist
LA	Outer aspect of left wrist
RL or N	Outer aspect of right ankle
LL or F	Outer aspect of left ankle
V1	4th intercostal space, just right of the sternum
V2	4th intercostal space, just left of the sternum
V3	Between leads V2 and V4
V4	5th intercostal space in the mid-clavicular line
V5	Horizontally level with V4 in the anterior axillary line
V6	Horizontally level with V4 in the mid-axillary line

The ECG leads can be grouped according to which aspect of the heart they represent. Leads I, aVL, and V4–6 look at the lateral border of the heart; leads II, III, and aVF look at the inferior surface of the heart; and leads V1–3 look at the anterior surface of the heart. Understanding the underlying anatomy then allows interpretation of the ECG according to specific cardiac structures. The right ventricle (RV) is anterior and inferior, meaning the anterior and inferior leads look at the RV. However, leads V1–2 also look at the 'anterior wall' of the left ventricle (LV), which anatomically is a superior structure lying under these leads. Meanwhile, the lateral leads look at the lateral cardiac border, which is largely composed of the lateral LV.

An ECG is printed onto graph paper consisting of 1 mm 'small' squares and 5 mm 'large' squares. The paper runs at 25 mm per second, and this enables a calculation of HR. A ventricular ECG event occurring every 25 mm, or five large squares, equates to one heart beat per second and, therefore, a HR of 60 beats per minute (bpm). The relationship between the number of large squares between ventricular events and the HR is described in Table 2. Since a standard ECG is recorded over 10 seconds, a useful trick for irregular heart rhythms is to count the ventricular events and multiply by six.

Table 2. The relationship between the R-R interval and the heart rate

R-R interval	Heart Rate (bpm)
1 large square	300
2 large squares	150
3 large squares	100
4 large squares	75
5 large squares	60
6 large squares	50

Whilst the x-axis on an ECG denotes time in seconds, the y-axis is a measure of the electrical signal in millivolts (mV). 1 mV will result in a 1 cm deflection, and there is always a calibration marker on an ECG to ensure this relationship is accurate (ECG 1). The magnitude of ECG deflections can provide insight into cardiac chamber sizes, although it must be understood this is only an electrical estimate of an imaging variable and therefore, there is opportunity for error. For example, large deflections may be seen in very thin individuals where there is limited soft tissue to filter the ECG signal from a structurally normal heart. Conversely, ECG signals may appear very small in patients with obesity, emphysematous lungs, or pericardial effusion where there is impaired transmission of electrical cardiac signals to the surface electrodes.

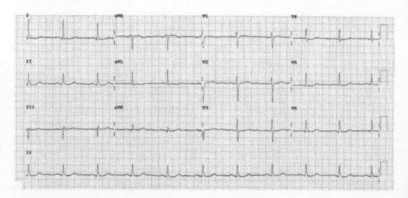

ECG 1. Normal sinus rhythm. Take particular note of the normal small r-waves in V1–2 and small q-waves in the lateral leads (I, aVL, and V5–6) due to septal depolarisation. There are also physiological U waves (most noticeable in V2) reflecting the heart rate. Note the rectangular calibration bars at the end of each line measuring 0.5 × 1 cm representing 0.2 seconds × 1 mV.

Normal cardiac conduction

Normal cardiac conduction arises within specialised pacemaker cells in the sino-atrial (SA) node in the right atrium before depolarising both atria and passing to the atrio-ventricular (AV) node near the junction of the atrial and ventricular septums. The AV node is composed of specialised conduction tissue, and there is a brief delay before the depolarisation wave passes to the ventricles via the Bundle of His. The Bundle of His lies within the interventricular septum and rapidly separates into two bundle branches to serve the two ventricles. The left bundle divides into two portions—the left anterior and left posterior fascicles—but also supplies septal fibres, which depolarise the interventricular septum from left to right. The left bundle fascicles and the right bundle branch develop into networks of specialised conduction elements, called Purkinje fibres, which penetrate deep into the ventricular myocardium and allow rapid spread of the depolarisation wave through the ventricles (Figure 2).

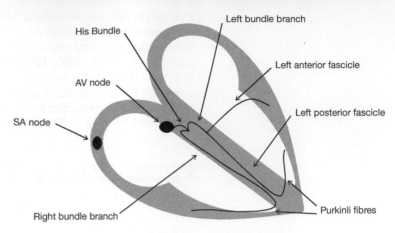

Fig. 2 The anatomical structures of the cardiac conduction system

Each phase of cardiac conduction, depolarisation, and repolarisation is denoted by separate deflections in the ECG, which are nominally labelled P, Q, R, S, T, and U by convention. The P-wave represents atrial depolarisation; the PR interval represents the time taken for the cardiac impulse to generate within the SA node, exit, travel to the AV node, and then pass to the His-Purkinje system; the QRS complex represents ventricular depolarisation while the T-wave arises from ventricular repolarisation. The Q-wave is the first negative deflection in a ventricular ECG event, an R-wave is a positive deflection, and an S-wave is a negative deflection after an R-wave. A normal QRS complex may be comprised of one, two, or all three of these waves. A ventricular complex without an R-wave is called a QS complex (Figure 3). Within a QRS complex, the dominant wave is denoted by uppercase and nondominant waves are in lowercase. U-waves occur immediately following T-waves and are small deflections (usually < 2 mm or < 25% of the T-wave height) in the same direction as the T-wave. The precise source of U-waves is unclear, but they often become visible at lower heart rates and are associated with hypokalaemia and digoxin therapy (ECGs 1 and 12).

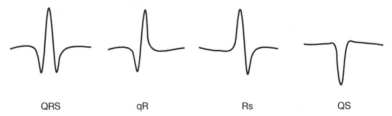

QRS   qR   Rs   QS

Fig. 3 Variations in QRS complexes. The dominant wave within a complex is denoted in capitals and smaller waves in lowercase.

In sinus rhythm, the SA node dictates the HR and each P-wave is followed by a single QRS complex and T-wave, representing coordinated atrial and ventricular contraction (ECG 1). By convention, normal resting HR is 60–100 bpm, resting HR < 60 bpm is termed bradycardia, and resting HR >100 bpm is tachycardia. However, there is significant physiological variance; for example, an athlete would be expected to have a resting bradycardia. Normal parameters for P, QRS, T and intervals are described in Table 3.

Table 3. Normal ECG parameters and intervals

ECG variable	Normal range
P-wave	< 2.5 mV in limb leads and < 1.5 mV in chest leads < 120 ms
PR interval	120–200 ms
QRS complex	< 120 ms
QT interval (corrected for heart rate, QTc = QT / √ RR)	350–440 ms in men 350–460 ms in women

It is worth examining how the QRS complex develops in more detail (Figure 4), as this will allow a better understanding of abnormal patterns. In the normal heart, the LV contains more mass than the RV and therefore exerts more effect on the overall electrical signal recorded on the ECG. In the anterior chest leads, there is normally no Q-wave but a small r-wave that represents depolarisation of the interventricular septum from left to right, towards leads V1–3. This is followed by depolarisation of the ventricles, and since the depolarisation vector of the LV is away from the anterior chest leads, these are predominantly negative complexes with large S-waves. Conversely, the interventricular septum depolarises on a vector away from the lateral chest leads (V4–6) while the dominant ventricular vector is towards these leads. Therefore, there is often a small q-wave followed by a dominant R-wave (ECG 1).

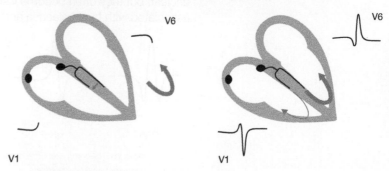

Fig. 4 The development of a normal QRS complex in the chest leads. In the left panel, septal depolarisation left-right creates a small r-wave in V1 and small q-wave in V6. In the right panel, depolarisation of the left ventricle exerts a dominant effect on the ECG, causing a large R-wave in V6 and large S-wave in V1.

The average direction of the electrical signal through the heart can provide a measure of the cardiac axis. The normal axis is between aVL (−30°) and aVF (+90°). The cardiac axis can be estimated by the relative deflections of the QRS complexes in leads I and II.

In a normal axis, the QRS complexes are positive in leads I and II as the normal axis will always be directed towards these leads. As the axis swings to the left (ECG 8b), lead I will remain positive but lead II becomes negative and the QRS complexes point in opposite directions and appear to be '**L**eaving' each other on the ECG. In right axis deviation (ECG 7), lead I becomes negative while lead II remains positive and the QRS complexes point towards each other and are described as '**R**eturning' (Figure 5). If both leads are negative, the axis is described as north-west, in relation to the quadrant on a compass, and is caused by extreme left or right axis deviation. North-west axes are commonly seen in patients with apical right ventricular pacing since the depolarisation vector is artificially generated from the RV apex and then travels in a retrograde fashion through the ventricles towards aVR.

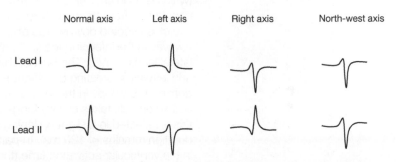

Fig. 5 Changes in QRS complexes in leads I and II in axis deviation. They are both upright in normal axis, "leaving" each other in left axis deviation and "returning" to each other in right axis deviation. A north-west axis causes negative complexes in both leads.

Common ECG abnormalities
Axis deviation

The diagnosis of abnormal deviations of cardiac axis has been described above. There are many causes (Table 4), but we will pay particular attention to disease of the left bundle fascicles. It is important to remember that left anterior fascicular block (LAFB) and left posterior fascicular block (LPFB) are diagnoses of exclusion; fascicle disease can mimic or hide MIs (ECG 8b and 9) and left ventricular hypertrophy (LVH).

Table 4. Causes of axis deviation

Left axis deviation	Right axis deviation
LVH	RVH
LBBB	PE / COPD / Cor pulmonale
Mediastinal shift	Mediastinal shift
LAFB	LPFB
Inferior MI	Lateral MI
Primum ASD	Secundum ASD
Pre-excitation	Pre-excitation
Hyperkalaemia	Hyperkalaemia
	Dextrocardia
	Normal variant (tall, slim individuals)

ASD, atrial septal defect; COPD, chronic obstructive pulmonary disease; LAFB, left anterior fascicular block; LBBB, left bundle branch block; LPFB, left posterior fascicular block; LVH, left ventricular hypertrophy; MI, myocardial infarction; PE, pulmonary embolus; RVH, right ventricular hypertrophy.

To understand the ECG findings in fascicular block, it is helpful to review the anatomical course of the fascicles in the heart. The fascicles are endocardial structures and activate myocardial depolarisation from the endocardium (inside surface) to the epicardium (outside surface). The anterior fascicle supplies the antero-lateral LV myocardium (anatomically superior and lateral), and the posterior fascicle supplies the inferior LV.

In LAFB (Figure 6), the LV depolarises via the posterior fascicle (which is an inferior epicardial structure); so, as the myocardium depolarises from the endocardial to epicardial surface, the initial vector is directed downwards and rightwards. This creates small r-waves in the inferior leads (II, III, aVF) and small q-waves in the lateral leads (I, aVL). The bulk of the LV then depolarises upwards and leftwards, creating dominant R-waves in the lateral leads and dominant S-waves in the inferior leads. The abnormal activation of the ventricle takes slightly longer to reach the lateral leads, and this is reflected in a slight widening of the QRS (although total QRS duration remains < 120 ms). In particular, there is a slight increase in the ventricular activation time (the time taken from the onset of QRS to the peak of the R-wave) in aVL. The abnormal ventricular activation can cause an increase in limb lead QRS voltages, which may be confused with LVH. For a diagnosis of LAFB, an inferior MI should be excluded, as this can also cause predominantly negative complexes in the inferior leads (Table 5).

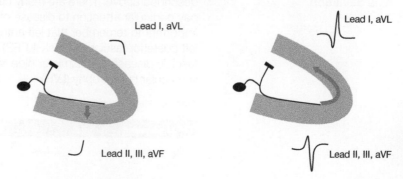

Fig. 6 The development of the lateral and inferior limb lead ECG changes in left anterior fascicular block. Initial LV depolarisation via the left posterior fascicle is downwards, creating a small r-wave inferiorly and small q-wave laterally (left panel). The bulk of the LV then depolarises towards the lateral leads, creating dominant inferior S-wave and lateral R-wave (right panel).

Table 5. Diagnostic criteria of fascicle block

LAFB	LPFB
Left axis deviation	Right axis deviation
qR in I and aVL	rS in I and aVL
rS in II and III	qR in II and III
Ventricular activation time > 45 ms in aVL	Ventricular activation time > 45 ms in aVF
Inferior MI and other causes of left axis deviation excluded	Lateral MI and other causes of right axis deviation excluded

LAFB, left anterior fascicular block; LPFB, left posterior fascicular block; MI, myocardial infarction

Pure LPFB (Figure 7) is quite rare since the posterior fascicle is a broad structure and not easily damaged in its entirety. In LPFB, the LV depolarises via the anterior fascicle (a superior and lateral epicardial structure) and the initial vector (as the myocardium depolarises outwards to the epicardium) is upwards and leftwards. This results in a small r-wave in the lateral leads and a small q-wave in the inferior leads. The remainder of the LV depolarises downwards and rightwards, causing dominant inferior R-waves and dominant lateral S-waves. Since the depolarisation wave takes longer to reach the inferior LV, there is slight prolongation of the time from QRS onset to peak R-wave in aVF. For a diagnosis of LPFB, lateral MI should be excluded as this can also cause a negative QRS complex in lead I (Table 5).

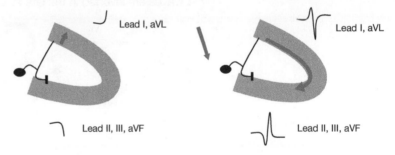

Lead I, aVL

Lead I, aVL

Lead II, III, aVF

Lead II, III, aVF

Fig. 7 The development of the lateral and inferior limb lead ECG changes in left posterior fascicular block. Initial LV depolarisation via the left anterior fascicle is upwards and lateral, creating a small r-wave laterally and small q-wave inferiorly (left panel). The bulk of the LV then depolarises towards the inferior leads, creating dominant lateral S-wave and inferior R-wave (right panel).

Bundle branch block

There are two main bundles of the His-Purkinje system, and conduction defects in these bundles result in left bundle branch block (LBBB) and right bundle branch block (RBBB). Since ventricular depolarisation follows a very abnormal path in both types, they share a common feature of causing a broad QRS (> 120 ms). For diagnosing bundle branch blocks, we concentrate on leads V1 and V6.

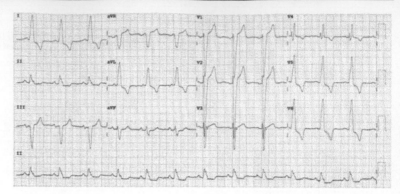

ECG 2. Sinus rhythm with normal axis, left bundle branch block (LBBB), and voltage criteria for left ventricular hypertrophy. Note how in LBBB the T-wave is opposite to the QRS direction.

In LBBB (ECG 2), depolarisation of the interventricular septum occurs in a reverse direction, from right to left, causing a small q in V1 and a small r in V6 (this is the opposite of the normal small q-waves often seen in the lateral leads on a normal ECG). Since the right bundle is intact, the RV depolarises before the LV, causing a small r-wave in V1 and small s-wave in V6 (Figure 8). The RV depolarisation often appears as only a notch in the QRS complex. The delayed depolarisation of the LV then causes a second S-wave in V1 and R-wave in V6. Left axis deviation is also often present, and T-waves are inverted in the lateral leads.

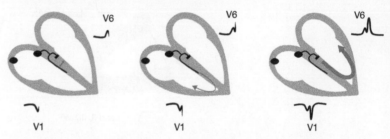

Fig. 8 QRS development in left bundle branch block. Septal depolarisation occurs right-left, via the right bundle, creating a small q-wave in V1 and r-wave in V6 (left panel). The right ventricle then depolarises creating a small positive deflection in V1 and a small negative deflection in V6 (middle panel). The left ventricle depolarises late, creating a dominant S-wave in V1 and R-wave in V6 (right panel).

In RBBB (ECG 7), depolarisation of the interventricular septum (from left to right) and LV are normal. Therefore, the initial stages of the QRS are relatively normal with a small initial r-wave in V1 and q-wave in V6 followed by a dominant S in V1 and R in V6. There is then an abnormally delayed depolarisation of the RV, occurring from left to right, causing a large second R-wave in V1 (RSR pattern) and wide, slurred S in V6 (Figure 9).

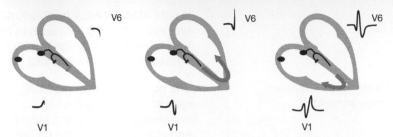

Fig. 9 QRS development in right bundle branch block. Depolarisation of the interventricular septum (left panel) and left ventricle occur normally, creating a rS in V1 and qR in V6. The right ventricle then depolarises late, creating a second R-wave in V1 and a deep slurred S-wave in V6 (right panel).

An easy acronym to remember the typical features of LBBB and RBBB is 'WiLLiaM MoRRoW' since in LBBB the QRS complexes in V1 and V6 are W and M shaped, respectively; while in RBBB, the QRS complexes in V1 and V6 are M and W shaped, respectively.

RBBB alone does not usually cause axis deviation since there is normal depolarisation of the LV, which exerts a dominant effect on cardiac axis. RBBB with axis deviation can be caused by concomitant fascicular block and is termed bifascicular block. Bifascicular block associated with a prolonged PR interval is often termed trifascicular block, although this is an anatomically incorrect description since block in all three fascicles would result in complete heart block.

Atrial chamber enlargement

The SA node is found in the superior free wall of the right atrium, which depolarises immediately before the left atrium. The atrial depolarisation wave therefore travels right to left, and since the left atrium sits posteriorly, there is also a posterior element to the left atrial vector. The P-wave on an ECG is an amalgamation of depolarisation of both atria, with the right atrium predominantly contributing to the early P-wave and the left atrium contributing to the later portion. A normal P-wave is positive in leads I and II, inverted in aVR, and biphasic in V1. The late negative portion of the P-wave in V1 represents the late posterior vector caused by left atrial depolarisation (Figure 10).

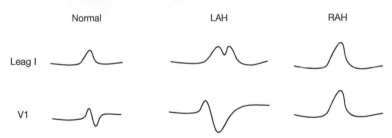

Fig. 10 P-wave morphology in normal atria, left atrial hypertrophy (LAH) and right atrial hypertrophy (RAH).

In left atrial hypertrophy (LAH), left atrial depolarisation is prolonged, which causes separation of the two components of the P-wave and a broadened, notched P-wave (P mitrale) in lead II (ECG 13). Prolongation of left atrial depolarisation also causes widening and deepening of the negative P-wave deflection in V1 (Figure 10).

In right atrial hypertrophy (RAH), right atrial depolarisation is prolonged, causing the peaks of the two components of the P-wave to overlie each other. This results in an increased amplitude or peaked P-wave (P Pulmonale) (Figure 10).

Ventricular chamber enlargement

The gold standard for measuring chamber mass is magnetic resonance imaging, but ventricular hypertrophy on imaging may not always be associated with chamber enlargement on ECG and vice versa. There are numerous ECG voltage criteria for chamber enlargement, but these are often associated with poor sensitivity or specificity (Table 6). Ventricular hypertrophy results in increased ventricular mass, which generates a larger electrical signal represented by taller or deeper R- and S-waves, respectively. Hypertrophied ventricles also result in prolonged depolarisation (resulting in increased ventricular activation times) and delayed repolarisation (resulting in ST depression and/or T-wave inversion or 'strain patterns').

Table 6. Sensitivity and specificity of commonly employed voltage criteria for left ventricular hypertrophy

ECG criterion	Sensitivity (%)	Specificity (%)
S V1 + R V5–6 > 35 mm	56	90
R aVL + 7.5 mm	23	97
R aVL + 11 mm	11	100
R I + S III > 25 mm	11	100

The diagnosis of LVH (ECG 2) is based on the presence of both voltage and nonvoltage criteria. Some voltage criteria are listed in Table 6, but the most familiar are the Sokolov-Lyon criteria (S-wave in V1 + tallest R in V5–6 > 35 mm). Nonvoltage criteria include a ventricular activation time > 50 ms in V5–6 or the presence of a strain pattern. Other supporting ECG findings in LVH include LAH and left axis deviation. Common causes of LVH are listed in Table 7.

Table 7. Common causes of ventricular hypertrophy

Left ventricular hypertrophy	Right ventricular hypertrophy
Hypertension	Chronic lung disease (COPD, pulmonary hypertension, PE)
Aortic stenosis	Pulmonary stenosis
Aortic regurgitation	Mitral stenosis
Mitral regurgitation	Pulmonary embolism
Hypertrophic cardiomyopathy	Hypertrophic cardiomyopathy
Normal variant (young, thin individuals)	Arrythmogenic right ventricular cardiomyopathy
Coarctation of the aorta	Congenital heart disease

Right ventricular hypertrophy (RVH) results in increased QRS amplitude in the right precordial leads (V1–3), which may be associated with ST depression or T-wave inversion due to strain. The diagnostic criteria are listed in Table 8, and supporting ECG findings include RAH and RV strain. The diagnosis of RVH in the context of RBBB is difficult, and there are no formalised criteria.

Table 8. Diagnostic criteria for right ventricular hypertrophy

Dominant R V1 > 7 mm or R/S ratio > 1
Dominant S V5–6 > 7 mm or R/S ratio < 1
QRS duration < 120 ms

Tachyarrhythmia

A tachyarrhythmia is a resting HR above 100 bpm caused by an abnormal cardiac rhythm. In ECG interpretation, tachyarrhythmias are classified into two groups: narrow complex tachycardia and broad complex tachycardia. We will review these two broad groups here.

Narrow complex tachycardia

Since narrow complex tachycardias involve ventricular activation through the normal His-Purkinje system, they must originate within the atria and are therefore often referred to as supraventricular tachycardia (SVT).

There are only five common types of SVT (Figure 11), and therefore, when faced with an ECG of narrow complex tachycardia, examining the P-wave and the QRS regularity will often easily lead to the correct diagnosis.

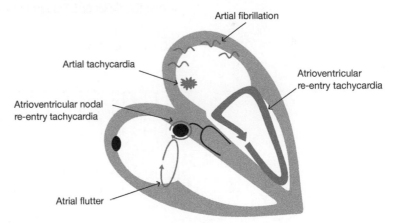

Fig. 11 Classification of supraventricular tachycardias

- Atrial fibrillation (AF). There is completely disorganised atrial activity, with P-waves replaced by an irregular baseline due to fibrillation waves, and QRS complexes occur in an irregularly irregular fashion (ECG 12).

- Atrial flutter. There is a self-perpetuating wave of atrial depolarisation usually circulating within the right atrium, causing regular, saw-toothed flutter waves at 300 bpm and QRS complexes every second, third, or fourth flutter wave (ECG 3).

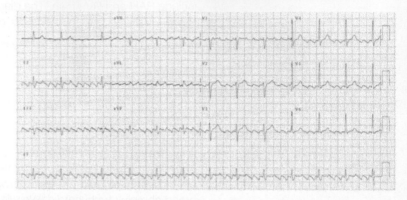

ECG 3. Atrial flutter with variable block. There are classical sawtooth flutter waves occurring at approximately 300 bpm (every one large square), most noticeable in the inferior leads.

- Atrial tachycardia. There is an abnormal atrial focus driving the ventricular rate. This rhythm can be difficult to distinguish from sinus tachycardia, but P-wave morphology and axis is usually abnormal. If the atrial focus is close to the AV node, a junctional tachycardia may occur and P-waves may be absent.
- Atrio-ventricular nodal reentry tachycardia (AVNRT). There is a rapid reentry circuit within the AV node resulting in simultaneous atrial and ventricular depolarisation. The P-wave is usually buried within the QRS or ST-segment (ECG 4).

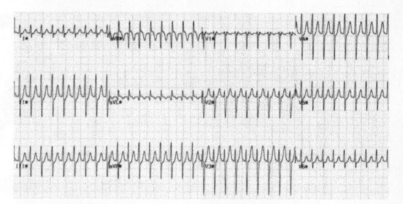

ECG 4. Atrioventricular nodal re-entry tachycardia (AVNRT). There is a fast (210 bpm), regular narrow complex tachycardia, and P-waves can be seen buried in the terminal portion of the QRS complex in lead I (may easily be mistaken for a second, small R-wave). The very close proximity of the QRS and P-waves implies near simultaneous depolarisation of atria and ventricles.

- Atrio-ventricular reentry tachycardia (AVRT). There is an accessory pathway bridging the atria and ventricles allowing antegrade conduction down the AV node (causing a narrow QRS) and retrograde conduction back to the atria via the accessory pathway. Since the depolarisation wave takes time to complete this circuit, the P-wave occurs after the QRS complex and is often buried within the T-wave. AVRT can occur with antegrade conduction to the ventricles via the accessory pathway, but this will result in ventricular depolarisation via an abnormal route and consequently a broad QRS (ECG 5b). In sinus rhythm, antegrade conduction via the accessory pathway produces a short PR interval (as the normal delay in the AV node is avoided) and the abnormal activation of the ventricles produces a slurred upstroke in the QRS called a delta wave (ECG 5a). The QRS complex is said to be pre-excited and can be associated with repolarisation abnormalities.

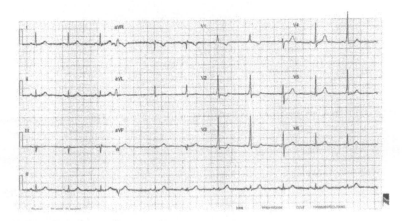

ECG 5a. Sinus rhythm with normal axis, short PR interval and broadening of the QRS with ST–depression due to pre-excitation. The delta wave represents ventricular depolarisation via an accessary pathway and is most obvious in the chest leads. Note that not all complexes are pre-excited (compare the QRS complexes in V4–6) as some QRS complexes conduct via the AV node and His-Purkinje system.

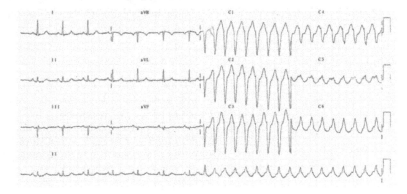

ECG 5b. This ECG is from the same patient as ECG 5a. There are seven sinus beats followed by a ventricular ectopic beat that conducts to the atria retrogradely through the atrioventricular node and then returns to the ventricles via the accessory pathway. This cycle repeats and triggers a broad complex tachycardia.

Broad complex tachycardia

A broad QRS complex (> 120 ms) is caused by abnormal ventricular depolarisation; either due to bundle branch block, an accessary pathway, or ventricular depolarisation having started in an abnormal focus within the ventricle itself (ventricular tachycardia [VT]). Broad complex tachycardia is therefore due to SVT with aberrancy or VT, and differentiating between the two can be challenging. However, there are a few pathognomonic ECG features that diagnose VT (ECG 6).

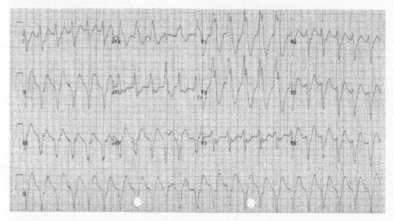

ECG 6. A broad complex tachycardia with multiple features of ventricular tachcardia. There is atrioventricular dissociation (a P-wave can be seen distorting the down slope of the second T-wave in lead I), a fusion beat (fourth QRS in aVR), QRS complexes are very broad (200 ms) with an atypical right bundle branch block pattern (taller first R-wave in V1-2), the axis is north-west, and aVR is positive.

- Atrio-ventricular (AV) dissociation. There is a higher ventricular rate than atrial rate (more QRS complexes than P-waves). This can only occur if the ventricular rate is autonomous and no longer under control of the SA node.
- Capture beats. There is an isolated narrow complex amongst a train of broad complexes. This represents a normally conducted P-wave via the AV node and an intact His-Purkinje system indicating there is no underlying bundle branch block. Therefore, the train of broad complexes are ventricular in origin (i.e. VT).
- Fusion beats. A normally conducted P-wave may fuse with a simultaneous ventricular beat causing a complex halfway between the appearance of a normal QRS and a broad complex.

If none of these features are present or obvious on an ECG, a number of other features may support the diagnosis of VT over SVT with bundle branch block.

- VT is more likely in patients with a prior history of MI.
- VT complexes are usually very broad (> 160 ms) due to a very abnormal path taken by the depolarisation wave from the VT focus.
- The time from R-wave onset to the nadir of the S-wave is prolonged (> 100 ms) in VT, again representing an abnormal activation path through the ventricle.
- A north-west axis and positive aVR are more common in VT, as the ventricles are depolarised in the opposite direction to normal conduction.

- The absence of typical RBBB or LBBB patterns suggests VT. For example, an RSR pattern in V1 with a taller first R-wave suggests VT (in RBBB the first R-wave is caused by septal depolarisation and is therefore smaller than the second R-wave, which is caused by depolarisation of the RV).
- SVT with aberrancy is more likely if previous ECGs demonstrate an accessory pathway or a bundle branch block with identical morphology to the broad complex tachycardia.

When in doubt, treat as VT.

Bradyarrhythmia

Bradycardia is a resting HR < 60 bpm and may be physiological (e.g. in athletes or during sleep), due to intrinsic conduction disease (e.g. heart block), or due to external influences (e.g. cholinergic or adrenergic-blocking medications). For the purpose of this chapter, we will concentrate on intrinsic conduction disease, which can occur at any point in the SA-AV-His-Purkinje pathway.

The normal HR is governed by the SA node, and sinus node disease may result in inappropriate or excessive sinus bradycardia and pauses either due to failure of the SA node to depolarise when expected or failure of the SA node to capture the surrounding atrial myocardium (sino-atrial exit block).

Disease at the level of the AV node will result in alteration in the PR interval or P-QRS relationship. This is often referred to as heart block (HB), of which there are three common types:

- 1st degree: Each P-wave is followed by a QRS complex, but the PR interval is prolonged (> 200 ms).
- 2nd degree: Not all P waves are followed by a QRS complex.
  - Mobitz Type I: There is progressive lengthening of the PR interval until a P-wave is 'dropped' and not followed by a QRS complex. The cycle then resets and repeats. This is also termed Wenkebach phenomenon and may be physiological in young people, especially at night. However, in the elderly it can be a sign of significant AV node disease and there may be a risk of inducing higher degrees of AV block, particularly with AV nodal blocking agents (e.g. beta-blockers, verapamil, diltiazem, amiodarone).
  - Mobitz Type II: The PR interval is constant, but there are intermittent dropped P-waves, usually occurring every second (2:1 HB) or third P-wave (3:1 HB).

- 3rd degree (ECG 7): There is complete dissociation of P-waves and QRS complexes due to complete block at the AV node (complete HB). The QRS rate is slower than the P-wave rate as the ventricular complexes are generated by an escape rhythm within the ventricular conduction system, which has a lower intrinsic automaticity rate compared to atrial tissue. If the escape rhythm originates high within the His-Purkinje system, the escape rhythm may consist of narrow QRS complexes (since onward ventricular depolarisation occurs via the normal conduction pathway) and only slightly reduced HR (40–50 bpm). The lower the escape rhythm in the His-Purkinje system, the broader and slower the QRS complexes and the higher the risk of progressing to asystole.

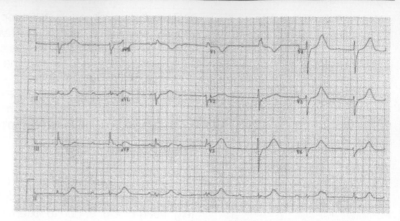

ECG 7. Complete heart block with right axis deviation and right bundle branch block (RBBB). The ventricular rate (43 bpm) is slower than the atrial rate (75 bpm), and there is no relationship between P and QRS complexes, indicating 3rd degree heart block. Lead I is negative, and lead II is positive (the QRS complexes are 'returning'), indicating right axis deviation. The QRS complexes are broad, positive in V1 with RSR pattern and a deep slurred S in V6 due to RBBB.

Acute ischaemia

Acute ischaemia results in abnormal myocyte cell surface polarity, which on an ECG is often represented by repolarisation abnormalities, including ST-segment deviation (elevation or depression) and T-wave inversion (although there are many other causes of ST-segment deviation and T-wave inversion [Table 9]). Historical descriptions suggest full-thickness infarction causes ST-elevation, subendocardial infarction causes only T-wave inversion, and ST-depression represents critical ischaemia. However, pathologically, these associations are not always correct.

Table 9. Causes of ST-elevation and T-wave inversion

ST-elevation	T-wave inversion
Myocardial infarction	Myocardial infarction
Normal variant (early repolarisation)	Normal (lead III, aVR, V1–2)
LVH	LVH and RVH
LBBB	LBBB and RBBB
Pericarditis	Cardiomyopathies
Myocarditis	Subarachnoid haemorrhage and raised ICP
Ventricular aneurysm	Persistent juvenile pattern
Hypothermia (J waves)	Pulmonary embolus
Hyperkalaemia	Electrolyte disturbance
Pulmonary embolus	Drugs
Subarachnoid haemorrhage and raised ICP	ECT
Cardiac trauma	

ECG evolution in acute ST-elevation myocardial infarction

ECG changes in acute ST-elevation MI can develop within minutes of symptoms, and initially there may be only hyperacute T-waves in the affected territory. This is followed by ST-elevation (ECG 8a), and pathological ST-elevation is defined in Table 10. The ST-segment is measured at the J-point, which is the junction between the end of the QRS complex and the start of the ST-segment. Some ST-elevation in the anterior leads can be normal in young people (early repolarisation), especially men and Afro-Caribbean's, and the ST-segment may be very difficult to interpret in the context of significant LVH and LBBB. In patients where ST-elevation does not meet criteria for acute MI, serial ECG monitoring is recommended, as the ST-segments may progress with time.

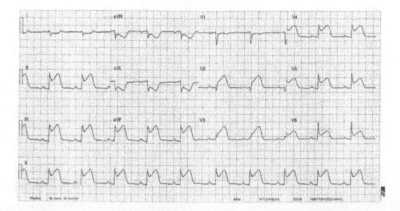

ECG 8a. Sinus rhythm with widespread inferolateral and anterior ST-elevation consistent with extensive myocardial infarction. There are reciprocal changes in aVR and aVL. The likely culprit is proximal occlusion of a large right coronary artery supplying the right ventricle (anterior and inferior changes) and infero-lateral left ventricle (inferior and lateral changes).

Table 10. ECG changes associated with acute ST-elevation MI and prior MI

Acute STEMI	Prior MI
New ST-elevation at the J point in two contiguous leads with cut-points > 0.1 mV in all leads except V2–3 where the following cut-points apply; > 0.2 mV in men > 40 years and > 0.25 mV in men 0.15 mV in women	Q-wave > 30 ms and > 0.1 mV deep or QS in any two leads of contiguous grouping in leads I, II, aVL, aVF, or V4–6
	Any Q-wave in V2–3 > 20 ms or QS in V2–3
	R wave > 40 ms in V1–2 and R/S > 1 with concordant positive T-wave in the absence of conduction defect

Without reperfusion of the culprit vessel (either spontaneous or following treatment), ST-elevation may persist for hours, during which time T-wave inversion and pathological Q-waves (Table 10) may develop (ECG 8b). After many hours, the ST-segment may normalise, leaving T-wave inversion or Q-waves that can be permanent (Figure 12). Extensive infarction, resulting in deep Q-waves, is often associated with a few millimetres of persistent ST-elevation, which can cause confusion if the patient represents with further chest pain at a later date. However, the presence of deep Q-waves indicates that the ECG changes are likely to be old and static (ECG 9).

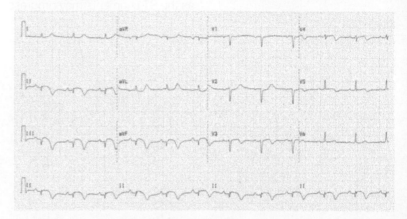

ECG 8b. This ECG is from the same patient as ECG 8a, taken 3 days after their myocardial infarction. Pathological Q-waves and T-wave inversion are seen in the inferior leads, and there is poor R-wave progression in V1–4 associated with T-wave inversion in V3–5. Note the left axis deviation, which is due to inferior infarction causing a deep Q-wave in lead II. There is also 1–2 mm residual ST-elevation, particularly in association with the inferior Q-waves, which may persist permanently.

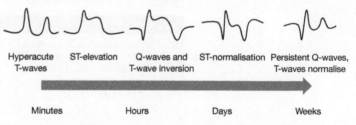

| Hyperacute T-waves | ST-elevation | Q-waves and T-wave inversion | ST-normalisation | Persistent Q-waves, T-waves normalise |

| Minutes | Hours | Days | Weeks |

Fig. 12 Evolutionary ECG changes during ST-elevation myocardial infarction

ST-elevation due to acute MI will usually be associated with reciprocal changes (ST-depression) in anatomically opposite leads. Therefore, a posterior ST-elevation MI presents with ST-depression and dominant R-waves in the anterior leads (V1–3) (which represent ST-elevation and Q-waves when viewed from a posterior aspect).

Localisation of a myocardial infarction

By remembering the relationship between cardiac structures and the surface electrodes, one can infer the coronary artery and territory affected by an acute or prior MI (ECG 9). There are three main coronary arteries, one on the right and two on the left. The right coronary artery (RCA) supplies the inferior surface of the heart (depicted by leads II, III, and aVF), which comprises the RV and inferior LV. The RCA can also supply a branch to the posterior surface of the LV. The left main coronary artery divides into two branches, the left anterior descending (LAD) and left circumflex (LCX) arteries. The LAD supplies the anterior LV and apex (leads V1–3) but also gives off diagonal branches that supply the lateral LV wall (leads I, aVL, V4–6). The LCX usually supplies the lateral (I, aVL, and V4–6) and sometimes posterior LV walls. However, these are only approximate guidelines, and significant normal anatomical variation can occur. In the cases of RV and posterior infarction, nonstandard electrodes applied to the right parasternal (V3R and V4R) or back (V7–9) can be useful.

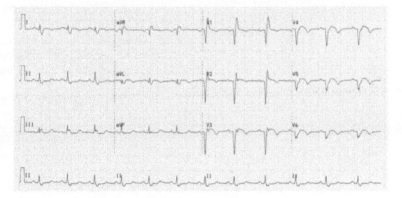

ECG 9. Sinus rhythm with right axis deviation, right bundle branch block (RBBB) and pathological Q-waves in the antero-lateral chest leads consistent with prior infarction in the left anterior descending artery. Note the QRS is broad and the initial R-wave expected in RBBB is missing as it is replaced by a Q-wave. There is also persistent 1–2 mm ST-elevation associated with the deep anterolateral Q-waves, and right axis deviation is caused by reduction of R-wave height in I and aVL due to lateral extension of the infarct.

**Miscellaneous conditions
Hyperkalaemia**

Hyperkalaemia (ECG 10) can cause ECG changes and lead to fatal ventricular arrhythmia. ECG changes can appear with serum potassium levels of > 6.5 mmol/L and become progressively more pronounced as the potassium elevates further. Initial ECG changes include peaked T-waves, and as hyperkalaemia progresses, P-waves flatten and the QRS complex and T-wave become broad. Eventually, QRS and T-wave prolongation can resemble a sine wave; this is usually a premorbid finding unless there is prompt treatment. Intravenous calcium gluconate will help to electrically stabilise the myocytes, while serum potassium is reduced with insulin-dextrose, calcium resonium, and dialysis, if appropriate.

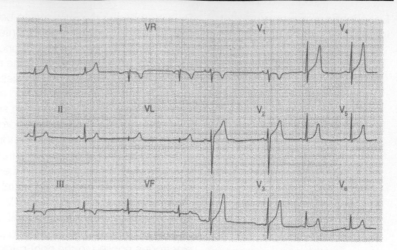

ECG 10. Sinus rhythm with normal axis and tall, tented T-waves due to hyperkalaemia

Hypokalaemia

Hypokalaemia (ECG 11) causes progressive diminution and eventual disappearance of T-waves, progressive increase in U waves, ST-segment depression, and 1st or 2nd degree AV block. Hypokalaemia can also promote ventricular ectopics, and severe potassium depletion leads to ventricular fibrillation.

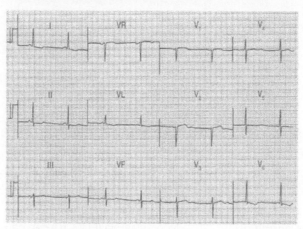

ECG 11. Sinus rhythm with normal axis, widespread flattened T-waves, and prominent U-waves in V4–6 due to hypokalaemia. Note the U-wave heights are disproportionate to the T-waves (normally < 25% of T-wave voltage).

Digoxin therapy

Digoxin is an AV nodal blocking agent (by augmenting vagal tone) and shortens atrial and ventricular refractory periods. Digoxin therapy therefore lowers heart rate, prolongs the PR interval (if in sinus rhythm), shortens the QT interval, and causes repolarisation abnormalities. The classical repolarisation abnormality is down-sloping or 'reverse tick' ST-segment depression, but J-point depression, biphasic T-waves, and prominent U-waves can also occur (ECG 12). It must be noted that these changes occur with digoxin therapy and do not represent digoxin toxicity.

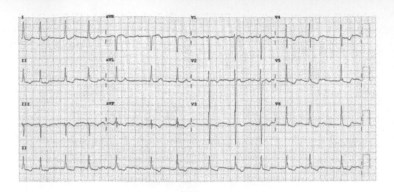

ECG 12. Atrial fibrillation with controlled ventricular rate, normal axis, and digoxin-effect. There are no discernable P-waves, the baseline is irregular due to fibrillation waves in the atria, and the ventricular rhythm is irregularly regular. There is down-sloping ('reverse tick') ST-depression in the inferolateral leads, biphasic T-waves, and prominent U-waves consistent with digoxin therapy. There are large R-waves in the lateral leads and deep S-waves anteriorly, which, when paired with the repolarisation abnormalities, could be confused for left ventricular hypertrophy. However, the ST changes are highly characteristic of treatment with digoxin rather than a strain pattern.

Electroconvulsive therapy

Electroconvulsive therapy (ECT) can cause ECG changes including arrhythmia and diffuse T-wave inversion, which can persist for many weeks (ECG 13). These changes may occur in patients without any prior history of cardiac disease. A number of mechanisms have been suggested, including myocardial ischaemia driven by post-ECT hypertension and tachycardia, and certainly, occult coronary disease has been demonstrated in patients with ECG changes post-ECT. Post-ECT ECG changes are also suggested to occur as a response to ECT-induced increase in sympathetic and adrenergic drive, and adrenaline-induced cardiomyopathy syndromes have been described following ECT. Baseline ECGs in all patients undergoing ECT are recommended. ECG 14 describes the stimulation of parasympathetic nervous system through direct neuronal stimulation of the hypothalamus to the vagal nerve, resulting in transient asystole.

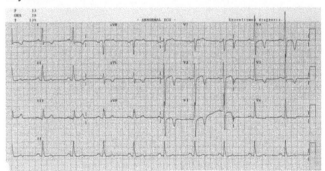

ECG 13. Sinus rhythm with normal axis, left atrial hypertrophy (LAH), and widespread anterolateral T-wave inversion in a patient following electroconvulsive therapy (ECT). The T-wave inversion may be secondary to ECT-induced increased sympathetic activity or unmasking of pre-existing coronary disease. The P-wave is also broad and notched in lead II (P-mitrale) and with borderline increase in the late negative component in V1, consistent with LAH.

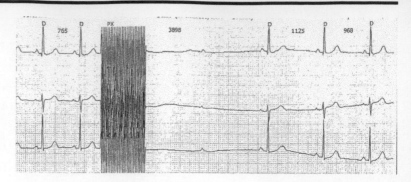

ECG 14. Stimulation of parasympathetic nervous system resulting in transient asystole immediately after ECT

Paediatric ECG

We thought we would include this topic as a few questions on paediatric ECG interpretation have been surfacing recently.

Comparison with adult ECG	• At birth, as the right ventricle is larger and thicker than the left ventricle, it produces an ECG picture of right ventricular hypertrophy—marked rightward axis, dominant R wave in V1, and T-wave inversions in V1–3.
	• Conduction intervals are shorter than adults due to the smaller cardiac size.
	• Heart rates are much faster in neonates and infants, decreasing as the child grows older.

Hence, the following electrocardiographic features are normal in children:
• Heart rate >100 beats/min
• Marked sinus arrhythmia
• Short PR interval (< 120 ms) and QRS duration (< 80 ms)
• Slightly peaked P waves (< 3 mm in height is normal if ≤ 6 months)
• Slightly long QTc (≤ 490 ms in infants < 6 months)
• T wave inversions in V1–3
• Rightward QRS axis > +90°
• Dominant R wave in V1
• RSR' pattern in V1

Normal QRS axis varies with age:
• 1 week–1 month: + 110° (range +30° to +180°)
• 1 month–3 months: + 70° (range +10° to +125°)
• 3 months–3 years: + 60° (range +10° to +110°)
• Over 3 years: + 60° (range +20° to +120°)
• Adult: + 50° (range −30° to 105°)

Intervals

PR Interval
• Short PR interval (< 120 ms)

QRS Duration
• QRS duration varies with age

QT Interval
• QT interval varies with heart rate
• Bazett's formula is used to correct the QT for HR:
• $QTc = QT$ measured $/ (\sqrt{R-R}$ interval)

Normal QTc
• Infants less than 6 months = < 0.49 seconds
• Older than 6 months = < 0.44 seconds

Waves and segments

P wave amplitude and duration
- Normal P-wave amplitude is < 3 mm (tall P waves = right atrial enlargement).
- Normal P wave duration is < 0.09 seconds in children and < 0.07 seconds in infants (wide P waves = left atrial enlargement).
- A combination of tall and wide P waves occurs in combined atrial hypertrophy.

QRS amplitude
High QRS amplitudes
- Ventricular hypertrophy
- Ventricular conduction disturbances

Low QRS amplitudes
- Pericarditis
- Myocarditis
- Hypothyroidism
- Normal newborns

ST segment
The normal ST is isoelectric. Elevation or depression is judged in relation to the TP segment.

Some ST changes may be normal:
- Limb lead ST depression or elevation of up to 1 mm (up to 2 mm in the left precordial leads).
- J-point depression: the J point (junction between the QRS and ST segment) is depressed without sustained ST depression, i.e. upsloping ST depression.

Others are **pathological**.

T Waves
The precordial T-wave configuration changes over time:
- For the first week of life, T waves are upright throughout the precordial leads.
- After the first week, the T waves become inverted in V1–3 (the 'juvenile T-wave pattern')
- This T-wave inversion usually remains until ~ age 8 (rarely into adulthood); thereafter, the T waves become upright in V1–3.

U waves
A U wave is a positive deflection at the end of a T wave.
Most common causes include:
- Hypokalaemia
- Normal finding at slower heart rates

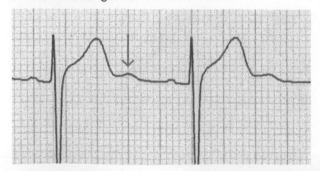

Supraventricular tachycardia	• Rapid regular, narrow complex tachycardia of 220–320/min in infants and 150–250 in older children. • The P wave is usually invisible. • Half of patients with SVT will have no underlying heart disease. • Almost 1/4 will have congenital heart disease and 1/4 will have WPW. • Avoid verapamil or β blockers in infants or children with SVT as they may cause profound AV block, negative inotropy, and sudden death.
Acute treatment: aims to induce AV nodal slowing	*Vagal manoeuvres* • Infants: Dipping face in ice cold water for up to 10 seconds; often effective. • Older children: carotid sinus massage, Valsalva manoeuvre (30–60 seconds), deep inspiration/cough/gag reflex, headstand. *Adenosine* • Half-life: < 1.5 seconds: transient AV nodal block as well as sinus node block, negative chronotrope, inotrope. • Side effects: flushing, nausea, dyspnea, bronchospasm are short lived. • Give 100 mcg/kg rapidly into a large vein. Repeat according to APLS guidelines. • Maximum total dose 12 mg. *Cardioversion* • Rapid deterioration of the 'SVT-stressed' myocardium may occur with anaesthesia. If shock is present, synchronous DC shock is indicated 0.5–2 J/kg (monophasic).
Chronic treatment	Conducted as an inpatient; either medical or surgical/catheter pathway ablation.

Risk scoring in anaesthesia and intensive care

ASA score	Scoring for assessing fitness before surgery

ASA I   Healthy person
ASA II   Mild systemic disease
ASA III   Severe systemic disease
ASA IV   Severe systemic disease that is a constant threat to life
ASA V   A moribund person who is not expected to survive
          without the operation
ASA VI   A declared brain-dead person for organ retrieval

NYHA classification for heart failure

I   Patients with cardiac disease but no limitation of physical activity. Ordinary physical activity does not cause fatigue, palpitation, dyspnoea, and angina.

II   Patients with cardiac disease with slight limitation of physical activity. Comfortable at rest but ordinary physical activity causes symptoms.

III Patients with cardiac disease with marked limitation of physical activity. Comfortable at rest but less-than-ordinary activity brings on symptoms.

IV Symptomatic at rest.

Canadian Cardiovascular Society (CCS) Classification of angina

0   Asymptomatic
I   Angina with strenuous exercise
II   Angina with moderate exertion
III   Angina with climbing one flight of stairs
IV   Inability to perform any physical activity without development of angina

Goldman's risk stratification (1977): Nine variables

- History:
  Age > 70 years   (5 points)
  Myocardial infarction within 6 months   (10 points)

- Cardiac examination:
  Signs of congestive heart failure:
  Ventricular gallop or raised JVP   (11 points)
  Significant aortic stenosis   (3 points)

- Electrocardiogram:
  Arrhythmia other than sinus or premature atrial
  contractions (7 points)
  Five or more premature ventricular contractions
  per minute (7 points)

- General Medical Conditions:
  $PO_2 < 60$ mmHg; $PCO_2 > 50$ mmHg; $K < 3$ mEq/L;
  $HCO_3 < 20$ mEq/L; Creatinine > 3 mg/dL (3 points)

- Operation:
  Emergency (4 points)
  Intraperitoneal, intrathoracic or aortic (3 points)

0 to 5 Points: Class I   1% Complications
6 to 12 Points: Class II   7% Complications
13 to 25 Points: Class III   14% Complications
26 to 53 Points: Class IV   78% Complications

CHADS2 and CHA2DS2 – VASc	Determines the risk of stroke in patients with atrial fibrillation receiving anticoagulation

CHADS2 score of 6 carries 18% risk

Congestive heart failure	1
Hypertension	1
Age ≥ 75	1
Diabetes	1
Stroke	2

Score 0 or 1	Low risk; use aspirin
Score ≥ 2	Use warfarin aiming for INR 2–3
Score ≥ 2/warfarin contraindicated	Consider referral

CHA2DS2 – VASc score of 1 carries 1.3% risk and 9 carries 15.2% risk

Congestive heart failure	1
Hypertension	1
Age ≥ 75	2
Diabetes	1
Stroke	2
Vascular disease	1
Age 65–75	1
Sex category (Female)	2

ACC/AHA (American College of Cardiology/American Heart Association)	Guidelines on cardiac risk stratification for non-cardiac surgery (2007)

Clinical predictors

- Major
  MI < 30 days
  Unstable angina
  Decompensated Congestive Heart Failure (CHF)
  Significant arrhythmias
  Severe valvular disease

- Intermediate
  Previous MI
  Mild angina
  Compensated CHF
  Diabetes mellitus
  Renal insufficiency

- Minor
  > Age
  Abnormal ECG
  Nonsinus rhythm
  Poor functional capacity
  History of stroke
  Uncontrolled hypertension

Surgical procedures

- High risk; cardiac risk > 5%
  Aortic and major vascular surgery
  Peripheral vascular surgery

- Intermediate risk; cardiac risk 1%–5%
  Intraperitoneal and intrathoracic surgery
  Carotid endarterectomy
  Head and neck surgery
  Orthopaedic surgery
  Prostate surgery

- Low risk; cardiac risk < 1 %
  Other simple procedures

Detsky's modified cardiac risk index (1986)

Age > 70 years	5
MI < 6 months	10
MI > 6 months	5
CCS angina class III	10
CCS angina class IV	20
Unstable angina < 6 months	10
Pulmonary oedema < 1 week	10
Pulmonary oedema > 1 week	5
Aortic stenosis	20
Arrhthymia	
- Nonsinus rhythm	5
- > 5 premature ventricular beats	5
Emergency operation	10
Poor general medical status	5

Class I	0–15 points	low risk
Class II	20–30 points	medium risk
Class III	> 31 points	high risk

Lee's revised cardiac index (1999): six variables

Easier and more accurate
1. History of ischaemic heart disease
2. History of congestive heart failure
3. History of cerebrovascular disease (stroke or transient ischaemic attack)
4. History of diabetes requiring preoperative insulin use

5. Chronic kidney disease (creatinine > 2 mg/dL)
6. Undergoing suprainguinal, vascular, intraperitoneal, or intrathoracic surgery

Risk for cardiac death, nonfatal myocardial infarction, and nonfatal cardiac arrest:
0 predictors = 0.4%, 1 predictor = 0.9%, 2 predictors = 6.6%, ≥3 predictors ≥ 11%

Functional capacity assessment (Metabolic Equivalent)

- Poor < 4 METS
  Activities of daily living,
  Walking 2 mph

- Moderate 4–7 METS
  Climbing a flight of stairs, cycling
  Walking 4 mph

- Excellent > 7 METS
  Jogging (10-min mile),
  Playing tennis

Recommended timing of noncardiac surgery following percutaneous coronary intervention (PCI), American College of Cardiology guidelines

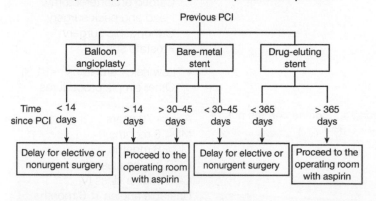

Proposed approach to management of patients with prior PCI

The RIFLE criteria for classification of Acute Kidney Injury

Class	GFR criteria	Urine output criteria
Risk	Creatinine × 1.5 or GFR decrease > 25%	Urine output < 0.5 mls/kg × 6 hours
Injury	Creatinine × 2 or GFR decrease > 50%	Urine output < 0.5 mls/kg × 12 hours
Failure	Creatinine × 3 or GFR decrease > 75%, creatinine > 4.0 mg/dl or acute rise of > 0.5 mg/dl	Urine output < 0.3 mls/kg × 24 hours or anuria × 12 hours
Loss	Complete loss of renal function for > 4 weeks	
End Stage Renal Disease	Complete loss of renal function for > 12 weeks requiring dialysis	

Ranson criteria for predicting severity in acute pancreatitis

Below are the criteria for gallstone pancreatitis (for nongallstone pancreatitis the values are different).

At admission:
Age in years > 70 years
White blood cell count > 18 000 cells/mm^3
Blood glucose > 12.2 mmol/L (> 220 mg/dL)
Serum AST > 250 IU/L
Serum LDH > 400 IU/L

Within 48 hours:
Serum calcium < 2.0 mmol/L (< 8.0 mg/dL)
Haematocrit fall > 10%
Oxygen (hypoxaemia PaO_2 < 60 mmHg)
BUN increased by 1.8 mmol/L or more (5 mg/dL or more) after IV fluid hydration
Base deficit (negative base excess) > 5 mEq/L
Sequestration of fluids > 4 L

If the score $\geq$ 3, severe pancreatitis is likely.
If the score < 3, severe pancreatitis is unlikely.

MELD score
Model for end-stage Liver Disease
MELD uses the patient's values for serum bilirubin, serum creatinine, and the international normalised ratio for prothrombin time (INR) to predict survival. The 3-month mortality is then calculated using a formula.

40 or more: 71.3% mortality
30–39: – 52.6% mortality
20–29: 19.6% mortality
10–19: 6.0% mortality
< 9: 1.9% mortality

WILSON score for difficult airway prediction	Weight
	> 90 kg 1
	> 110 kg 2
	Head and neck movement 0–2
	Jaw movement 0–2
	Receding mandible 0–2
	Buck teeth 0–2

Total = Maximum 10 points
Total of $\geq$ 3 predicts 75% of difficult intubations, while a total of $\geq$ 4 predicts 90% of difficult intubations.

Mallampati classification

Patient sits upright with head in neutral position. Mouth open as wide as possible with tongue extended to maximum.
Classed according to what structures are visible
Class I: hard palate, soft palate, uvula, and tonsillar pillars
Class II: hard palate, soft palate, uvula
Class III: hard palate, soft palate
Class IV: hard palate

May fail to predict over 50% of difficult intubations.

Cormack & Lehane grading

Used to grade the view at laryngoscopy
Grade I: visualization of entire laryngeal aperture
Grade II: visualization of posterior part of the laryngeal aperture
Grade III: visualization of epiglottis only
Grade IV: not even the epiglottis is visible

Glasgow Coma Score (GCS)

Eyes Verbal Motor scores provide systematic way of assessing head injury patients and are affected by alcohol and sedation.

Scoring systems commonly used in ICU **Therapeutic Intervention Scoring System (TISS)**	Estimates severity of illness and quantifies burden of work for ICU staff by daily collection of interventions and treatments. It is a good indicator of nursing and medical work but a poor measure of severity of illness.
Acute Physiology, Age, and Chronic Health Evaluation Systems (APACHE I-IV)	I: 1981 II: 1985 (most widely used in the world, 12 variables, score of 0–71, worse values in first 24 hours in ICU, limited by derivation from an historical data set) III: 1991 (score of 0–299, 16 variables, improved prognostication, improved discrimination and calibration) IV: 2006 (large data set, more variables included, more accurate, only used in US)
Simplified Acute Physiology Score (SAPS 1-3)	SAPS 1 (French ICUs, solely looked at physiology) SAPS 2 (1993, European and North American, added chronic health conditions, greater calibration and discrimination) SAPS 3 (2005, around the world, 20 variables—prior to admission, at admission, acute physiological derangement)
Mortality Prediction Model I (MPM I)	Variables at admission and during first 24 hours, computes a hospital risk of death from the absence or presence of factors in a logistic regression equation.
Mortality Prediction Model II (MPM II)	It is based on the same data set as SAPS 2.
POSSUM (1991)	12 acute physiological parameters (surgery and severity of surgery). It is a useful tool for surgeons who need a risk adjustment tool. P-POSSUM: Portsmouth: predicts hospital mortality more accurately V-POSSUM: vascular surgery Cr-POSSUM: colon cancer resection
Sequential Organ Failure Assessment (SOFA)	The SOFA score is used to determine the extent of a person's organ function or rate of failure. The score is based on six different scores for respiratory, cardiovascular, hepatic, coagulation, renal and neurological systems.
Confusion Assessment Method for the Intensive Care Unit (CAM-ICU)	The CAM was developed in 1990 to aid in delirium assessment by nonpsychiatric personnel. It was modified to the CAM-ICU in 2001 for use in mechanically ventilated ICU patients not able to verbalise. The four major criteria to assess delirium include acute mental status change, inattention, disorganized thinking, and altered level of consciousness. The CAM-ICU was prospectively tested in 96 mechanically ventilated patients with a sensitivity of 93% and a specificity of 98% for predicting the presence of delirium.

Preoperative Risk Stratification and Optimisation

The fundamental aim of anaesthesia is to enable a patient to undergo safe surgery. In order to achieve this aim, the patient must be as 'fit' as possible for surgery. This entails identifying potential risks to patients in the perioperative period and, where possible, correcting abnormal physiology to minimise those risks.

Preoperative Risk Stratification

Why is risk stratification important?

- To inform patient consent: providing a patient with some hard numbers regarding surgical risk. This may help them decide whether to undergo surgery.
- To inform clinical decision making: Again, accurately quantifying risk helps clinicians decide whether the benefits of surgery outweigh the risks.
- Benchmarking performance: Comparing actual postoperative mortality/morbidity with that predicted from risk scoring tells hospitals whether their surgical outcomes are better or worse than expected and how they compare with other institutions.

How do we risk-stratify patients?

1. **Functional assessment**
   a. Subjective (patient-reported): Exercise tolerance > 4 METS (metabolic Equivalents), i.e. climbing one flight of stairs, light housework.
   b. Duke Activity Status Index: Reflects activities of daily living.
   c. Incremental Shuttle Walk Test: Patient walks back and forth between two points, getting gradually faster until limit of exertion is reached.
   d. Cardiopulmonary exercise testing (CPET): Patient exercises on a bike, while measurements of ECG, HR, BP and expired gases are taken.
      - Anaerobic threshold (AT) and VO_2 peak correlate closely with ability to increase oxygen delivery in the postoperative period and hence to meet the metabolic demands of the neuroendocrine 'stress response' to surgery.
      - AT < 11 ml O_2/kg/min or VO_2 peak < 15 ml O_2/kg/min puts patient in the high-risk category.

2. **Risk prediction models (estimate risk for an individual patient)**
   a. EuroSCORE (cardiac surgery): Patient data is inputted on an online algorithm, which then calculates patient-specific risk.
   b. POSSUM (Physiology and Operative Severity Score for enUmeration of Mortality) and P-POSSUM (Portsmouth predictor modification)

- Involves 12 physiological variables (HR, BP, cardiac and respiratory signs, etc) and 6 intra-operative variables (peritoneal soiling, blood loss, urgency, etc.)
- Requires intraoperative information, hence unable to provide patient-specific risk preoperatively.

3. Risk scores

a. ASA-physical status (I-V): Doesn't correlate linearly with postoperative mortality or morbidity but provides a simple, widely understood comparator for describing the severity of a patient's systemic disease.
b. Goldmann cardiac risk index: Risk of postoperative cardiac events, published in 1977. Additive score using nine variables.
c. Lee's revised Cardiac risk score: Designed to improve on Goldmann, this is easier to use and more accurate.
d. Surgical Risk Scale - three variables: ASA score, surgical severity, and surgical urgency: It is as accurate as P-POSSUM in predicting mortality.

Preoperative Optimisation

- Preoperative optimisation is a strategy of manipulating cardiac output preoperatively to achieve supranormal oxygen delivery. (A target DO_2 of 600 mL/min is commonly quoted.) The practice was born out of several studies from the 1980s (mainly those of Bland and Shoemaker) showing that, among patients undergoing high-risk surgery, mortality and morbidity were higher in patients who incurred a postoperative 'oxygen debt' due to inability to increase tissue oxygen delivery.
- Several RCTs of 'supranormal' vs 'normal' DO_2 have confirmed a significantly lower mortality rates in patients who achieved 'supranormal' DO_2.
- Other possible 'targets' were also studied (e.g. $ScVO_2$—Central venous Oxygen saturation), but no strong evidence of a survival benefit was found.
- Robust risk stratification tools are key to identifying those 'high-risk' patients most likely to benefit from preoperative optimisation. Cardiopulmonary exercise testing is one risk stratification tool that reliably identifies patients with limited cardiorespiratory reserve and has been employed to select patients for preoperative optimisation. However, risk stratification tools may soon play an important role in deciding which surgical patients warrant perioperative intensive care.
- Surgical urgency and availability of local resources (e.g. ICU beds, CPET testing) will dictate the feasibility of investigating and correcting abnormal physiology preoperatively.

Respiratory

- Ensuring a patent airway and giving supplemental oxygen is the first step in treating hypoxaemia.
- Further measures may include NIV or IPPV, management of fluid overload, and initiating treatment of bronchospasm or chest infection.
- Chest physiotherapy may have a role in clearing secretions and expanding lung bases.

Cardiovascular

- Haemodynamic optimisation may require fluid resuscitation, management of arrhythmia, invasive haemodynamic monitoring, and/or vasopressor/inotropic support.
- Targeted haemodynamic optimisation (i.e. to a specific cardiac output/VO_2) has been shown to improve outcome.

Renal

- Correct any electrolyte abnormalities.
- Ensure adequate renal perfusion; measuring hourly urine output via a urinary catheter is helpful (and prevents the possibility of 'post-renal' acute kidney injury from urethral obstruction).

Haematological

- Correct any coagulopathy—may require FFP, cryoprecipitate, platelets, or other blood products.
- Transfuse to specific Hb target. It is interesting to note that the TRICC trial—'Transfusion Requirements In Critical Care'—shows no difference in outcome between 'conservative' (targeting Hb > 7 g/dL) and 'liberal' (targeting Hb > 9 g/dL) transfusion strategy.

Miscellaneous

- Warning if patient is hypothermic (remember... hypothermia is bad for several reasons):
  - impairs platelet and clotting factor function
  - depresses cardiac contractility and is pro-arrhythmic
  - may increase oxygen consumption via shivering
  - impairs wound healing
- Pain relief to attenuate sympathetic response (regional blocks are extremely useful, e.g. femoral or fascia iliaca blocks for fractured neck of femur patients).

In summary, the evidence is reasonably convincing that postoperative mortality and morbidity are more common in 'high-risk' patients with poor cardiorespiratory reserve who cannot sustain an increase in DO_2. However, 'goal-directed haemodynamic preoptimisation' is extremely costly and resource-intensive, since it requires ICU admission before surgery as well as afterwards. Such resource constraints have restricted its uptake in the NHS.

Further reading

1. Davies SJ, Wilson RJT. Preoperative optimization of the high-risk surgical patient. *British Journal of Anaesthesia*. 2004; **93**(1): 121–8.
2. Hebert PC, et al. A multicenter, randomized, controlled clinical trial of transfusion requirements in critical care. *The New England Journal of Medicine*. 1999; **340**(6): 409–417.

Compilation of important trials in anaesthesia and intensive care

GALA trial (2007)

Carotid endarterectomy: general or local anaesthesia?

Randomised multicentre trial from 2001 to 2007.

N = 3500

Postoperative evaluations were made by a stroke physician or neurologist at 1 month after surgery, blinded to anaesthetic technique.

Major perioperative outcomes after CEA are similar between RA and GA. This does not mean that anaesthetic technique is unimportant, because GA or RA performed well (or badly) contributes to good (or bad) outcome.

Perceived advantages and disadvantages of GA and RA for CEA

General anaesthesia

Advantages:
Immobility
Potential for neuroprotection
Controlled ventilation and CO_2
Attenuated stress response

Disadvantages:
Lack of direct neurological monitoring during surgery
Intraoperative hypotension
Postoperative hypertension
Increased rate of shunt use
Delayed recovery from GA may mask postoperative neurological complications

Regional anaesthesia

Advantages:
Allows direct real-time neurological monitoring
Avoids the risks of airway intervention
Reduced shunt rate
Allows arterial closure at 'normal' arterial pressure: may reduce risk of postoperative haematoma

Disadvantages:
Risks associated with performing blocks (deep cervical plexus blockade)
Patient stress/pain causing increased risk of myocardial ischaemia
Restricted access to airway during surgery
Requires cooperative patient, able to lie flat
Risk of requirement to convert to GA during surgery

Perioperative cerebral ischaemia monitors
Used to detect cerebral ischaemia, thromboembolism, or both. These are often used to identify patients who need a vascular shunt during surgery.

Awake testing	Using simple tasks for the patient to perform to assess the signs for cerebral ischaemia, it monitors the neurological function directly.
Stump pressure	The stump pressure distal to the carotid clamp reflects the perfusion pressure around the circle of Willis and is a specific measure of ischaemia. It is a nonsensitive measure of cerebral ischaemia but cannot identify emboli, and it reflects only cortical, not deeper structure, ischaemia.
Transcranial Doppler	A Doppler probe is placed on the petrous temporal bone allowing measurement of middle cerebral artery flow, which monitors both flow and emboli. The problems are that these are operator-dependent and the acoustic window is not found in many patients.
EEG	EEG is affected by cerebral ischaemia but not emboli and is difficult to interpret as GA can alter the signal.
Somatosensory evoked potentials	Thought to be no more sensitive or specific compared with EEG and it cannot identify emboli.
Near-infrared spectroscopy (NIRS)	NIRS measures arterial, venous and capillary oxygenation producing a regional cerebral oxygenation (rSO_2) value. It has a high negative predictive and poor positive values for cerebral ischaemia. The problems are interference from noncerebral blood flow and light.
EVAR Trial 1 (2005)	EVAR had an ongoing 3% better aneurysm-related survival than open repair but no demonstrable all-cause mortality. The continuing need for interventions mandates ongoing surveillance and longer follow-up for detailed cost-effectiveness evaluation.
EVAR Trial 2 (2005/2010)	EVAR had a considerable 30-day operative mortality in patients deemed unfit for open repair of their aneurysm. EVAR did not improve longer-term survival and was associated with a need for continued surveillance and reinterventions, at substantially increased cost. Thus, for these sick patients the emphasis had shifted towards improving patient fitness before considering EVAR, particularly in terms of cardiac, respiratory, and renal function.

PROWESS trial (2001)

Randomised, double-blind, placebo-controlled trial, published in 2001, the Recombinant Human Activated **PRO**tein C **W**orldwide **E**valuation in **S**evere **S**epsis (PROWESS) trial randomised 1,690 adults with severe sepsis to either drotrecogin alfa or placebo. The study was halted early after its second interim analysis revealed a statistically significant survival benefit with the drug.

Treatment with drotrecogin alfa activated significantly reduces mortality in patients with severe sepsis and may be associated with an increased risk of bleeding.

ADDRESS, RESOLVE, and ENHANCE and PROWESS-SHOCK trials demonstrated that the drug conferred no survival benefit in patients with high-risk septic shock.

PACMAN study (2004)

It was a multicentre RCT of PA catheter effectiveness involving 65 adult ICUs in the United Kingdom conducted to determine if use of the PA catheter results in decreased mortality.

Insertion of a PA catheter confers no excess risk but also offers no survival benefit to the critically ill patient.

PROSEVA trial (2013)

(Prone Positioning in Severe Acute Respiratory Distress Syndrome) Multicentre, prospective, controlled trial, randomising patients with severe ARDS to undergo prone-positioning sessions of at least 16 hours or to be left in the supine position.

N = 366

In patients with severe ARDS, early application of prolonged prone-positioning sessions significantly decreased 28-day and 90-day mortality.

NICE-SUGAR trial (2009)

The **N**ormoglycemia in **I**ntensive **C**are **E**valuation-**S**urvival **U**sing **G**lucose **A**lgorithm **R**egulation

Randomised 6,104 patients in medical and surgical ICUs to receive either intensive glucose control with insulin therapy or conventional glucose level.
A higher mortality rate with intensive glucose control.

CRASH 1 (2006)

Corticosteroid **R**andomisation **A**fter **S**ignificant **H**ead injury

A large simple placebo-controlled trial, among adults with head injury and impaired consciousness, of the effects of a 48-hour infusion of corticosteroids on death and neurological disability.

N = 10 000

The study showed a significant increase in number of deaths in patients given steroids compared with patients who received no treatment. The significant increase in deaths with steroids suggests that steroids should no longer be routinely used in people with traumatic head injury.

CRASH 2 (2010)

Clinical **R**andomisation of an **A**ntifibrinolytic in **S**ignificant **H**aemorrhage
Effects of tranexamic acid on death, vascular occlusive events, and blood transfusion in trauma patients with significant haemorrhage.

N = 20 000

Tranexamic acid safely reduced the risk of death in bleeding trauma patients in this study and should be considered for use in such patients.

CRASH-3 (current)

Tranexamic acid for the treatment of significant traumatic brain injury: study protocol for an international randomized, double-blind, placebo-controlled trial.

OSCILLATE Trial (2013)

It is a multicentre RCT where adults with new-onset moderate-to-severe ARDS were randomly assigned to high-frequency oscillation ventilation (HFOV) or to a conventional ventilation strategy; in both groups high airway pressures were used to maintain maximum lung recruitment.

The trial was stopped after 548 of the planned 1,200 patients because the use of HFOV resulted in a 12% increase of in-hospital mortality.

The early use of a similar HFOV protocol in all ARDS patients is likely to lead to a worse outcome compared to usual care and should therefore be avoided.

OSCAR trial (2013)

Study to compare HFOV treatment group or the control group, in which the patients were treated with conventional ventilation.

N = 795

The results showed that there was no significant difference between the two treatment groups, with 41.7% mortality in the HFOV group and 41.1% mortality in the control group.

CALORIES Trial (current)

A phase III, open, multicentre, randomised controlled trial comparing the clinical and cost-effectiveness of early nutritional support in critically ill patients via the parenteral versus the enteral route.

ARDS
Old definition of ARDS:
1. Acute onset of hypoxemia with PaO_2/FiO_2 ratio $\leq$ 200 mm Hg
2. Bilateral infiltrates on chest X-ray
3. No evidence of left atrial hypertension

Problems with old definition:
- No explicit criteria for defining 'acute'
- PaO_2/FiO_2 ratio is sensitive to changes in ventilator settings
- High inter-observer variability in interpreting chest X-rays
- Difficulties identifying/ruling out cardiogenic or hydrostatic pulmonary oedema

Berlin definition (2012)

ARDS is an acute diffuse, inflammatory lung injury, leading to increased pulmonary vascular permeability, increased lung weight, and loss of aerated lung tissue with hypoxemia and bilateral radiographic opacities, associated with increased venous admixture, increased physiological dead space, and decreased lung compliance.

ARDS is categorized as being mild, moderate, or severe.

Mild: PaO_2/FiO_2 of 200–300 mmHg (27% mortality)
Moderate: PaO_2/FiO_2 of 100–200 mmHg (32%)
Severe: PaO_2/FiO_2 of $<$ 100 mmHg (45%)

HEMODIAFE study (2006)

A multicentre RCT randomized 184 patients to intermittent haemodialysis (IHD) and 175 patients to continuous veno-venous hemodiafiltration (CVVHDF).

CVVHDF and IHD may be used interchangeably for the critically ill patient in ARF.

RECORD trial (2008)

(**RE**gulation of **C**oagulation in **OR**thopedic Surgery to Prevent **D**eep Venous Thrombosis and Pulmonary Embolism)
The study looked at the effectiveness of Rivaroxaban in preventing VTE after hip and knee arthroplasty, comparing it with Enoxaparin.

N = 9,000

Significant reductions in venous thromboembolism (VTE) after knee replacement surgery with comparable rates of bleeding.

ENIGMA 1 (2007)

Evaluation of **N**itrous oxide **I**n the **G**as **M**ixture for **A**naesthesia
This trial compares the use of nitrous oxide-free or nitrous oxide-based anaesthesia in over 2,000 patients having major surgery.

Administration of nitrous oxide was associated with increased long-term risk of MI but not death and stroke.

ENIGMA 2 (current)

Evaluation of nitrous oxide anaesthesia and cardiac morbidity after major surgery.

TRICC trial (1999)

Transfusion **R**equirements **I**n **C**ritical **C**are.
Restrictive transfusion in critically ill does not result in increased mortality and is superior to liberal transfusion strategy with exception of patients with AMI/unstable angina.

SHOT trial

Serious **H**azards **O**f **T**ransfusion
Reports wrong blood/components infusion.

SABRE
Serious **A**dverse **B**lood **R**eactions and **E**vents

POISE trial (2008)	The POISE study highlights the increased risks of stroke and all-cause mortality associated with the perioperative administration of β-blocking drugs.

N = 8,351

More deaths and stroke on β blocker group and less MI than non-β-blocker group.

Perioperative β-blockade should be prescribed only on an individual patient basis after due consideration has been given to their possible benefits and hazards.

POISE-2 trial

Clinical trial focused on major cardiovascular complications in noncardiac surgery. The trial looks at the efficacy and safety of low-dose clonidine versus placebo and also low-dose aspirin versus placebo in patients with atherosclerotic cardiovascular disease.

N = 10 000

Low-dose clonidine increased rates of 'clinically important hypotension' and nonfatal cardiac arrest after noncardiac surgery. Patients given aspirin after noncardiac surgery had a higher risk of major bleeding than the patients who did not receive aspirin.

The Collaborative Eclampsia trial (1995)

This is an international multicentre randomised trial comparing standard anticonvulsant regimens.

N = 1,687

Women allocated to Magnesium Sulphate had a lower risk of recurrent convulsions and maternal mortality.

MAGPIE trial (2002)

Magnesium Sulphate, compared with placebo, seems to be better for the prevention of eclampsia and may reduce maternal mortality.

NAP 1

Supervisory role of consultant anaesthetists

NAP 2

Place of mortality and morbidity review meetings

NAP 3 (2009)

The Third National Audit Project (NAP3) is the largest prospective study recording the incidence of complications after central neuraxial blocks (CNBs).

Paraplegia and death   1 in 54 500
Overall death   < 1 in 100 000

NAP 4 (2011)

Major complications of airway management in the UK.

The data suggests the incidence of death and brain damage from airway management during general anaesthesia is low, but it may be because of under reporting. It therefore provides an indication of the lower limit for incidence of such complications.

NAP 5 (current)

NAP 5 report focuses on failure of general anaesthesia in the UK – Accidental awareness during general anaesthesia (AAGA)

Findings:
1. Estimated incidence ~1:19,000 anaesthetics, ~1:8,000 when neuromuscular blockade was used and ~1:136,000 without it. Caesarean sections and cardiothoracic surgeries had the highest risks.
2. AAGA occurred more commonly during induction and emergence, contributed by the use of thiopentone, rapid-sequence induction, obesity, neuromuscular blockade, failure to use a nerve stimulator, difficulties with airway management, and interruption in anaesthetic delivery when transferring the patient from anaesthetic room to theatre (the 'gap').
3. Also drug errors and communication failure due to human factors, inadequate use of specific depth of anaesthesia monitoring are suggested to have led to AAGA.

Recommendations:
The committee has made 64 recommendations stressing the importance of safe conduct of anaesthesia, clear documentation, robust incident reporting, discussing risk of AAGA in the preoperative period, use of nerve stimulators, adequate patient follow up, and insists the need for improving knowledge in TIVA and monitoring depths of anaesthesia.

NAP 6 (future)

Perioperative anaphylaxis

Compilation of causes of blood and electrolyte imbalance

Electrolyte abnormalities
Hyponatraemia

Plasma sodium < 135 mmol/L

Excessive intake (urine sodium < 10 mmol/L)
- IV administration of sodium deficient fluids
- TURP syndrome
- Excessive drinking

Reduced excretion (Urine sodium > 20 mmol/L)
- SIADH
- Drugs—chlorpropamide, oxytocin

Water excess with smaller sodium excess
(urine sodium < 10 mmol/L)
- Cardiac failure
- Hepatic failure
- Nephrotic syndrome

Water deficiency with greater sodium deficiency
- Renal loss
- Diuretic therapy
- Hypoadrenalism
- Salt-losing nephritis
- Renal tubular acidosis
- Vomiting and diarrhoea
- Pancreatitis

Redistribution of water/sodium
- Redistribution of water from intracellular to extracellular compartment (e.g. hyperglycaemia)
- Pseudohyponatraemia (e.g. in hyperlipidaemia)

Hypernatraemia

Plasma sodium > 145 mmol/L

Sodium excess (urine sodium > 20 mmol/L)
- Cushing's syndrome
- Hyperaldosteronism
- Iatrogenic (e.g. hypertonic saline)

Water depletion
- Diabetes insipidus
- Insufficient water intake
- Insensible water loss

Sodium deficiency with greater water deficiency
- Renal loss (e.g. osmotic diuresis)
- Vomiting, diarrhoea
- Adrenocortical deficiency

Hypokalaemia

Plasma potassium < 3.5 mmol/L

Reduced intake (e.g. IV fluids without potassium supplementation)

Excessive losses

Renal
- Solute diuresis
- Diuretic therapy
- Hyperaldosteronism
- Cushing's syndrome
- Diuretic phase of acute renal failure

Movement of potassium into cells
- Alkalosis
- Drugs (e.g. insulin)

Hyperkalaemia

Plasma potassium > 5.5 mmol/L

Increased intake (e.g. IV fluids, rapid blood transfusion)

Decreased renal output
- Renal failure
- Adrenocortical insufficiency
- Drugs (e.g. ACE inhibitors, potassium-sparing diuretics)

Movement of potassium out of cells
- Trauma, Crush syndrome, malignant hyperthermia, rhabdomyolysis
- Acidosis
- Action of suxamethonium

Artefactual (e.g. haemolysed blood sample)

Hypercalcaemia

Plasma calcium level > 2.6 mmol/L

Hyperparathyroidism

Malignancy—both primary and bony metastasis

Increased intake (e.g. milk alkali syndrome)

Vitamin D metabolic disorders
- Hypervitaminosis D (vitamin D intoxication)
- Idiopathic hypercalcaemia of infancy
- Rebound hypercalcaemia after rhabdomyolysis

Disorders related to high bone-turnover rates
- Hyperthyroidism
- Prolonged immobilization
- Thiazide use
- Vitamin A intoxication
- Multiple myeloma

Renal failure

Adrenocortical insufficiency

Hypocalcaemia	Plasma calcium < 2.2 mmol/L

Hypocalcaemia

Plasma calcium < 2.2 mmol/L
- Decreased parathyroid hormone
- Decreased Vitamin D activity (e.g. intestinal malabsorption, liver disease, chronic renal failure)
- Increased calcium loss (e.g. chelating agents, calcification of soft tissues)
- Decreased ionised calcium (e.g. alkalosis)

Hypermagnesaemia

Normal magnesium level is 0.7 to 1.1 mmol/L
- Renal failure
- Excessive intake
- Lithium therapy
- Hypothyroidism
- Addison disease
- Laxative/antacid abuse
- Adrenocortical insufficiency

Hypomagnesaemia

Decreased intake
- Starvation
- Alcohol dependence
- Total parenteral nutrition

Redistribution
- Hungry bone syndrome
- Treatment of diabetic ketoacidosis
- Alcohol withdrawal syndromes
- Refeeding syndrome
- Acute pancreatilis

Increased gastrointestinal loss
- Diarrhoea
- Vomiting and nasogastric suction
- Gastrointestinal fistulas

Hyperphosphataemia

Plasma phosphate > 1.4 mmol/L
Increased intake
- Diet
- IV administration
- Excess vitamin D

Increased release from cells/bones
- Diabetes mellitus
- Starvation
- Rhabdomyolysis
- Malignancy
- Renal failure

Factitious (e.g. haemolysis)

Decreased excretion
- Hypoparathyroidism
- Renal failure
- Excess growth hormone secretion

Hypophosphataemia

Mild
- Hyperparathyroidism
- Osteomalacia
- Increased carbohydrate metabolism
- Haemodialysis
- Acute alkalosis

Severe
- Ketoacidosis
- TPN and refeeding after starvation
- Chronic alcoholism/withdrawal

Acidosis

Metabolic
Increased acid production
- Ketone bodies (e.g. DKA)
- Lactate (e.g. in shock, exercise)

Acid ingestion (e.g. Salicylate poisoning)

Failure to excrete hydrogen ion
- Renal failure
- Distal renal tubular acidosis
- Carbonic anhydrase inhibitors

Loss of bicarbonate
- Diarrhoea
- GI fistula
- Proximal renal tubular acidosis

Respiratory
Increased arterial PCO_2 secondary to alveolar hypoventilation

Anion gap

The anion gap is the difference between primary measured cations (Na^+ and K^+) and the primary measured anions (Cl^- and HCO_3^-) in serum. This test is most commonly performed in patients who present with altered mental status, unknown exposures, acute renal failure, and acute illnesses.
Anion Gap = $(Na^+ + K^+) - (Cl^- + HCO_3^-)$.

The normal value for the serum anion gap is 8–16 mEq/L.
The anion gap increases when organic anions increase (e.g. in lactic acidosis, ketoacidosis) and does not increase in acidosis due to loss of bicarbonate or intake of hydrochloric acid.

High anion gap metabolic acidosis
Accumulation of organic acids or impaired H^+ excretion
- Lactate
- Toxins
- Ketones
- Renal
- Lab tests to consider = lactate, glucose, creatinine and urea, urinary ketones, serum levels of methanol, ethanol, paracetamol, salicylates, and ethylene glycol

Normal anion gap metabolic acidosis
Loss of HCO_3^- from extracellular fluid
- GI causes—diarrhoea/vomiting, fistulae (pancreatic, ureters, biliary, small bowel, ileostomy)

Low anion gap
- Nonrandom analytical errors (increased Na^+, increased viscosity, iodide ingestion, increased lipids)
- Decrease in unmeasured anions (albumin, dilution)
- Increase in unmeasured cations (multiple myeloma, hypercalcaemia, hypermagnesemia, lithium overdose)

Blood abnormalities
Polycythaemia

Primary
- Polycythaemia rubra vera

Secondary—With an appropriate increase in erythropoietin
- High altitude
- Respiratory disease
- Cyanotic heart disease
- Heavy smoking

Secondary—With an inappropriate increase in erythropoietin
- Renal cell carcinoma
- Hepatocellular carcinoma
- Massive uterine fibroma

Relative
- Stress polycythaemia
- Dehydration
- Burns

Anaemia

Etiological classification
- Impaired RBC production
- Excessive destruction
- Blood loss

Morphological classification
- Macrocytic anaemia
- Microcytic hypochromic anaemia
- Normochromic normocytic anaemia

Etiological classification
Impaired RBC production
- Abnormal bone marrow
  - Aplastic anaemia
  - Myelofibrosis

- Essential factors deficiency
  - Iron deficiency anaemia
  - B12 deficiency
  - Folate deficiency
  - Erythropoietin deficiency, as in renal disease

- Stimulation factor deficiency
  - Anaemia in chronic disease
  - Anaemia in hypothyroidism and hypopituitarism

Excessive destruction
- Intracorpuscular defect
  - Membrane: hereditary spherocytosis
  - Enzyme: G6PD deficiency
  - Haemoglobin: thalassemia, haemoglobinopathies

- Extracorpuscular defect
  - Mechanical: microangiopathic haemolytic anaemia
  - Infective: Clostridium tetani
  - Antibodies: SLE
  - Hypersplenism

Blood loss
- Acute: trauma, acute GI bleed
- Chronic: parasitic infestation, chronic NSAIDS

Morphological classification
Macrocytic /megaloblastic anaemia
MCV > 94; MCHC > 31
- Vitamin B12 deficiency: Pernicious anaemia
- Folate deficiency: Nutritional megaloblastic anaemia
- Drug-induced abnormal DNA synthesis: anticonvulsant, chemotherapy agents, etc.

Microcytic hypochromic anaemia
MCV < 80; MCHC < 31
- Iron deficiency anaemia: chronic blood loss, dietary inadequacy, malabsorption, increased demand, etc.
- Abnormal globin synthesis: thalassaemia

Normocytic normochromic anaemia
MCV 82–92; MCHC > 30
- Blood loss
- Increased plasma volume
- Hypoplastic marrow
- Endocrine: hypothyroidism, adrenal insufficiency
- Renal and liver disease

Thrombocytopenia

Platelet count is less than 100×10^9/L

Decreased production
- Bone marrow depression by drugs, infection
- Vitamin B12/folate deficiency
- Paroxysmal nocturnal haemoglobinuria
- Alcoholism

Shortened survival
- Immune (e.g. autoantibodies, drugs such as heparin, malignancy)
- Nonimmune: DIC, cardiopulmonary bypass

Abnormal distribution
- Hypersplenism
- Hypothermia

ECG changes	**Hyperkalaemia**

Hyperkalaemia

5.5–6.5 mmol/L—repolarisation problems
- Peaked T waves

6.5–7 mmol/L—progressive paralysis of atria
- Flattening of P waves
- Long PR interval

7–9 mmol/L—conduction defects and bradycardia
- Prolonged QRS interval
- Conduction block (bundle branch blocks, fascicular blocks)
- Sinus bradycardia or slow AF
- Sine wave appearance (preterminal rhythm)

> 9 mmol/L—cardiac arrest
- Asystole
- Ventricular fibrillation

Hypokalaemia

Mild to moderate
- Tall and wide P wave
- Prolonged PR interval
- T wave flattening and inversion
- ST depression
- Prominent U waves

Severe
- Supraventricular and ventricular ectopics
- AF, atrial flutter, atrial tachycardia
- VT, VF, and Torsades de Pointes

Hypercalcaemia
- Shortening of the QT interval
- J waves in severe hypercalcaemia
- VF arrest

Hypocalcaemia
- Prolonged QTc prolongation by prolonging the ST segment
- Torsades de pointes and atrial fibrillation in severe cases

Hypermagnesaemia
- Bradycardia
- Prolonged PR, QRS, and QT intervals
- Complete heart block and asystole at higher concentrations

Hypomagnesemia
- Prolonged PR, QRS, and QT interval
- Flattened T wave
- Prominent U waves
- ST depression
- Atrial/ventricular arrhythmias

ECG changes of hypomagnesemia resemble that of hypokalaemia.
ECG changes of hypermagnesemia resemble that of hyperkalaemia.

Hypothermia
- Osborne Waves (J waves)
- Prolonged PR, QRS, and QT intervals
- Ventricular ectopics
- Atrial fibrillation
- Sinus bradycardia
- Cardiac arrest due to VT, VF, or asystole
- Shivering artefact

INDEX

A

AAAQIP, 126

AABCDS acronym, 340–1

α adrenoceptor blockers, 214

ABCDE - BIT approach to chest x-rays, 324–5

abdomen, 20–21

abdominal aortic aneurysm, 120–6

Abdominal Aortic Aneurysm Quality Improvement Project (AAAQIP), 126

α blockers, 145

abscess, epidural, 192–3

absolute humidity, 253

ACC/AHA cardiac risk stratification for non-cardiac surgery, 374–5

accidental awareness during general anaesthesia (AAGA), 389

ACE-i, 180, 181

acetylcholinesterase (AChE), 250

acidaemia, 67

acidosis, 394–5

acoustic neuroma, 342

acromegaly, 244–5; anaesthetics of, 245; diagnosis and treatment of, 244–5

active humidification, 253

active scavenging system for pollution in the operating theatre, 183

acute cervical spine subluxation, 258–63

acute chest syndrome, 265

acute coronary syndrome, 172

acute glaucoma, 47–48

acute ischaemia, 362

acute kidney injury, 376

acute pain in caudal block, 138

acute pancreatitis, 376–7

Acute Physiology, Age, and Chronic Health Evaluation Systems (APACHE I-IV), 378

acute rejection by denervated heart, 211

Acute Renal Failure Trial Network (ATN), 219

acute respiratory distress syndrome (ARDS), 385–7

adenohypophysis, 240

adenosine, 371; and supraventricular tachycardia, 231

ADH stimulating water reabsorption, 246

adolescents and parent-guardian consent issues, 76

adrenergic neuron blockade, 214

adults' anatomy of caudal epidural space, 141

aero-digestive colonisation, 249

AHI. See apnoea-hypopnoea index (AHI)

air bronchogram, 326

air space opacification, 328

airway, 388; in acromegaly, 244; in cervical spine subluxation, 262; in chest x-rays, 325; for cholesteatoma, 304; control with ingested foreign body, 109; in fractured mandible, 127; in micro laryngoscopy, 162; predicting difficulties, 377; in rheumatoid arthritis, 132

alcoholic hepatitis, 177, 178

alcoholic liver disease, 177–8

alkylating agents, 58

allodynia, 314

American College of Cardiology, 376

American College of Chest Physicians, 44

American Society of Anesthesiologists (ASA), 373

American Thoracic Society, 247

Ametop, 40

amniotic fluid embolism, 45–46; management of, 46; risk factors for, 46

Amsorb, 61

Amsorb Plus, 61

anaemia, 395–6; of chronic disease, 301; in gastro-oesophageal reflux disease, 187–8; normocytic, 95; preoperative, 301–3

anaesthesia: and autonomic dysfunction, 97; cardiac risk scoring system, 307–8; caudal, 138–9; for cholesteatoma, 305; for dentistry, 77; for Eisenmenger's syndrome, 102–3; hypotensive, 213–14; on intraocular pressure, 48; lowering blood pressure during, 213; for lung resection, 42–44; for mastoidectomy, 216; to minimize hyperreflexia, 202; nitrous oxide based, 387; for Parkinson's disease, 30–32; risk scoring in, 373–8; for sickle cell disease, 265; for superior vena cava obstruction (SVCO), 297–9; trials in, 383–9; for Wolff-Parkinson-White (WPW) syndrome, 79–80

anaesthetic equipment and magnetic resonance imaging, 34

anaesthetic gas pollution, 182–3

anaesthetic monitoring factors, 35

anaesthetics: for acromegaly, 245; administering

during electroconvulsive therapy, 16; for aortic stenosis in a pregnant patient, 158–9; for baby delivery, 145–6; for cardiomyopathy, 197–8; for complete heart block, 8–9; for cranial nerves monitoring, 83; for cystic fibrosis, 235; for diabetic ketoacidosis (DKA), 68–70; for electroconvulsive therapy, 15; for end-stage liver failure, 179; for epilepsy, 4; for foreign body, 40; for laparoscopic procedures, 56; and magnetic resonance imaging, 34; for myotonic dystrophy, 105; for obstructive sleep apnea (OSA), 5–6; for patient with permanent pacemaker, 9–10; for pulmonary hypertension (PHT), 284; during scoliosis surgery, 115, 117; and serotonin syndrome, 114; toxicity causing seizures, 70–71

anaesthetising: for bleeding tonsil, 272; in cancer patients, 60; for cardiac risk patients, 308; for cervical spine subluxation, 260; children with learning difficulties, 77; for corrective bronchopleural fistula (BPF) surgery, 278; for debridement and spinal cord injury, 201; for denervated heart for a noncardiac surgery, 210–11; for endovascular aneurysm repair (EVAR), 124; for food bolus removal, 109; for fractured mandible, 128–9; for fundoplication, 188–9; lung transplant patient for subsequent surgery, 212; for micro laryngoscopy, 161–2; for permanent pacemaker, 269; for rheumatoid arthritis, 132–3; for scoliosis surgery, 117; valve replacements patient having surgery, 227

analgesia: for cholesteatoma, 305; for corrective bronchopleural fistula (BPF) surgery, 278; for endovascular aneurysm repair (EVAR), 125; for fundoplication, 190; in intrauterine fetal death, 99; multimodal for hypospadias surgery, 138

anatomy: caudal block, 138–41; coronary circulation, 172–6; cranial nerve monitoring, 82–84; intraosseous anatomy, 310–13; liver and spleen, 20–25; mediastinum, 108–9; paravertebral block, 276–81; pituitary, 240–6; pleura, 204–8; spinal cord blood supply, 52–55

aneurysm, 384

angina: classification of, 373; managing in pregnant patient with aortic stenosis, 159

angioedema due to ACE-i, 181

angiotensin-converting enzyme inhibitor (ACE-i), 180–1

angiotensin I, 181

angiotensin II, 181

angiotensinogen, 181

anion gap, 95–96, 394–5

ankylosing spondylitis, 342

anterior cerebral artery, 111

anterior cerebral circulation, 110

anterior interventricular artery (AIVA), 174

anterior interventricular artery infarct, 174

anterior mediastinum, 108

anterior mediastinum mass, 326

anterior pituitary gland, 240–1

anterior spinal artery (ASA), 52, 54, 116

antero posterior (AP) projection in chest x-rays, 323

antibiotics: for intrauterine fetal death, 100; and valve replacements patient having surgery, 228

anticholinergics, 31, 32

anticholinesterases, 250–2; classification of, 250–1; indications for, 250

anticoagulants and bridging, 317–18

anticoagulation, 317–18; complications of renal replacement therapy, 219; managing during pregnancy, 160; and stroke risk, 374

anticonvulsant regimens, 388

antidepressants and Parkinson's disease, 32

antidiuretic hormone and diabetes insipidus, 245–6

antiemesis for cholesteatoma, 305

antiemetics and Parkinson's disease, 32

anti-epileptic drugs (AEDs), 4

antihypertensives and Parkinson's disease, 32

anti-metabolites, 58

antiplatelet agent for secondary post myocardial infarction, 180

antipsychotics and Parkinson's disease, 32

antisialogouges, 40

antitumor antibiotics, 59

aortic cross clamping, 54

aortic diastolic pressure (ADP), 175

aortic stenosis, 152–60, 260; blood flow in, 154–5; causes, 155; classification of, 155; impact of pregnancy, 155, 157–60; pathophysiology, 156; surgical interventions for, 160; symptoms and signs, 155

aortic surgery, 54–55

aortic valve, 338

aortic valve area, 154

aortic valve replacement (AVR), 160, 223

APACHE I, 378

APACHE II, 378

APACHE III, 378

APACHE IV, 378
aplastic sickling crisis, 264
apnoea-hypopnoea index (AHI), 3–4
apnoea physiology, 85–86
apnoea test, 85–86
apnoeic oxygenation, 85
ARDS, 385–7
arrhythmias: caused by tricyclic antidepressant
    drugs, 148; causes of, 78; in Wolff-
    Parkinson-White (WPW) syndrome, 80
arterial blood gas, 3, 66, 94, 95
arterial oxygen content, 302
arterial supply, 110, 242
arteria radicularis magna, 52
arteries in the spinal cord, 52
artery of Adamkiewicz, 52, 116
arthritis, rheumatoid, 130–3
ASA-physical status, 380
ASA score of fitness before surgery, 373
ASA syndrome, 55
aspiration, 38–41, 249
aspiration pneumonia, 248
aspirin: in noncardiac surgery, 388; for secondary
    post myocardial infarction, 180
asystole, risk of, 9
atelectasis, 328–9
Atlanto-axial subluxation, 131
Atlanto occipital alignment, 340
atrial chamber enlargement, 355–6
atrial fibrillation (AF), 80, 357
atrial flutter, 358
atrial tachycardia, 358
atrio-ventricular (AV) dissociation, 360
atrio-ventricular nodal reentry tachycardia
    (AVNRT), 358
atrio-ventricular reentry tachycardia (AVRT), 359
atropine on denervated heart, 210
atypical agents for Parkinson's disease, 31
atypical pneumonia, 247
autonomic dysfunction in Guillain Barre
    syndrome, 97
autonomic dysreflexia, 200–2; anaesthetic
    considerations, 201–2; drugs for, 202
autonomic hyperreflexia, 201–2
autonomic innervation of the heart, 209
AV nodal slowing, 371
awake fibreoptic intubation (AFOI), 262
awake testing, 384
A waves in intracranial pressure
    waveforms, 91–92
axillary brachial plexus block, 69
axis deviation in ECG, 351–3

B
baby delivery and use anaesthetics, 145–6
β adrenoceptor blockers, 213
baralyme, 61
barium lime, 61
basal metabolic rate (BMR), 12
basic metabolic demand (VO_2), 86
β blockers, 145, 214; for secondary prevention
    post myocardial infarction, 180; and
    stroke, 388
Becker's muscular dystrophy, 106
behavioural management of complex regional pain
    syndrome (CRPS), 315
Berlin definition (2012) of ARDS, 387
Berlin questionnaire, 5
bicarbonate, 394
bilateral airspace disease, 130
bilateral hilar lymphadenopathy, 296
bipolar diathermy, 10
biventricular pacemaker, 338
bleeding: in endovascular aneurysm repair (EVAR),
    125; in end stage hepatic disease, 177
bleeding tonsil, 271–3
blocked left coronary artery, 172
blood: and blood:gas coefficient, 88; coagulability
    in valve replacements patient having
    surgery, 225–6; coronary, 173–6; loss, 396;
    loss during scoliosis surgery, 117; loss in
    post-tonsillectomy, 272; manifestation in
    rheumatoid arthritis, 132; reduction in to
    manage intracranial pressure, 90–91; in
    stenosis, 154–5; supply to the pleura, 204;
    and treating raised intracranial pressure, 111
blood filter for epidurals, 193
blood:gas coefficient, 87
blood imbalance, 395–7
blood pressure: during anaesthesia of a pregnant
    patient with aortic stenosis, 158; in
    Cushing's reflex, 90; lowering during
    anaesthesia, 213; lowering to induce
    hypotension, 213
blood supply: of pituitary gland, 242; of spinal cord,
    52–55, 116
blood transfusion. See transfusion
blue spells, 101
BMR, 12
bolus dose in target controlled infusion (TCI), 286
bone: in chest x-rays, 325; infusion of fluids,
    311–13; parts of, 312; vascular supply
    of, 313
bone cement, 228
bone cement implantation syndrome (BCIS), 228–9

bone marrow toxicity due to nitrous oxide, 182
bone-modifying drugs, 58
bony landmarks, 340
BPF, 276
bradyarrhythmia, 361–2
bradycardia: during electroconvulsive therapy, 16; during fundoplication, 190
brain injury, 386
brain natriuretic peptide (BNP), 307
brainstem and preconditions for testing, 85
brainstem death, 26–29; organ donation, 29; physiological changes in, 26; testing, 85
brainstem evoked auditory potential (BAEP), 82–83
brain tissue and treating raised intracranial pressure, 111
breakthrough pain, 60
breath, shortness of, 303
breathing noise, 297
breathing system and absorption of carbon dioxide, 61–63
British Committee for Standards in Haematology (BCSH), 318
British Pacing and Electrophysiology Group, 269
British Thoracic Society, 44
British Thoracic Society Pleural disease guideline 2010, 206
broad complex tachycardia, 360–1
bronchodilators, 169
bronchopleural fistula (BPF), 276–8; anaesthetizing for corrective surgery, 278; diagnosis and causes of, 277; surgical treatment of, 278; ventilating patients with, 277
broncho pleural leak, 277
bronchoscopes, 41
bronchoscopy, 41
Bruce Protocol, 123
β thalassemia, 267
bundle branch block, 353–5
Bundle of His, 348
B waves in intracranial pressure waveforms, 91–92

C
caffeine in inadvertent dural puncture, 135
calcium, 392, 393
calcium channel blocker, 181
calcium-modulating drugs for complex regional pain syndrome (CRPS), 316
CALORIES trial (current), 386
CAM-ICU, 378
Canadian Cardiovascular Society (CCS) classification of angina, 373

cancer: analgesia in, 60; and blood transfusion, 302; drugs used in, 58–60; pain, 139
cannulation, intravenous, 189–90
capacity, mental, 75–76
capillaries in portal circulation, 242
capture beats, 360
carbamylated enzyme complex, 250
carbon dioxide: absorption in the breathing system, 61–63; increased during a laparoscopic procedure, 56; increased intra-operatively, 56
carbon monoxide formed by soda lime, 62
cardiac arrest, 196, 198; induced by magnesium, 146; preventing, 217
cardiac catheterisation techniques, 154–5
cardiac conduction, normal, 348–52
cardiac cycle, 175–6
cardiac death and organ donation, 29
cardiac diseases as contraindications in pregnancy, 156–7
cardiac failure, 226
cardiac manifestations of myotonic dystrophy, 104
cardiac output, 292, 302; manipulating, 380–1; monitoring, 289–92
cardiac output monitor, 290–1
cardiac risk: for abdominal aortic aneurysmaneurysm, 122; stratification, 306–8, 374–5
cardiac status assessment, 306–7
cardiac surgery risk prediction models, 379
cardiac toxicity from chemotherapy drugs, 59
cardiogenic oedema, 333
cardiomyopathy, 194–9; ECG, 198–9; hypertrophic, 195–6; pathophysiology of, 196; treatment, 196–7
cardiopulmonary exercise testing (CPET), 123, 125, 126, 303, 307
cardiovascular compromise, 57
cardiovascular disease during pregnancy, 152–60
cardiovascular system: factors in cardiac output, 381; impact of hypothermia, 254; manifestation in acromegaly, 244; manifestation in rheumatoid arthritis, 132; manifestation in scoliosis, 115; manifestation in tricyclic antidepressant drug poisoning, 147; preserving for organ donation, 28; problems with gas insufflation, 56
cardioversion, 371; for supraventricular tachycardia, 232
care bundles in the intensive care unit, 73–74
cartilaginous space, 341

catheter, 385; complications of renal replacement therapy, 219; pulmonary floatation, 340

caudal anaesthesia, 138–9

caudal block, 138–41; additive drugs used in, 140–1; complications of, 141; indications of, 138–9; performing, 140–1

caudal epidural space, 141

causalgia, 315

central DI, 245

central line, 340

central line bundle, 73

centrally acting drugs, 214

central nervous system manifestation of tricyclic antidepressant drug poisoning, 147

central neuraxial blocks (CNBs), 388

central venous pressure (CVP), 289

cerebral autoregulation, 111

cerebral blood flow, 111

cerebral circulation, 110–1

cerebral herniation, 26

cerebral ischaemia, 384

cerebral metabolic rate of oxygen ($CMRO_2$), 111

cerebral oedema, 89

cerebral perfusion pressure, 111

cerebral spinal fluid: analysis, 94, 96; leakage in inadvertent dural puncture, 135; and managing intracranial pressure, 91; and treating raised intracranial pressure, 111

cerebrospinal fluid pressure (CSFP), 54

cervical plexus, 298–9

cervical plexus blocks, 298–9

cervical spine fracture, 200

cervical spine injury, 165

cervical spine radiographs, 340–1

cervical spine subluxation, 258–63; airway management, 262; anaesthetizing, 260; extubating, 263; in prone position, 263

cervical spondylosis, 341

CHADS2 score, 374

CHA2DS2 - VASc score, 374

chemical determinants of coronary circulation, 175

chemotherapy drugs, 59

chemotherapy for lymphoma, 300

chest drainage system, 207–8, 340

chest drain insertion, 206–8; anatomy of, 206–8; role of ultrasound, 206

chest radiograph for COA, 156

chest x-rays, 323–7; for abdominal aortic aneurysm, 121, 123; for bronchopleural fistula (BPF), 276; for cervical spine subluxation, 259, 261; in epileptic, 3; for foreign body aspiration, 39; for

fundoplication, 186; for Guillain Barre syndrome, 98; for lung resection, 42; lungs, 328–35; for mediastinal mass, 294; for pneumothorax, 237; projections of importance, 323; for pulmonary hypertension (PHT), 283–4; for rheumatoid arthritis, 130–1; of valve replacements patient having surgery, 223, 224

Cheyne-Stokes breathing pattern, 89, 90

Child-Pugh score, 178–9

children: anatomy of caudal epidural space, 141; dehydration in, 310; and fundoplication, 186–91; obtaining consent from those with parental responsibility, 76

Children Act (1989), 76

chloride channel impacting mucus in cystic fibrosis, 233

cholesteatoma, 304–5, 343

chronic bronchitis, 168

chronic glaucoma, 47–48

chronic liver disease, 178

chronic obstructive pulmonary disease (COPD), 168–70; complications, 169; diagnosing, 168–9; managing, 169–70

chronic pain in caudal block, 139

chronic regional pain syndrome, 314–16

chronic rejection by denervated heart, 211

chronic thromboembolic pulmonary hypertension, 282

Circle of willis, 110

circle system for carbon dioxide absorption, 63

circulation factors and equilibrium of inhaled agents, 88

circumflex artery infarct, 174

circumflex branch in left coronary artery, 174

cirrhosis, 177

clearance in target controlled infusion (TCI), 286

Clinical Randomisation of an Antifibrinolytic in Significant Haemorrhage, 386

clonidine, 140–1; in noncardiac surgery, 388

closed-angle glaucoma, 47–48

COA, 156

coagulation during amniotic fluid embolism, 46

coarctation of aorta (COA), 156

Collaborative Eclampsia trial (1995), 146, 388

colligative properties, 150

colloid osmotic pressure, 150

community-acquired pneumonia, 247

compartment model for target controlled infusion (TCI), 286

compensation phase of ICP elastance curve, 90

complete heart block, 7–10; airway and breathing, 9; anaesthetizing, 8; intraoperatively, 8–9
complex regional pain syndrome (CRPS), 314–16
Compound A, 62
compound motor action potentials (CMAPs), 73
computerized tomography. See CT
COMT inhibitors, 31
Confusion Assessment Method for the Intensive Care Unit (CAM-ICU), 378
congenital bicuspid valve, 156
consent forms, 76
consent issues, 75–77
context sensitive half time (CSHT), 287
continuity equation for determining aortic valve area, 154
continuous arteriovenous haemofiltration (CAVHF), 218
continuous renal replacement therapy (CRRT), 218
continuous venovenous haemodiafiltration (CVVHDF), 218, 387
continuous venovenous haemofiltration (CVVH), 218
Control of Substances Hazardous to Health (COSHH), 183
convection and heat loss, 255
COPD, 168–70
Corinaud's classification, 22
Cormack & Lehane grading, 377
corneal reflex, 49
coronary angiography, 307
coronary arteries, 172–6
coronary blood supply and the ventricles, 175
coronary circulation, 172–6; arterial supply, 173–5; blockage of arteries, 172–3; determinants of, 175–6; difference between systemic circulation and, 176
coronary perfusion pressure (CoPP), 175
coronary sinus, 174
corrected flow time (FTc), 292
Corticosteroid Randomisation After Significant Head injury, 385
cranial nerve monitoring, 82–84
CRASH 1 (2006), 385
CRASH 2 (2010), 386
CRASH-3 (current), 386
creatine level in intrauterine fetal death, 100
critical illness myopathy (CIM), 72–73
critical illness neuromyopathy (CINM), 72–73
critical illness polyneuropathy (CIP), 72–73
CRPS type 1, 315
CRPS type 2, 315
CSF. See cerebral spinal fluid

CSF glucose, 96
CSF protein, 96
C3/4 spinal cord injury, 201
C spine, 341–2; x-ray, 131
CT: of abdomen, 20–21; criteria for adult trauma patients, 164; of the head, 342–3; for mediastinal mass, 295
Cushing's reflex, 90
C1 vertebra, 131
C2 vertebra, 131
C waves in intracranial pressure waveforms, 91–92
cyanotic heart disease, 101
cyanotic spells, 101
cystic fibrosis, 233–5; anaesthesia for, 235; impact on organs, 233–4
cystic fibrosis transmembrane regulator (CFTR), 233
cytotoxic drugs, 58–59

D
day-care dentistry and general anaesthesia, 77
dc cardioversion for supraventricular tachycardia, 231–2
debridement, 68, 69; of ankle pressure, 201
decompensated phase of ICP elastance curve, 90
decompensation in end stage hepatic disease, 177
deep vein thrombosis (DVT), 6
dehydration in children, 310
denervated heart, 209–12; immunosuppressant therapy, 211–12; long-term health issues, 212; physiology of, 210; rejection, 211
dentistry and general anaesthesia, 77
depolarising neuromuscular blocking agents (DMB), 320
dermatome, 20
desflurance, 87
Detsky's modified cardiac risk index (1986), 375
diabetes insipidus (DI), 245–6
diabetic ketoacidosis (DKA), 66–71; anaesthetics for, 68–70; fluids for, 68; management of, 67–68
diaphragm in chest x-rays, 325
diaphysis, 312
diarrhoea in children, 310
diastolic pressure time (DPTI), 176
diathermy, 10
dicrotic notch, 290
diffusing capacity of the lung for carbon monoxide, 43
digoxin therapy, 366–7
2,3 diphosphoglycerate (DPG), 302
direct sympathomimetics, 210

disc space, 341
diuretics, 145, 214
DLCO, 43–44, 123
DNAR status of patient, 228
Dobutamine Stress Echo, 123
donation after brainstem death (DBD), 29
donation after cardiac death (DCD), 29
do not attempt resuscitation (DNAR) status of
    patient, 228
dopamine, 30
dopamine agonists, 31
dopamine precursors, 31
Doppler, 291–2; for diagnosing valvular heart
    disease, 153–5
double burst stimulation, 320
double lumen tube (DLT), 44
doxazosin, 145
Dragersorb, 61
drain in chest drainage system, 207
driving pressure in a jet ventilator, 163
drugs: for acromegaly, 245; causing pleural
    effusion, 205; to change pH of gastric
    contents, 249; for chronic obstructive
    pulmonary disease (COPD), 169;
    complications of renal replacement therapy,
    219; for dysreflexia, 202; and equilibrium of
    inhaled agents, 88; hypotensive, 213–16;
    and impact on rheumatoid arthritis, 132;
    for organophosphate poisoning, 252; for
    Parkinson's disease, 31–32; poisoning
    of tricyclic antidepressants (TCA), 147;
    precipitating serotonin syndrome, 114;
    for secondary prevention, 180–1; used in
    caudal block, 140–1; used in malignancy,
    58–60
dry bulb hydrometer, 254
dry cough due to ACE-i, 181
dual chamber pacemaker, 338–9
dual platelet therapy for secondary post myocardial
    infarction, 180
Duchene muscular dystrophy, 106
Duke Activity Status Index, 123
dural puncture, inadvertent, 134–6; use of epidural
    blood patch (EDP), 135–6
dynamic fluid responsiveness, 289
dysreflexia, autonomic, 200–2
dystrophy, myotonic, 104–6

E
early reversible inhibition anticholinesterases, 250
ECG: for abdominal aortic aneurysm, 121, 122;
    abnormalities, 351–62; for anaesthetists,
345–71; for aortic stenosis, 153–4;
    associated with myocardial infarction,
    175; for cardiomyopathy, 194–5, 198–9;
    for cervical spine subluxation, 258–60;
    changes reflected in, 397; in complete heart
    block, 7–8; construction of, 346–8; digoxin
    therapy, 366–7; electroconvulsive therapy,
    15, 367–8; electrode positioning, 346–7;
    hyperkalaemia, 217, 365–6; hypokalaemia,
    366; in myocardial infarction, 363–4;
    paediatric, 369–71; and supraventricular
    tachycardia, 230; of valve replacements
    patient having surgery, 223, 224; variables,
    350; in Wolff-Parkinson-White (WOW)
    syndrome, 78–79
ECG 7, 361
ECHO, 307; for cervical spine subluxation, 259,
    261; for HCM, 195; of valve replacements
    patient having surgery, 225; for valvular heart
    disease, 153–5
echocardiogram. See ECHO
eclampsia, 388
ECT. See electroconvulsive therapy
Eisenmenger's syndrome, 101–3
ejection fraction (EF), 227
electrical cardioversion for supraventricular
    tachycardia, 231–2
electric shocks for supraventricular tachycardia,
    231–2
electrocardiogram. See ECG
electroconvulsive therapy, 14–17, 367–8;
    administering anesthetics, 16; anaesthetic
    issues of, 15; bradycardia in, 16; drug
    therapy influencing anesthetics for, 17;
    how is performed, 14; indications for, 14;
    physiological effects, 15; preoperative
    patient assessment, 16
electrode positioning in an ECG, 346–7
electrolyte imbalances, 391–5
electromyogram, 83
electromyography, 73
embolism, amniotic fluid, 45–46
emboli theory, 228
EMLA, 40
emphysema, 168, 335
end expiratory pressure (EEP) limit in a jet
    ventilator, 163
endocardial viability, 176
endocrine: and impact of acromegaly, 244; and
    impact of hypothermia, 255; impact of
    myotonic dystrophy, 104; management for
    organ donation, 28

endothelial dysfunction in preeclampsia, 143
endotracheal intubation, 109
endotracheal tube, 340
endovascular aneurysm repair (EVAR), 120, 124–6
end-stage liver disease, 177–9
energy for electric shocks for supraventricular
        tachycardia, 231–2
energy requirements of the critically ill, 12
enhanced recovery, 302
ENIGMA 1 (2007), 387
ENIGMA 2 (current), 387
enteral nutrition, 12
epidural abscess, 192–3; incidence of, 192;
        preventing, 192; symptoms and
        managing, 193
epidural anaesthesia, 192
epidural block *versus* thoracic paravertebral
        block, 281
epidural blood patch (EBP) for inadvertent dural
        puncture, 135–6
epidural filter, 193
epidural veins, 54
epilepsy: anaesthetic implications for, 4; in
        health history, 2–6; induction and airway
        management, 6
epiphyseal plate, 312
epiphysis, 312
epithelial tissue, 240
Epworth sleepiness scale, 5
equilibrium of inhaled agents, 88
European Resuscitation Council (ERC), 310
European Society of Parenteral and Enteral
        Nutrition (ESPEN), 12
EuroSCORE, 379
Evaluation of Nitrous oxide In the Gas Mixture for
        Anaesthesia, 387
evaporation and heat loss, 255
EVAR Trial 1 (2005), 384
EVAR Trial 2 (2005/2010), 384
exchange transfusion in sickle disease, 266
exercise ECG, 123
extradural haematoma, 165
extrinsic cardiomyopathy, 195
extubation: in cervical spine subluxation, 263; in
        endovascular aneurysm repair (EVAR), 125;
        and fundoplication, 191
exudates, 205
eye manifestation in rheumatoid arthritis, 132
eye pain, postoperative, 47–49

F
facial manifestations of myotonic dystrophy, 104

facial nerve, 83, 84, 305
Faraday's cage, 36
fascicle block, 351–3
fast-track surgery, 302
fatty liver, 21
feeds, absorbing of, 13
femur fracture surgery, 222
fetal death, intrauterine, 99–100
FEV1, 43–44
FEV1/FVC ratio, 261
filter needles for epidurals, 193
filters, epidural, 193
filtration for renal replacement therapy, 218
Final FRCA examination, radiology for, 323–43
fitness before surgery, 373
fixed rate insulin infusion, 68
fluid filter for epidurals, 193
fluid management for organ donation, 29
fluid responsiveness, dynamic, 289
fluids: for diabetic ketoacidosis (DKA), 68; infusion
        into the bone, 311–13; in the pleural space,
        334; shift in preeclampsia, 143
food bolus removal, 109
forced expired volume (FEV), 168
forced vital capacity (FVC), 168
foreign body: anaesthetics for, 109; aspiration,
        38–41
fractionated heparin, 317
fracture mandible, 127–9
fracture of neck of femur, 222–9, 317–18
Fraser guidelines, 76
frequency of breaths in a jet ventilator, 163
fresh frozen plasma (FFP), 318
fresh gas flow (FGF), 62
functional assessment, 379
functional capacity assessment, 123, 306, 376
functional endoscopic sinus surgery (FESS), 78
functional residual capacity (FRC), 86
fundoplication, 186–91; anaesthetizing, 188–9;
        intravenous cannulation, 189–90
fusion beats, 360

G
GALA trial (2007), 383
gallstone pancreatitis, 376–7
ganglion-blocking drugs, 214
gas/air embolism, 57
gas exchange in HFJV, 163
gas induction for mediastinal mass, 299
gas insufflation, 56–57
Gasserian ganglion, 84
gastric contents' pH, 249

gastro-intestinal manifestations: of cystic fibrosis, 234; of hypothermia, 255; of myotonic dystrophy, 104; of sickle cell disease, 265

gastro-oesophageal reflux disease, 186

general anaesthesia: advantages and disadvantages of, 383; for baby delivery, 135–6; failure of, 389; for mediastinal mass, 298–9; to minimize hyperreflexia, 202; for myotonic dystrophy, 105; in pregnant patients with aortic stenosis, 158; for Wolff-Parkinson-White (WPW) syndrome, 79–80

General Dental Council, 77

generalised lymphadenopathy, 296

genitourinary manifestations of sickle cell disease, 265

GH and control of release, 243–5

gigantism, 244

Gillick competence, 76

Glasgow Coma Score (GCS), 377

glaucoma, 47

glucocorticoids for complex regional pain syndrome (CRPS), 316

glucose control with insulin therapy, 385

glucose-6-phosphate dehydrogenase (G6PD) deficiency, 267–8

GOLD guidelines for diagnosing COPD, 168–9

Goldmann cardiac risk index, 380

Goldman's risk stratification, 373–4

G6PD deficiency, 267–8

gram-negative organisms causing ventilator associated pneumonia (VAP), 238

grommets, 230

growth hormone (GH) and control of release, 243–5

Guillain Barre syndrome, 94–98; autonomic dysfunction, 97; diagnosing, 94–96; ICU related problems, 98; intubation of patient, 97; managing, 97–98; treatment options, 97

H

haematological system: in cardiac output, 381; impact of hypothermia, 255; impact of sickle cell disease, 265

haematological toxicity from chemotherapy drugs, 59

haematoma, extradural, 165

haemodiafiltration for renal replacement therapy, 218

haemodialysis, 387; for renal replacement therapy, 218

haemodynamic changes during amniotic fluid embolism, 46

haemofiltration for renal replacement therapy, 218

haemoglobin level in hypoxia, 86

haemoglobin S (HbS), 264–6

haemolytic sickling crisis, 265

hair hygrometer, 253

half-life in target controlled infusion (TCI), 287

Harris Benedict equation, 12

Haversian canals, 313

HbS, 264–6

head, computed tomography of, 342–3

headache: caused by intracranial pressure, 89; post-dural puncture headache (PDPH), 134–5; postpartum, 135

head injury, 127–9, 164–7, 385; hypothermia in, 167; intubation for, 165; patient transfer of, 166–7

health-care associated pneumonia, 247

heart: autonomic innervation of, 209; and contraindications of organ donation, 27; denervated, 209–12; in pulmonary hypertension (PHT), 282–4; sympathetic stimulation of, 209; x-rays, 325

heart block (HB), 361–2

heart cardiomegaly, 336

heart disease: classification of, 307; cyanotic, 101

heart failure, 226–7; classification of, 373

heart murmur, 194

heart rate, 292

heart ratio relating to R-R interval, 347

heart transplant, 209–10

heat, 254; loss in operating theatre, 255–6; and moisture exchanger/filter (HMEF), 193

hemiarthroplasty, 226

HEMODIAFE study (2008), 219, 387

heparin, 317–18; for managing anticoagulation during pregnancy, 160

hepatic acinus, 23

hepatic arterial buffer response (HABR), 24

hepatic artery, 23

hepatic blood flow, 24

hepatic encephalopathy, 177, 178

hepatic sinusoids, 22

hepatocytes, 22

hepatorenal syndrome (HRS), 178

hepatotoxicity from chemotherapy drugs, 59

hereditary spherocytosis, 266

Herring bodies, 241

high-frequency jet ventilation (HFJV), 163

high-frequency oscillation ventilation (HFOV), 386

hilar lymphadenopathy, 296

Hilar mass, 327

hoarseness and micro laryngoscopy, 161–3

Hodgkin's lymphoma, 300

hormonal determinants of coronary circulation, 176
hormones for malignancy, 59
hospital-acquired pneumonia (HAP), 247
HRS type 1, 178
HRS type 2, 178
5-HT2 receptors, 112
5-HT3 receptors, 112
5-HT6 receptors, 112
5-HT7 receptors, 112
humidification, 253
humidity, 253–4; measuring, 253–4; types of, 253
Hunter Criteria for serotonin syndrome, 113
hydralazine, 145
hydrogen ion, 394
5-hydroxytryptamine. See serotonin
hygrometer, 253–4
hyperalgesia, 315
hyperbaric oxygen for complex regional pain
        syndrome (CRPS), 316
hypercalcaemia, 392, 397
hyperglycaemia, 67
hyperinflation, 40
hyperkalaemia, 217, 300, 365–6, 392, 397; in
        tumour lysis syndrome (TLS), 59
hypermagnesaemia, 146, 393, 397
hypernatraemia, 391
hyperparathyroidism, 392
hyperphosphataemia, 393; in tumour lysis
        syndrome (TLS), 59
hyperreflexia, autonomic, 201–2
hypertension: with dysreflexia, 202; managing in
        pregnant patient with aortic stenosis, 159;
        during pregnancy, 142, 144–5; pulmonary,
        282–4
hypertonic cardiomyopathy (HCM), 195–9;
        anaesthetic considerations, 197–8; ECG,
        198–9; inheritance of, 195; treatment, 196–7
hyperuricaemia in tumour lysis syndrome (TLS), 60
hypocalcaemia, 393, 397; in tumour lysis syndrome
        (TLS), 60
hypokalaemia, 392, 397
hypomagnesaemia, 95, 393, 397
hyponatraemia, 188, 391–2
hypophosphataemia, 394
hypospadias surgery, 138
hypotension: caused by tricyclic antidepressant
        drug, 148; due to ACE-i, 181; inducing, 213;
        in scoliosis surgery, 117
hypotensive anaesthesia, 213–14, 305; problems
        with, 214
hypotensive drugs, 213–16
hypothalamic hormones, 241

hypothalamo-hypophyseal portal system, 242
hypothermia, 254–5, 397; in a head injury patient,
        167; in scoliosis surgery, 117
hypotoxcity during fundoplication, 190
hypoxemia and pulmonary hypertension, 282
hypoxia, 86

I

ICD, 270
ICP elastance curve, 90
ICU-acquired weakness (ICUAW), 72–74
ICU care bundles, 73–74
ICU scoring systems, 378
ICU weakness, 72–74
IGF-1, 243
IgG as treatment for Guillain Barre syndrome, 97
IMCA service, 76
immunoglobulin for complex regional pain
        syndrome (CRPS), 316
immunosuppressants, 58
immunosuppressant therapy of denervated heart
        for a noncardiac surgery, 211–12
implantable cardiac defibrillator (ICD), 270, 338–9
implants and magnetic resonance imaging, 34
inadvertent dural puncture, 134–6
incomplete triflascicular block, 260–1
incremental shuttle walk test, 123
indirect sympathomimetics, 210
induced hypotension, 213
infection in end stage hepatic disease, 177
inferior vena cava, 54
infusion, target controlled, 285–8
ingested foreign body, 109
inhalational agents for scoliosis surgery, 117
inhalational induction: for anaesthesia of a bleeding
        tonsil, 272–3; and volatile agents, 87
inspiration in chest x-rays, 324
inspiratory to expiratory (I:E) ratio in a jet
        ventilator, 163
insulin dependent diabetes mellitus, 66–71
insulin infusion, 68
intensive care, trials in, 383–9
intensive therapy unit. See ITU
intercostal drain in pneumothroax, 206
intercostal space and chest drain insertion, 207
intermittent haemodialysis (IHD), 218, 387
internal carotid artery, 110
international normalized ratio in valve replacements
        patient having surgery, 225–6
interstitial lung disease, 332
interstitial opacification, 328
intervals in paediatric ECG, 369

intervention in chest x-rays, 325
intracranial neoplasms, 242
intracranial pressure, 26; causes, 89; managing, 90–91, 111; measuring, 91; during patient transfer, 166–7
intracranial pressure elastance curve, 90
intracranial pressure waveforms, 91–92
Intralipid, 71
intra-obdiminal pressure, 54
intraocular pressure (IOP), 47–48
intraosseous anatomy, 310–13
intraosseous needle insertion, 310–11
intrauterine fetal death, 99–100; causes of, 100; incidence of, 100
intrauterine growth retardation in preeclampsia, 143
intravenous cannulation for fundoplication, 189–90
intravenous rapid sequence induction for anaesthesia of a bleeding tonsil, 273
intrinsic cardiomyopathy, 195
intubation: for cholesteatoma, 304; in Guillain Barre syndrome patient, 97; in a head injury patient, 165; for ingested foreign body, 109
irreversible inactivation by organophosphorus compounds, 251
ischaemia, 196; in the spinal cord, 54, 116
isoflurane, 87
ITU, nutrition in, 11–13
IUGR, 143
IV induction agents for scoliosis surgery, 117

J
jet ventilation, 163
jet ventilator, 163
joints in rheumatoid arthritis, 132

K
Kerley lines, 326
ketamine, 140–1
ketonaemia, 67
kidney and contraindications of organ donation, 27
kidney injury, acute, 376

L
labetalol, 144
laminar flow, 184
laparoscopic procedure, 56–57; advantages and disadvantages of, 57; anaesthetic issues for, 56; contraindications, 56
laryngeal mask airway (LMA), 304
laryngeal nerve damage, 161
laryngoscopy, 161–3, 377
larynx: lesions in, 162; nerve supply of, 161

laser surgery on the larynx, 162
lateral decubitus projection in chest x-rays, 323–4
lateral projection in chest x-rays, 323–4
learning difficulties: anaesthetizing those with, 77; and consent issues, 75; in health history, 2–6
Lee's revised cardiac index (1999), 375–6, 380
Le Fort fractures, 128
left anterior fascicular block (LAFB), 351–3
left atrial enlargement, 337
left atrial hypertrophy (LAH), 355–6
left axis deviation in ECG, 351
left bundle branch block (LBBB), 353–5
left coronary artery, 174
left heart disease and pulmonary hypertension, 282
left lower lobe collapse, 329, 331
left posterior fascicular block (LPFB), 351–3
left tension pneumothorax, 333
left upper lobe collapse, 329
left upper lobe consolidation, 331
left ventricle and coronary blood supply, 175
left ventricular and diastolic pressure (LVEDP), 175
left ventricular enlargement, 337
left ventricular hypertrophy (LVH), 195, 337, 356
left ventricular outflow tract (LVOT), 154
lesions in larynx, 162
LiDCO™, 291
light reflex, 49
Light's criteria, 205
lipid solubility and oil:gas coefficient, 88
lithium influencing anesthetics for electroconvulsive therapy, 17
lithium lime, 61
litholyme, 61
liver: anatomy of, 20–25; blood supply of, 23–24; and contraindications of organ donation, 27; fatty, 21; lesions, 22; manifestation in rheumatoid arthritis, 132; types of divisions of, 22–23
liver disease, 177–9; alcoholic, 177–8; pathophysiology of, 177–8
loading dose in target controlled infusion (TCI), 286
lobar consolidation, 330–2
lobules of the liver, 23
local anaesthetic: for mediastinal mass, 298; for myotonic dystrophy, 105
long bone, 312
Lord Scarman's test, 76
lower lobe consolidation, 331
low molecular weight heparin (LMWH), 317; for anticoagulation during pregnancy, 160
low QRS ampitudes, 370

LUL, 329, 331
lumbar epidural analgesia, 139
Lundberg A waves, 91–92
Lundberg B waves, 91–92
Lundberg C waves, 91–92
lung cancer, 261
lung collapse, 328–9
lung diseases and pulmonary hypertension, 282
lung function tests, 43–44; for abdominal aortic
        aneurysm, 121, 123; for cervical spine
        subluxation, 260, 261
lung resection: anaesthesia for, 42–44; pain relief,
        44; preassessment of, 43
lungs: and contraindications of organ donation, 27;
        lobar consolidation, 330–2; x-rays, 328–35
lung transplant and anaesthetizing for subsequent
        surgery, 212
Luscombe and Owens formula, 187
lymphadenopathy, 296–7
lymphocytosis, 295–6
lymphoma and chemotherapy, 300

M
macroadenomas, 242
macrocytic/megaloblastic anaemia, 188, 396
magnesium, 393; in hypomagnesaemia, 95
magnesium-induced cardiac arrest, 146
magnesium sulphate, 388; for preeclampsia, 145–6
magnetic resonance imaging, 33–36
MAGPIE trial (2002), 146, 388
malignancy and drugs, 58–60
Mallampati classification, 377
malnutrition, 12
MAO-B inhibitors, 31
MAOIs, 114; influencing anesthetics for
        electroconvulsive therapy, 17
Marsh Model for target controlled infusion (TCI),
        287–8
massive transfusion, 125
mass spectrometry measuring humidity, 254
mastoidectomy, 216, 304
maternal mortality of pregnant patients with cardiac
        diseases, 157
maternal risk factors for preeclampsia, 143
mean arterial pressure (MAP), 54; in normotensive
        patient, 215
mean corpuscular Hb concentration (MCHC), 188
mean corpuscular volume (MCV), 188
mediastinal mass, 294–300, 326; anaesthesia for,
        297–9; complications of, 297
mediastinum, 108–9; in chest x-rays, 325
mediators theory, 229

medical management of complex regional pain
        syndrome (CRPS), 315
Medisorb, 61
MELD score, 377
mental capacity, assessing, 75–76
Mental Capacity Act 2005, 75
metabolic acidosis, 67, 394–5
metabolic determinants of coronary circulation, 175
Metabolic Equivalent (METs), 306, 376
metastasis, preventing and treating, 58–59
methotrexate, 59
methyldopa, 144
Meyer Overton hypothesis, 88
microadenomas, 242
microcytic hypochromic anaemia, 188, 396
micro laryngoscopy and hoarseness, 161–3
micro laryngoscopy tube, 162
middle cerebral artery, 111
middle mediastinum, 108
middle mediastinum mass, 327
miliary tuberculosis, 335
6-minute walk test, 123
miscarriage due to nitrous oxide, 182
mitral valve, 338; replacement, 223
Mobitz Type I heart block, 361
Mobitz Type II heart block, 361
Model for End-Stage Liver Disease (MELD) score,
        178, 377
monoamine oxidase inhibitors. See MAOIs
monoclonal antibodies for malignancy, 59
monpolar diathermy, 10
Monroe-Kellie theory, 89
morbidity: in gas/air embolism, 57; of pregnant
        patients with cardiac diseases, 157
Mortality Prediction Model I (MPM I), 378
Mortality Prediction Model II (MPM II), 378
motor-evoked potential, 83
motor sign of chronic regional pain
        syndrome, 314
MPM I, 378
MPM II, 378
MRI. See magnetic resonance imaging
mucus in cystic fibrosis, 233
multimodal analgesia, 138
muscular dystrophies, 104–6
musculoskeletal manifestations of sickle cell
        disease, 265
myasthenia gravis, 96
myocardial infarction, 174–5; ECG evolution in,
        363–4; localisation of, 365; secondary
        prevention post, 180–1
myocardial oxygen consumption, 176

myogenic autoregulation of coronary circulation, 175
myotonic dystrophy, 104–6
myringotomy, 230

N
NADPH in G6PD deficiency, 267–8
NAP 1, 388
NAP 2, 388
NAP 3 (2009), 388
NAP 4 (2011), 388
NAP 5 (current), 389
NAP 6 (future), 389
narrow complex tachycardia, 357–9
nasogastric tube, 340; position of, 11
NASPE/BPEG classification of pacemakers, 269
National Audit Project. *See* NAP
National Institute of Clinical Excellence. *See* NICE
National Patient Safety Agency guideline. *See* NPSA guideline
near-infrared spectroscopy (NIRS), 384
neck of femur fracture, 222–9, 317–18
neck pain, 258–63
needles for intraosseous insertion, 311
neoplasms, intracranial, 242
nephrogenic DI, 245
nerve conduction studies, 73
nerves: monitoring peripheral nerves, 319–21; stimulating, 319–21
nerve stimulator, 319
nerve supply of scrotum and penis, 138
nervous system in rheumatoid arthritis, 132
neural determinants of coronary circulation, 176
neural tissue, 241
neuraxial block, 192
neurohypophysis, 241
neurological function during scoliosis surgery, 116
neurological manifestations: of acromegaly, 244; of hypothermia, 255; of myotonic dystrophy, 104; of sickle cell disease, 265
neuromuscular block, 83
neuromuscular blocking agents, 320
neuromuscular functioning, 319
neurosurgery and monitoring cranial nerves, 83
neurotoxicity: from chemotherapy drugs, 59; from nitrous oxide, 182
New York Heart Association (NYHA), 307
NICE, 247
NICE guidelines for diagnosing COPD, 168–9
NICE-SUGAR trial (2009), 385
nifedipine, 144
Nissen's fundoplication, 189

nitrous oxide: based anaesthesia, 387; effects of, 182
NMDA antagonists for complex regional pain syndrome (CRPS), 316
nodular opacification, 328
noise while breathing, 297
noncardiac surgery following percutaneous coronary intervention (PCI), 376
noncardiogenic oedema, 333
nondepolarising neuromuscular blocking agents (NDMB), 320
Non-Hodgkin's lymphoma, 300
nonreceding motor block after epidural anaesthesia, 192
normal cardiac conduction, 348–52
normal QTc interval in paediatric ECG, 369
normocytic anemia, 95
normocytic normochromic anaemia, 188, 396
Normoglycemia in Intensive Care Evaluation-Survival Using Glucose Algorithm Regulation, 385
North American Society of Pacing and Electrophysiology, 269
nosocomial pneumonia, 247
NPSA guideline on nasogastric tube, 11
nutrition: in ITU, 11–13; requirements in healthy person, 12
NYHA classification of heart failure, 227, 373

O
obesity, consequences of, 224
obstructive HCM, 196
obstructive sleep apnea (OSA), 4–6; anaesthetic implications, 5–6; complications of, 5; risk factors, 5; scoring systems for screening, 4–5
ocular causes of eye pain, 47
oedema, 332–3; of chronic regional pain syndrome, 314
oesophageal Doppler, 291
oesophagus, 109
oil:gas partition coefficient, 88
oncotic pressure, 150
one-bottle chest drainage system, 207
open-angle glaucoma, 47–48
operating theatre: heat loss in, 255–6; pollution in, 182–4
opoids: in caudal block, 140; for scoliosis surgery, 117
opportunistic pneumonia, 248
OPSI. *See* overwhelming post-splenectomy infections (OPSI)

orbital causes of eye pain, 47
organ donation: contraindications, 27; preservation of organs, 28–29
organophosphate poisoning, 251–2
organophosphorus compounds, 251
OSA. See obstructive sleep apnea (OSA)
OSCAR trial (2013), 386
OSCILLATE trial (2013), 386
osmolality, 149
osmolarity, 149–50; calculation of estimated, 149; conditions affecting, 150; defined, 149; difference between estimated and calculated, 150; measurement of, 150
osmole, 149
osmometers, 150
osmosis, 149
osmotic pressure, 149
outflow obstruction in hypertrophic cardiomyopathy (HCM), 196
overwhelming post-splenectomy infections (OPSI), 25
oxygen: in apnoeic oxygenation, 85; delivery, 302, 380–1; desaturation, 4; dissociation curve in sickle cell disease, 266
oxygenation, 384; during the apnoea test, 85; apnoeic, 85
oxygen extraction ratio, 176

P
PA catheter, 385
pacemaker, 9, 338–9; anaesthetic implications for patient with permanent, 9–10; classification of, 10
pacemaker, permanent, 269–70; preventing malfunction during surgical diathermy, 269–70; types of, 269
pacing for heart block, 8–9
PACMAN study (2004), 385
paediatric ECG, 369–71
pain: after thoracotomy, 279; in caudal block, 138–9; chronic regional pain syndrome, 314–16; in paravertebral block (PVB), 280
pain control: for fundoplication, 190; in post-dural puncture headache (PDPH), 135
pain relief: for cardiac output, 381; for lung resection, 44
paired posterior spinal arteries (PSA), 52
palpitations, 78
pancreas and contraindications of organ donation, 27
pancreatitis, predicting severity of, 376–7
PaO$_2$ and sickling, 265

paravertebral block (PVB), 276–81
paravertebral space (PVS), 279
parental responsibility and obtaining consent, 76
parent-guardian issues with adolescents, 76
parietal membranes, 204
Parkinsonism, 30–31
Parkinson's disease, 30–32
paroxysmal supraventricular tachycardia, 80
passive humidification, 253
passive scavenging system for pollution in the operating theatre, 183
patent airway, 86
paternal risk factors for preeclampsia, 143
pathogens causing ventilator associated pneumonia (VAP), 248
patient positioning in scoliosis surgery, 117
patient transfer, handling, 165–7
peak velocity (PV), 292
peanuts as a foreign body, 40
penetration in chest x-rays, 324
penis, nerve supply of, 138
percussion pacing, 8
percutaneous balloon aortic valvuloplasty (PBAV), 160
percutaneous coronary intervention (PCI) and noncardiac surgery, 376
percutaneous tracheostomy, 98
pericardial effusion, 335
perioperative cerebral ischaemia monitors, 384
perioperative pulmonary complications, 170
peripheral autonomic system and tricyclic antidepressant drug poisoning, 147
peripheral nerve monitoring, 319–21
peripheral nerve stimulator, 319
peritoneal dialysis for renal replacement therapy, 218
permanent pacemaker, 269–70
peroperative anaphylaxis, 389
pethidine and Parkinson's disease, 32
pharmacology: anaesthesia in Parkinson's disease, 30–32; anticholinesterases, 250–2; anticoagulants and bridging, 317–18; drugs for malignancy, 58–60; drugs for secondary prevention, 180–1; hypotensive drugs, 213–16; serotonin, 112–14; target controlled infusion, 285–8; tricyclic antidepressants, 147–8; volatile agents, 87–88
pharmacology-induced stress testing, 123
phase I block, 321
phase II block, 321
phosphate, 393–4

physical management of complex regional pain syndrome (CRPS), 315

physics: cardiac output monitoring, 289–92; humidity/temperature, 253–6; intracranial pressure monitoring, 89–92; magnetic resonance imaging, 33–35; monitoring in scoliosis surgery, 115–17; osmolarity, 149–50; peripheral nerve monitoring, 319–21; renal replacement therapy, 217–19; scavenging, 182–4; sodalime, 61–63

physiology: apnoea physiology, 85–86; brainstem death, 26–29; cerebral circulation, 110–11; chronic regional pain syndrome, 314–16; denervated heart, 209–12; liver disease, 177–9; pneumoperitoneum, 56–57; preeclampsia, 142–6; pulmonary hypertension, 282–4

Physiology and Operative Severity Score for enUmeration of Mortality (POSSUM), 379–80

pial arterial plexus, 52

pituitary adenoma, 343

pituitary apoplexy, 240

pituitary gland, 240–2; blood supply of, 242; venous drainage, 242

pituitary hormones, 240–1

pituitary tumours, 240; types and clinical manifestations, 242–3

placental blood flow in preeclampsia, 143

placentation, abnormal, 142–3

plant alkaloids, 58

plateau waves, 91

pleura, 204–8; blood supply of, 204; innervated, 204

pleural aspiration, 206

pleural capillaries, 205

pleural effusion, 334; drugs causing, 205; pathogenesis, 205; two-bottle drainage system, 208

pleural fluid, 204–5

pleural pressure and impact of pneumothorax, 206

pleural space, 204–5

plexus, 54

pneumomendiastinum, 98, 334

pneumonia: types, 247–8; ventilator associated, 247–9

pneumopericardium, 334

pneumoperitoneum, 21, 56–57

pneumothorax, 41, 236–8, 333; impact on pleural pressure, 206; intercostal drain in, 206; one-bottle drainage system, 207; spontaneous, 238; tension, 237; three-bottle drainage system, 208

POISE-2 trial, 388

POISE trial (2008), 388

poisoning by organophosphates, 251–2

pollution in the operating theatre, 182–4

polycythaemia, 395

polysomnogram, 3

portal circulation, 242

portal hypertension in end stage hepatic disease, 177

portal vein, 23, 242

Portsmouth predictor modification, 379–80

positioning of body during laparoscopic surgery, 57

POSSUM, 378–80

post-dural puncture headache (PDPH), 134–5

posterior cerebral artery, 111

posterior cerebral circulation, 110

posterior inferior cerebellar artery (PICA), 52

posterior interventricular artery (PIVA), 173

posterior mediastinum, 108

posterior mediastinum mass, 327

posterior pituitary gland, 241

posterior spinal arteries, 116

postero anterior (PA) projection in chest x-rays, 323

post myocardial infarction, secondary prevention, 180–1

postoperative eye pain, 47–49

postoperative ventilation during scoliosis surgery, 117

postpartum headache, 135

post-tonsillectomy bleeding, 271–3

potassium, 392; high levels indicated in ECG, 217; treating high levels following chemotherapy, 300

P-POSSUM, 379–80

prazosin, 145

pre-dentate space, 131

preeclampsia, 142–6; definition, 142; managing, 144; pathophysiology of, 142–3; risk factors for development of, 143

pregnancy: and aortic stenosis, 152–60; associated risk factors for preeclampsia, 143; as contraindications with cardiac conditions, 156–7; and diabetic ketoacidosis, 66–71; hypertension during, 142, 144–5; impact on valvular diseases, 155; and magnetic resonance imaging, 34; managing anticoagulation during, 160; and preeclampsia, 142; shortness of breath in, 45

preoperative anaemia, 301–3

preoperative optimisation, 380–1
preoperative risk stratification, 379–81
preoxygenation, 86
pressure determinants of coronary circulation, 175
pressure gradients in aortic valve area, 154–5
primary cardiomyopathy, 195
PR interval in paediatric ECG, 369
P RIP acronym for chest x-rays, 323–4
procedure related complications of renal
        replacement therapy, 219
projections in chest x-rays, 323
prone position for cervical spine subluxation, 263
Prone Positioning in Severe Acute Respiratory
        Distress Syndrome, 385
propofol for total intravenous anaesthesia
        (TIVA), 285
PROSEVA trial (2013), 385
prosthetic valves, 338
prosthetic valve thrombosis, 160
protein creatinine ratio in preeclampsia, 142
proteinuria in preeclampsia, 142
prothrombin complex concentrate, 318
PROWESS trial (2001), 385
psychosocial management of complex regional
        pain syndrome (CRPS), 315
Pugh's modification of Child's criteria, 178–9
pulmonary arterial hypertension (PAH), 282
pulmonary artery pressure (PAP), 282
pulmonary capillary wedge pressure (PCWP), 282
pulmonary changes during amniotic fluid
        embolism, 46
pulmonary congestion in pregnant patient with
        aortic stenosis, 159
pulmonary embolism, 338
pulmonary fibrosis, 130, 332
pulmonary floatation catheter, 340
pulmonary hypertension (PHT), 282–4; anaesthetics
        of, 284; classifications of, 282; due to
        lung diseases and/or hypoxemia, 282;
        pathophysiology, 282–3; symptoms and
        diagnosis of, 283; treatment of, 284; with
        unclear multifactorial mechanisms, 282
pulmonary oedema, 332
pulmonary opacification, 328
pulmonary toxicity from chemotherapy drugs, 59
pulmonary tuberculosis, 335
pulmonary vasculature and pulmonary hypertension
        (PHT), 282–4
pulmonary venous hypertension due to left heart
        disease, 282
pulse power analysis, 291
pulse pressure, 290, 291

pulse volume recording. See PVR
pulsus paradoxus, 289
pupillary reflex, 49
Purkinje fibres, 348
PVR, 102–3
P wave amplitude, 370

Q
QRS amplitude, 370
QRS axis in paediatric ECG, 369
QRS complexes, 349–51
QRS duration interval in paediatric ECG, 369
QT interval in paediatric ECG, 369
quenching in magnetic resonance imaging, 36

R
radiation and heat loss, 255
radicular artery, 54
radicular veins, 54
radiology: of the cervical spine, 340–2; of the chest,
        323–7; for the Final FRCA, 323–43; of the
        head, 342–3; of the heart, 336–9; of lungs,
        328–37; of tubes and lines, 340
Randomised Evaluation of Normal versus
        Augmented Level (RENAL), 219
Ranson criteria for predicting acute pancreatitis,
        376–7
rate constant in target controlled infusion (TCI), 287
rate modulation function, 269
rate of infusion in target controlled infusion
        (TCI), 286
Recombinant Human Activated **PRO**tein C
        Worldwide **E**valuation in **S**evere **S**epsis
        trail, 385
RECORD trial (2008), 387
red blood cells: destruction, 266; diseases of
        the membrane, 266; disorders, 266–7; in
        gastro-oesophageal reflux disease, 187–8;
        structure of, 266
red cell morphology diseases, 264–8
red marrow, 313
refeeding syndrome, 13
reflex sympathetic dystrophy, 315
regional anaesthesia: advantages and
        disadvantages of, 383–4; for baby delivery,
        145–6; for cystic fibrosis, 235; to minimize
        hyperreflexia, 202; in rheumatoid arthritis,
        132–3; for Wolff-Parkinson-White (WPW)
        syndrome, 80
regional techniques of complex regional pain
        syndrome (CRPS), 315
Regnault's hygrometer, 254

REgulation of Coagulation in ORthopedic Surgery to Prevent Deep Venous Thrombosis and Pulmonary Embolism, 387
reinforced LMA, 304
rejection by denervated heart, 211
relative humidity, 253
remifentanil in mastoidectomy, 216
renal effect with gas insufflation, 57
renal factors in cardiac output, 381
renal haemofiltration filters, 193
renal impairment due to ACE-i, 181
renal management for organ donation, 29
renal manifestations of sickle cell disease, 265
renal replacement therapy (RRT), 217–19; complications of, 219; instituting, 217–18; role in sepsis, 219; types of, 218
renal system: impact of hypothermia, 255; manifestation in rheumatoid arthritis, 132
renal toxicity from chemotherapy drugs, 59
renin-angiotensin-aldosterone system drugs, 214
reproductive system impacted by cystic fibrosis, 234
resite to manage inadvertent dural puncture, 134
respiration and heat loss, 255
respiratory distress symptoms in children, 39, 41
respiratory rate in a jet ventilator, 163
respiratory swing, 289
respiratory system: in cardiac output, 381; with gas insufflation, 56–57; impacted by acromegaly, 244; impacted by cystic fibrosis, 233; impacted by hypothermia, 255; impacted by myotonic dystrophy, 104; impacted by rheumatoid arthritis, 132; impacted by sickle cell disease, 265; in patients with scoliosis, 115; preserving for organ donation, 28
respiratory tract and humidification, 253
resuscitation for bleeding tonsil, 272
rheumatoid arthritis, 130–3, 341–2
RIFLE criteria for acute kidney injury, 376
right apical simple pneumothorax, 333
right atrial enlargement, 336
right atrial hypertrophy (RAH), 355–6
right axis deviation in ECG, 351
right bundle branch block (RBBB), 353–5
right coronary artery, 173–4
right coronary artery infarct, 174
right lower lobe collapse, 329
right lower lobe consolidation, 330
right middle lobe collapse, 328
right middle lobe consolidation, 330
right upper lobe collapse, 328
right upper lobe consolidation, 330

right ventricle and coronary blood supply, 175
right ventricular enlargement, 336–7
right ventricular hypertrophy (RVH), 356
risk prediction models, 379–80
risk scores, 380
risk scoring in anaesthesia and intensive care, 373–8
risk stratification, 379–81
Rivaroxaban, 387
RLL, 329, 330
RML, 328, 330
rotation in chest x-rays, 324
Royal College of Anaesthetists, 77
R-R interval relating to heart rate, 347
RRT. See renal replacement therapy
RUL, 328, 330

S
SABRE, 387
sacral canal, 139
sacral hiatus, 139
sacrum, 139
SAD CHIN acronym, 332
SAPS 1, 378
SAPS 2, 378
SAPS 3, 378
scavenging, 182–4; for pollution in the operating theatre, 183–4
Schnider Model for target controlled infusion (TCI), 287–8
scoliosis, 115–17
scoliosis surgery: monitoring in, 115–17; neurological function during, 116
scrotum, nerve supply of, 138
secondary cardiomyopathy, 195
secondary prevention after a myocardial infarction, 180–1
sedative premedication, 5
segmental branches of arteries, 52
seizures caused by local anaesthetic toxicity, 70–71
selective serotonin reuptake inhibitors (SSRIs), 114; influencing anesthetics for electroconvulsive therapy, 17
sensory nerve action potentials (SNAPs), 73
sensory sign of chronic regional pain syndrome, 314
sepsis, 385; and renal replacement therapy, 219
sepsis care bundle, 73
Sequential Organ Failure Assessment (SOFA), 378
Serious Adverse Blood Reactions and Events, 387
serotonergic agents, 114
serotonin, 112–14

serotonin receptors, 112
serotonin syndrome, 112–13
serotonin toxicity, 112
serum osmolality, 245–6
serum potassium levels following chemotherapy, 300
sevoflurance, 87
shortness of breath, 303; in pregnancy, 45
SHOT trial, 387
SIADH, 246
sickle cell disease, 265
Sickledex test, 264
sickle disease, 264
sickle trait, 264
sickling, 265
sickling crises, 264–5
silhouette sign, 326
Simplified Acute Pulmonary Score (SAPS), 378
single chamber pacemaker, 338
sinus rhythm, 348, 354, 359
six-hour bundle, 74
skin manifestation in rheumatoid arthritis, 132
sleep studies in epileptic, 3
sliding scale insulin, 68
smoking and shortness of breath, 303
sodalime, 61–63
soda lime: accuracy of colour indicator for usage, 63; granule size, 62; harmful products of, 62
sodium, 391–2; low levels in gastro-oesophageal reflux disease, 188
sodium nitroprusside, 215
SOFA, 378
soft tissue, 341
somato sensory evoked potentials (SSEPs), 83, 116, 384
specialist nurse for organ donation (SN-OD), 28
spherocytosis, hereditary, 266
spinal catheter to manage inadvertent dural puncture, 134
spinal chord ischaemia, 54
spinal cord, 52–55; blood supply of, 54, 116; protection during thoracoabdominal aneurysm repair, 54–55
spinal cord injury, 201
spinal cord ischaemia, 116
spinal cord perfusion pressure (SCPP), 54
spinal veins, 54
spine fracture, 200
spine x-ray for cervical spine subluxation, 259, 261
spirometry, 168
spleen: anatomy of, 20–25; functions of, 24
splenic sequestration sickling crisis, 264

splenomegaly, 24
spontaneous and triggered electromyographic (EMG) responses, 116
spontaneous miscarriage due to nitrous oxide, 182
spontaneous pneumothorax, 238
SSRIs. See selective serotonin reuptake inhibitors (SSRIs)
Stagnara wake-up test, 116
Starling's force, 205
statin for secondary prevention post myocardial infarction, 180
steatosis, 177
ST-elevation, 362
ST elevation myocardial infarction (STEMI), 180, 363–4
stenosis. See aortic stenosis
steroids and their side effects, 59
STOP BANG questionnaire, 4
stress testing, 307
stridor, 297
stroke and β-blocking drugs, 388
stroke volume (SV), 289, 292
stroke volume variation (SVV), 289
ST segment, 370
stump pressure, 384
sub-axial subluxation, 131
substance abuse due to nitrous oxide, 182
sudden cardiac arrest, 196, 198
Sudek's atrophy, 315
sudomotor sign of chronic regional pain syndrome, 314
superficial cervical plexus block, 298–9
superior hypophyseal artery, 242
superior mediastinum, 108
superior vena cava obstruction (SVCO), 297
supine projection in chest x-rays, 323
supramaximal stimulus, 319
supraventricular tachycardia (SVT), 230–2, 357, 371
surgery: for acromegaly, 244; affected by cerebral circulation, 110; monitoring cranial nerves during, 82; risk for abdominal aortic aneurysm, 122; scoliosis, 115–17; on valve replacements patient, 222–9
surgical diathermy in those with permanent pacemakers, 269–70
Surgical Risk Scale, 380
surgical techniques of complex regional pain syndrome (CRPS), 315
sustained low-efficiency dialysis (SLED) for renal replacement therapy, 218
SVR, 102–3

sweat glands impacted by cystic fibrosis, 234
sweat test for cystic fibrosis, 233
sympathetic storm, 26
syncope managing in pregnant patient with aortic stenosis, 159
syndrome of inappropriate ADH secretion, 246
syndrome with marked vasodilation and relative hypovolaemia, 26
systemic circulation, 176
systemic vascular resistance. See SVR
systolic uptake, 290

T
tachyarrhythmia, 80, 357–61
tachycardia, 357–61; supraventricular, 230–2
target controlled infusion (TCI), 285–8; compartment model, 286; models for, 287–8; pharmacokinetics of, 286
TCA. See tricyclic antidepressants (TCA)
temperature, 254–6; measuring, 256
temporary pacing, 9
tension pneumothorax, 237
tension time (TTI), 176
teratogenicity due to nitrous oxide, 182
thalassemia, 267
Therapeutic Intervention Scoring System (TISS), 378
thoracic paravertebral block for open thoracotomy, 280–1
thoracoabdominal aneurysm repair, 54–55
thoracostomy tube, 237
thoracotomy, 44; pain after, 279; thoracic paravertebral block for, 280–1
three-bottle chest drainage system, 208
thrombocytopenia, 396
thromboembolism, 384; in valve replacements patient having surgery, 226
thromboprophylaxis, 317–18
tibia, 311–12
time constant in target controlled infusion (TCI), 287
TISS, 378
tissue: in chest x-rays, 325; and managing intracranial pressure, 91
tonic-clonic seizure, 14
tonicity, 150
tonsil, bleeding, 271–3; anaesthetizing, 272
topoisomerase inhibitors, 58
top-up for advertent dural puncture, 134
total intravenous anaesthesia (TIVA), 285
trachea in chest x-rays, 325
Train of Four (TOF), 83, 320
tranexamic acid, 386

transcatheter aortic valve implantation (TAVI), 160
transcranial Doppler, 384
transcranial motor evoked potentials (Tc-MEPs), 116
transcutaneous external pacing, 8
transducers measuring humidity, 254
transfusion: for anaemia, 302; in cancer patients, 302; massive, 125
Transfusion Requirements In Critical Care, 387
transoesophageal pacing, 8
transplanted heart. See denervated heart
transudates, 205
trauma patients, assessing and treating, 164–7
trials in anaesthesia and intensive care, 383–9
TRICC trial (1999), 381, 387
tricyclic antidepressants (TCA), 147–8
triflascicular block, 260–1
trigeminal nerve, 83–84
trophic sign of chronic regional pain syndrome, 314
tubes and lines in radiographs, 340
tubing used in carbon dioxide absorption, 63
tumor, mediastinal, 294–300
tumour lysis syndrome (TLS), 59–60, 300; preventing, 60
T10 vertebra, 20
T6 vertebra and hyperreflexia, 201
T waves, 370; inversion, 362
T1 weighted image, 34
T2 weighted image, 34
two-bottle chest drainage system, 208
Type 1 diabetes mellitus, 66–71

U
ultrasound in chest drain insertion, 206
underwater seal for pneumothorax, 237
unfractionated heparin (UFH), 317; for managing anticoagulation during pregnancy, 160
U waves, 370

V
vagal manoeuvres, 371
vagal nerve stimulator, 4
vagus nerve, 83, 108; supplying nerves to the larynx, 161
valve replacements patient having surgery, 222–9; identification of valves, 225; normalizing INR, 225–6
valves, prosthetic, 338; identification of in patient, 225
valve thrombosis, 160
valvular heart disease, 152–60; diagnosing, 153–5; impact of pregnancy on, 155

VAP, 247–9
variable rate intravenous insulin infusion (VRIII), 68
vascular supply of the bone, 313
vasoconstriction in preeclampsia, 143
vasodilators, 214, 215
vasomotor sign of chronic regional pain
        syndrome, 314
vaso-occusive sickling crisis, 264
vasopressin-2 receptors, 246
veins in the spinal cord, 54
venous drainage, 54, 174; of pituitary gland, 242
venous thromboembolism (VTE), 387
ventilation, 386; for chronic obstructive pulmonary
        disease (COPD), 169; and equilibrium of
        inhaled agents, 88; and fundoplication,
        191; in managing intracranial pressure,
        90–91; minimizing duration of, 249; in
        the operating theatre, 184; for patients
        with bronchopleural fistula (BPF), 277;
        postoperative during scoliosis surgery, 117
ventilator associated pneumonia (VAP), 247–9;
        features of, 248; preventing, 249; risk
        factors for, 248
ventilator care bundle, 73
ventricles in pulmonary hypertension (PHT), 282–4
ventricular chamber enlargement, 356–7
ventricular hypertrophy (LVH), 351–3
ventricular septal defect (VSD), 156
ventricular tachycardia (VT), 360–1
vertebra, 20
vertebral alignment, 340
vertebral artery, 52, 110

video-assisted thoracoscopic surgery
        (VATS), 278
visceral membranes, 204
vitamin K, 318
volatile agents, 87–88; and circulation factors, 88;
        and drug factors, 88; equilibrium of, 88; and
        ventilation factors, 88
Volkmann canals, 313
volume of distribution (Vd) in target controlled
        infusion (TCI), 286
vomiting in children, 310
VSD with blue spells, 101

W
warfarin, 317–18; for managing anticoagulation
        during pregnancy, 160; reversing the effect
        of, 318
warming factors in cardiac output, 381
warm ischaemia time (WIT), 29
water: in hyponatraemia, 391; reabsorption
        stimulated by ADH, 246
watershed effect, 54, 116
waves and segments in paedriatic ECG, 370
weaning from mechanical ventilation, 72
weight estimation for children, 187
wet bulb hydrometer, 254
WHO risk stratification, 157
WiLLiaM MoRRoW acronym, 355
WILSON score for difficult airway prediction, 377
Wolff-Parkinson-White (WPW) syndrome, 78–80;
        anaesthesia, 79–80; arrthymias in, 80; ECG
        in, 78–79; treatment of, 79